AF743792

Horizons in Neuroscience Research

nova
science publishers
www.novapublishers.com

Horizons in Neuroscience Research

Horizons in Neuroscience Research. Volume 47
Andres Costa and Eugenio Villalba (Editors)
2022. ISBN: 978-1-68507-832-4 (Hardcover)
2022. ISBN: 978-1-68507-918-5 (eBook)

Horizons in Neuroscience Research. Volume 46
Andres Costa and Eugenio Villalba (Editors)
2022. ISBN: 978-1-68507-679-5 (Hardcover)
2022. ISBN: 978-1-68507-728-0 (eBook)

Horizons in Neuroscience Research. Volume 45
Andres Costa and Eugenio Villalba (Editors)
2021. ISBN: 978-1-68507-509-5 (Hardcover)
2022. ISBN: 978-1-68507-517-0 (eBook)

Horizons in Neuroscience Research. Volume 44
Andres Costa and Eugenio Villalba (Editors)
2021. ISBN: 978-1-68507-072-4 (Hardcover)
2021. ISBN: 978-1-68507-085-4 (eBook)

Horizons in Neuroscience Research. Volume 43
Andres Costa and Eugenio Villalba (Editors)
2021. ISBN: 978-1-53619-705-1 (Hardcover)
2021. ISBN: 978-1-53619-710-5 (eBook)

Horizons in Neuroscience Research. Volume 42
Andres Costa and Eugenio Villalba (Editors)
2020. ISBN: 978-1-53618-787-8 (Hardcover)
2020. ISBN: 978-1-53618-802-8 (eBook)

More information about this series can be found at
https://novapublishers.com/product-category/series/horizons-in-neuroscience-research/

Andres Costa and Eugenio Villalba
Editors

Horizons in Neuroscience Research

Volume 48

nova
science publishers
www.novapublishers.com

Copyright © 2022 by Nova Science Publishers, Inc.

All rights reserved. No part of this book may be reproduced, stored in a retrieval system or transmitted in any form or by any means: electronic, electrostatic, magnetic, tape, mechanical photocopying, recording or otherwise without the written permission of the Publisher.

We have partnered with Copyright Clearance Center to make it easy for you to obtain permissions to reuse content from this publication. Simply navigate to this publication's page on Nova's website and locate the "Get Permission" button below the title description. This button is linked directly to the title's permission page on copyright.com. Alternatively, you can visit copyright.com and search by title, ISBN, or ISSN.

For further questions about using the service on copyright.com, please contact:
Copyright Clearance Center
Phone: +1-(978) 750-8400 Fax: +1-(978) 750-4470 E-mail: info@copyright.com.

NOTICE TO THE READER

The Publisher has taken reasonable care in the preparation of this book, but makes no expressed or implied warranty of any kind and assumes no responsibility for any errors or omissions. No liability is assumed for incidental or consequential damages in connection with or arising out of information contained in this book. The Publisher shall not be liable for any special, consequential, or exemplary damages resulting, in whole or in part, from the readers' use of, or reliance upon, this material. Any parts of this book based on government reports are so indicated and copyright is claimed for those parts to the extent applicable to compilations of such works.

Independent verification should be sought for any data, advice or recommendations contained in this book. In addition, no responsibility is assumed by the Publisher for any injury and/or damage to persons or property arising from any methods, products, instructions, ideas or otherwise contained in this publication.

This publication is designed to provide accurate and authoritative information with regard to the subject matter covered herein. It is sold with the clear understanding that the Publisher is not engaged in rendering legal or any other professional services. If legal or any other expert assistance is required, the services of a competent person should be sought. FROM A DECLARATION OF PARTICIPANTS JOINTLY ADOPTED BY A COMMITTEE OF THE AMERICAN BAR ASSOCIATION AND A COMMITTEE OF PUBLISHERS.

Additional color graphics may be available in the e-book version of this book.

Library of Congress Cataloging-in-Publication Data

ISBN: 979-8-88697-230-6
ISSN: 2159-113X

Published by Nova Science Publishers, Inc. † New York

Contents

Preface

The first chapter of this book reviews the main inflammatory processes described for ischemic stroke. In the second chapter, the authors discuss the development, functionality, myelination, pathologies, and molecular regulation of SC motility, further elucidating the significant role that migration plays in the repair of damaged nervous tissue. In Chapter 3, the distal components along with the sensitive receptors and the interconnectivity relevant to the nociception focusing on the modulatory role of the thalamus are examined. In Chapter 4, the origin, development, functionality, physiology, and pathology of astrocytes, further expanding on the significant roles that migration plays in the repair of damaged nervous tissue is looked at. In Chapter 5, the molecular mechanism of the attack of the HSV-1 genome on the cytoskeleton of brain neurons, leading to Alzheimer's symptoms, and the mechanism of restoration of the cytoskeleton by GMS, are reviewed. Next, the main evidence in literature in order to better understand and define the risks for patients undergoing neurosurgical procedures and taking aspirin is defined. The most common neurosurgical procedures are reviewed, elective or in emergency, summarizing the most important and recent literature evidence about the topic. The authors also try to collect and describe data not only about the hemorrhagic risk, but also about the thrombo-embolic one. In Chapter 7, a case series involving three traumatic brain injury (TBI) participants who underwent resting-state functional MRI scanning and neuropsychological assessments at two-time points is discussed, at one-month and twelve-month post-TBI. Longitudinal studies of TBI can reveal important information regarding the reorganization of the functional aspect of the brain. Untreated head injuries can take a long time to heal, affecting their physical and cognitive activities. The chapter focuses on neuropsychological performance and reorganization in functional connectivity. The authors of Chapter 8 exclusively concentrates on the influence of physical exercise on improvements in cognition and memory. The last chapter reviews the effects of deep breathing exercises on stress reduction.

Chapter 1 - Gravitational mass spectroscopy was used non-invasively and in vivo to study the molecular mechanism of the early stage of Alzheimer's disease in a 70-year-old probationer. An idea about the causes of the disease was obtained and the mechanism of its occurrence was established. A method for rapid non-invasive treatment is proposed.

Chapter 2 - Long it has been recognized the thalamus as the entry gate to the brain for the sensory input transmission from the periphery. In the relay of the nociceptive input to a painful sensation a combination of processes in the periphery, spinal cord and brain are involved, but not completely understood. The thalamus has a very rich nuclear organization; more than 20 nuclei have been identified, and it can be classified from an evolutionary perspective, from the interconnectivity of the fibers and from the cytoarchitectonic and anatomic-functional organization. The thalamic nuclei of the medial line conform two independent endogenous systems that exert some control over the nociceptive input: the medial dorsal nucleus that participates in the descendent facilitation of the development of mechanical allodynia, and the ventral medial that specifically mediates the descendent inhibition of thermal hyperalgesia. More recently, the periventricular nucleus, located in the medial line, has been recognized to have modulatory effects in the nociceptive pathway. In this way the thalamus along with other areas of the cerebral cortex play a crucial role in the integration of the sensitive information. The interconnectivity of the cortico-thalamic projections prompts a complex network of communication that paired with the several neurotransmitters result in the integration of the painful response. In the present chapter, the authors will discuss the distal components along with the sensitive receptors and the interconnectivity relevant to the nociception focusing on the modulatory role of the thalamus.

Chapter 3 - Physical exercise is a bodily movement caused by skeletal muscles with the expenditure of energy. It helps a person to stay energetic throughout the day. It activates the physiological systems of the body by acting on the heart and lungs, reduces stress and anxiety, and causes improvements in mood as well. This review exclusively concentrates on the influence of physical exercise on improvements in cognition and memory. Literature reports support the association that exercise activates brain plasticity by stimulation of growth factors that develop new connections between brain cells. Many researchers found evidence that hippocampal neurogenesis starts to diminish with aging, and this could be partially opposed by exercise in mouse models. Human studies also added support to this association that aerobic and neuromotor exercises increased memory performance in elderly subjects with improvements in short-term memory and long-term memory.

Chapter 4 - Astrocytes are abundant glial cells that exhibit highly diversified physiological roles in healthy and diseased nervous systems. They also play significant roles in various cell processes of the central nervous system (CNS) that actively participate in neuronal regulation for functional regeneration and repair of brain or spinal cord injuries. Astrocytes are specialized to assist in the reduction of damaged tissue surrounding the injury site and simultaneously stitch back the disrupted blood brain barrier (BBB) in support of neural tissue and maintenance of brain homeostasis. Astrocytes use a popular cell-to-cell communication mechanism to respond to various signaling molecules. A glial scar is the result of astrocytes' migration to the target site and their extensive proliferation to prevent further damage to cells. During reactive astrogliosis, astrocytes tend to upregulate and downregulate the expression of various proteins required for cell migration and repair, like glial fibrillary acidic protein (GFAP), $\alpha v\beta 3$, integrin, fibronectin, aquaporin (AQP)-4, Rho GTPases, syndecan-4 proteoglycan, connexin (Cx) 43, Cx30, and hemichannels (HCs), which are critical for migration. Astrocytes thrive at injury sites during brain or spinal cord injuries and assist the process of neuronal survival. In this review, the authors will discuss the origin, development, functionality, physiology, and pathology of astrocytes, further expanding on the significant roles that migration plays in the repair of damaged nervous tissue. Astrocyte migration is critical for performing several functions during both physiological and pathological conditions.

Chapter 5 - Schwann cells (SCs) myelinate neurons in the peripheral nervous system (PNS), thereby facilitating saltatory conduction via the myelination of axons, as well as digesting damaged axons and subsequently forming a tube-like structure to guide neural regeneration. During neural injury, Schwann cells migrate, proliferate, and assist the impaired neurons at injury site by engulfing damaged myelin and axon endings, and forming an endoneural tube connecting the neural cell body to the ends. They also secrete several neural growth factors promoting axon elongation. Motility and migration of Schwann cells are critical for remyelination of neurons after neural injury. SCs are reprogrammed by their dedifferentiation and activation, further initiating neural repair functionality, which results in down regulation of myelin genes and upregulation of trophic factors, thereby leading to the removal of damaged myelin. In this review, the authors will discuss the development, functionality, myelination, pathologies, and molecular regulation of SC motility, further elucidating the significant role that migration plays in the repair of damaged nervous tissue.

Chapter 6 - In this chapter, the authors discuss a case series involving three traumatic brain injury (TBI) participants who underwent resting-state functional MRI scanning and neuropsychological assessments at two-time points, at one-month and twelve-month post-TBI. Longitudinal studies of TBI can reveal important information regarding the reorganization of the functional aspect of the brain. Untreated head injuries can take a long time to heal, affecting their physical and cognitive activities. This chapter focuses on neuropsychological performance and reorganization in functional connectivity. The authors discuss work with participants who are in the sub-acute and chronic phases of TBI without intervention. Despite no rehabilitation being given, neuropsychological scores appeared to have the potential to improve over time, although lower scores in a few domains were recorded. Functional connectivity (FC) reveals alteration in the Default Mode Network (DMN) connectivity with other regions. Additionally, there is an alteration in FC within temporal regions involved in working memory and visual processing, as well as between visual areas and superior temporal areas involved in sound processing. Findings from a case series showed that neuropsychological performance and FC alterations at the onset of TBI can still improve without intervention but at a slower rate. Several studies show that cognitive training approaches promote better recovery than the no-intervention group. Rehabilitation or treatment is needed to help people recover quickly and get back to their normal lives.

Chapter 7 - Breathing is a subconscious phenomenon that needs to be accurately regulated. Improper breathing patterns can lead to improper exchange of oxygen and carbon dioxide transport at the alveolar level. There are two types of breathing patterns: Diaphragmatic (abdominal) breathing and Thoracic (chest) breathing. Chest breathing is characterized by an upward and outward movement of the chest wall. Abdominal Breathing is purely a diaphragmatic breathing; the diaphragm moves down and flattens, sucking the air into the lungs during inspiration and the diaphragm moves down pushing the abdominal wall out during expiration. Deep Breathing exercises are techniques that can help a person to relax, and to make a person feel comfortable. Deep breathing exercise is one of the effective and best ways to reduce the stress level in the body. Breathing exercises in the form laughter, paced breathing, abdominal breathing, yoga breathing is found to be beneficial. Deep breathing exercises are a part of relaxation strategy. It calms down the mind and balances your hormones- lowering down cortisol levels, increasing endorphin rush in the body. It helps to give a better sleep-in case of insomnia. Stress may invoke many cardiovascular problems, anxiety depression, immunosuppression and many pathological changes in the body. Deep breathing is considered as one of the best ways to lower stress in the body. They encourage full oxygen exchange at lung and tissue level and also it is a beneficial import and export of incoming oxygen for outgoing carbon dioxide. This effect can slow the heartbeat and lower or stabilize blood pressure.

Chapter 8 - Aspirin has always represented a sword of Damocles for surgeons, especially for neurosurgeons. On one hand, its discontinuation could be dangerous for patients with a high thromboembolic risk; on the other hand, its antiplatelets effects could significantly increase the risk of intra or post-procedural bleedings. In this chapter the authors will review the main evidence in literature in order to better understand and define the risks for patients undergoing neurosurgical procedures and taking aspirin. The authors will describe most common neurosurgical procedures, elective or in emergency, summarizing the most important and recent literature evidence about the topic. The authors will also try to collect and describe data not only about the hemorrhagic risk, but also about the thrombo-embolic one. The authors hope this chapter will constitute a practical guide for everyday practice in neurosurgery.

Chapter 9 - Inflammation plays crucial roles in the pathogenesis of atherosclerosis, which can result in thromboembolic events and different stroke subtypes such as large artery or cryptogenic ischemic stroke. Furthermore, both the blood flow withdrawal and the subsequent blood flow reperfusion that follows the ischemic events elicit inflammatory processes. This inflammatory response plays a dual role in stroke pathology: the initial response aims to fight the damaged tissue, while the continuous inflammatory activity after stroke exacerbates the neural damage. The inflammatory process involves a complex cellular and molecular response that includes not only the intrinsic cells in the brain (glia, neurons, vascular endothelium) but the involvement of the peripheral cells (macrophages, neutrophils, dendritic cells, lymphocytes) at different times after stroke eliciting, among other effects, a complicated sequence of cytokines that control the evolution of the inflammation and blood-brain barrier permeability. Different non-invasive imaging techniques such as computed tomography angiography, computed tomography perfusion, or magnetic resonance imaging, among others, allow following the atherosclerotic plaque instability and the neuroinflammatory progression.

Chapter 1

Epilepsy and Alzheimer's: Molecular Mechanism, Diagnostics and Treatment. History of One Mistake

Kristina Zubow[1,*], Anatolij Zubow[2,†] and Viktor Anatolievich Zubow[1,‡]

[1]R&D, Zubow Consulting (NPO), Germany

[2]Department Telecommunication Networks Group, TU Berlin, Germany

Abstract

Gravitational mass spectroscopy was used non-invasively and in vivo to study the molecular mechanism of the early stage of Alzheimer's disease in a 70-year-old probationer. An idea about the causes of the disease was obtained and the mechanism of its occurrence was established. A method for rapid non-invasive treatment is proposed.

Keywords: human brain, epilepsy, Alzheimer's disease, paresis, HSV-I/2, nucleosome, treatment, gravitational mass-spectroscopy

Introduction

The molecular mechanism of the occurrence and development of Alzheimer's disease is not known (https://ru.wikipedia.org/wiki/ Alzheimer's Disease). In

* Corresponding Author's Email: kristinazubow@gmail.com.

† Corresponding Author's Email: Heide-Lore@zubow.de.

‡ Corresponding Author's Email: anatolij.zubow@tu-berlin.de.

In: Horizons in Neuroscience Research. Volume 48

Editors: Andres Costa and Eugenio Villalba

ISBN: 979-8-88697-230-6

© 2022 Nova Science Publishers, Inc.

this work, we will consider the initiation of the disease as a result of the infiltration and attack of the herpes virus (HSV-1) in the neurons of the human brain during an erroneous surgical operation and the development of the process in the postoperative, long period [1]. The main diagnostic method used is non-invasive gravitational mass spectroscopy (GMS) *in vivo* mode [2]. This method is based on the analysis of the states of atomic nuclei clusters (ANC) in the gravitational noise of the brain [2].

The aim of this work was to study the molecular mechanism of the attack of the HSV-1 genome on the cytoskeleton of brain neurons, leading to Alzheimer's symptoms, and the mechanism of restoration of the cytoskeleton by GMS.

Topology of Brain Chromosomes as an Ensemble of Dominant Local Functions

It has recently become clear [2] that the main "violin," the main control organ of the entire neural network of the human body, is played by ensembles of chromosomes of different parts (functions) of the brain (https://ru.wikipedia.org/wiki/Brodmann'scytoarchitectonic_fields). Chromosomes are built from helical structures and are powerful accumulators of potential energy [3]. They interact with each other by means of resonance with ensembles of oscillators of the same type and subordinate to them in the chromosomes of the cells of the entire human body remotely. This field of resonance is known as the bio field. The above can be represented by a diagram, Figure 1. According to it, an ensemble of oscillators with a higher potential energy forces analog ensembles with a lower potential energy to oscillate in the forced mode (https://www.youtube.com/watch?v=HmmYtopGx7Y). Such oscillators in chromosomes include ANC in nucleosomes (https://ru.wikipedia.org/wiki/Nucleosome), protein coils in their octamers, DNA loops, as well as coils built from nucleosomes in solenoid constructions topology of chromosomes (https://en.wikipedia.org/wiki/Solenoid_(DNA), Figure 2. From this logic, it follows that ANC ensembles in brain chromosomes remotely change their counterparts, for example, in muscle neurons. That is, it is a channel for transmitting information through the resonance field. Violation of it should cause short-term disturbances in the functioning of the nervous system, for example, in the form of epileptic pathologies.

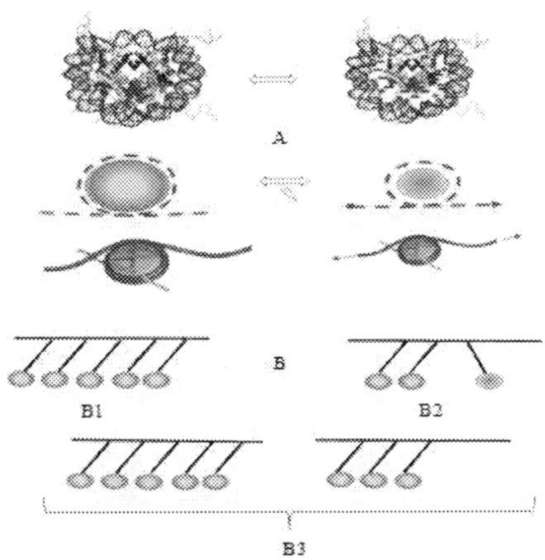

Figure 1. Models of nucleosomes (histone) memory cells in chromosomes and distance interactions of sub ensembles built from them. A – mechanical deformations of the octamer (changes in the conformations of protein coils) in nucleosomes under the influence of DNA helix tension, with the generation of a piezoelectric signal (https://ru.wikipedia. org/wiki/Piezoelectric_effect). B is the distance interaction of histone sub ensembles, like pendulums, with analogues of the surroundings, B1 is a harmonic oscillator of 5 histone pendulums (example) with a higher potential energy than the analog oscillator at a distance B2, B2 is an inharmonic oscillator of 3 histone pendulums (example) with less potential energy than B1. B3 is the resulting harmonic oscillator, as a result of forcing weak B2 by strong B1 and minimizing the potential energy of oscillation in the new pendulum.

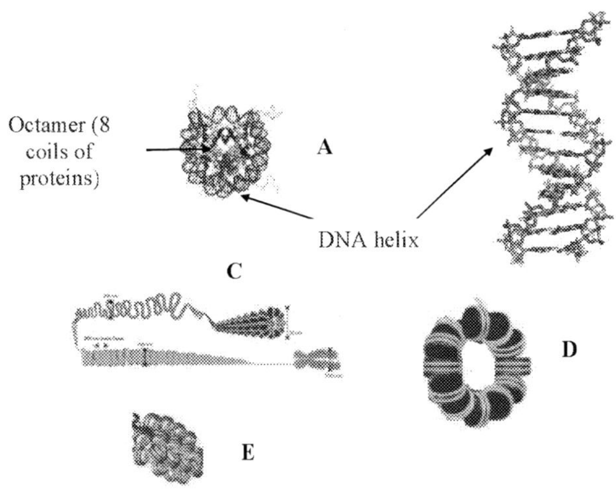

Figure 2. Models: nucleosome (**A**, https://en.wikipedia.org/wiki/Nucleosome), DNA helix (**B**, https://de.wikipedia.org/wiki/Desoxyribonukleins%C3%A4ure), solenoid (**C**), one turn of 12 nucleosomes in it (**D**, [4]), E - a group of turns of 6 nucleosomes in each (https://www.gida.de/testcenter/biologie/bio-dvd048/aufgabe_04.htm).

Thus, there is a fundamental possibility of resonant control of the chromosomes of the local functions of the brain by the topologies of analogue chromosomes in the neurons of other organs of the body.

Medical History

The object of the study was taken (in 2021) probant-70 (70 years old) with a diagnosis of "Flappy left facial-brachial hemiparesis with suspected recurrence of WHO grade II astrocytoma, immediately after resection 11/1999, epilepsy." As a result of an erroneous diagnosis (hematoma after hitting the doorknob on the right temple, with a gust of wind), the patient (probant-70) was treated (1999, Berlin), as already with glioblastoma (surgery, radiation and chemotherapy). This led to damage to the blood-brain barrier and the penetration of the HSV-1 virus into the neurons of the brain. Over the next 20 years there was a progressive anemia of the left side of the body (arm, leg), as well as muscular dystrophy of the obturator muscle of the bladder and manifestations of herpes in the genital part of the body. Further, over the past 2 years (until 2022), the head of the probationer was subjected to MRT (5 times) and X-ray scanning (4 times), which, of course, had a negative energy effect on the topology of chromosomes in brain neurons.

Material and Method

Gravitational mass spectroscopy (GMS) was chosen as a method of passive diagnostics and treatment [2]. The method makes it possible to register ANC oscillations in the range from 200 to 4 billion Daltons, to determine their conformational state and interaction with the surroundings in short scanning times (up to 10 s). ANCs form the so-called long-range order (LRO, https://www.sciencedirect.com/topics/materials-science/long-range-order) in the cytoskeleton. At the same time, the gravitational noise (GN) of the Universe forms potential pits with many energy minima in which the formation of molecular ANC is allowed. ANC that do not fall into these pits have no right to exist, they are quickly destroyed, being in an unstable, metastable state with a high level of potential energy. The gravitational sensor was placed in the left ear of the probant-70 or the donor-12 (source of GN), Figure 3. GMS spectra were obtained using the first Zubow equation [2], the

Zubow force constant (***Z***) was taken for the ANC of nucleosomes and octamers of protein coils 6.45E-12 N/m (https://ru.wikipedia.org/wiki/Nucleosome), and for loops of DNA ***Z*** = 6.528E-12 N/m and for the HSV-1 virus genome 6.48125E-12 N/m. Positive values of Δf are characteristic of loose clusters and domains; they reflect the energy fraction of ANC in the entire ensemble of studied masses; negative values of Δf reflect the same, but for dense coils. Average mass of ANC $M_{GMS} = \sum abs(\Delta f \cdot m)$. N is the number of signals from ANC in the spectrum, D_c is the part of signals from dense ANC. Scanning time from 10 s. A probant without pathologies was chosen as a GN donor. Figure 3 shows a schematic diagram of the GMS method.

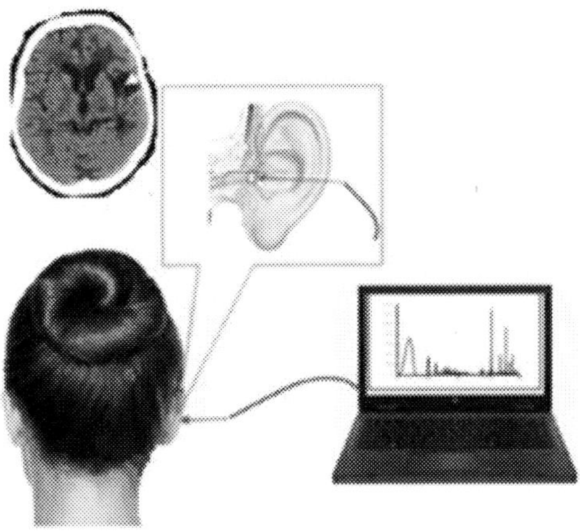

Figure 3. Schematic diagram of scanning gravitational noise from ANC in the cytoskeletal structure of the human brain using the GMS method. The arrow on the MRT indicates the site of impact (hematoma).

Gravitational Noise and Shock Waves

Shock waves (SW), as a mass impulse in gravitational noise (GN), have a strong effect on molecular, tense systems, for example, structures of buildings, ships, oil platforms, spiral mechanisms, etc. [2]. By GN we mean the noise arising from the equilibrium dynamics of freely oscillating protons (FOPs) with neutrinos (Figure 4). The more FOPs in the ANC, the more intense the dynamics of such an equilibrium, the clearer and more individual the signals in the GMS spectra. In this case, the energy of GN shock waves is the result of a shift in the equilibrium of FOPs and protons, whose oscillations are loaded with absorption neutrinos, Figure 4.

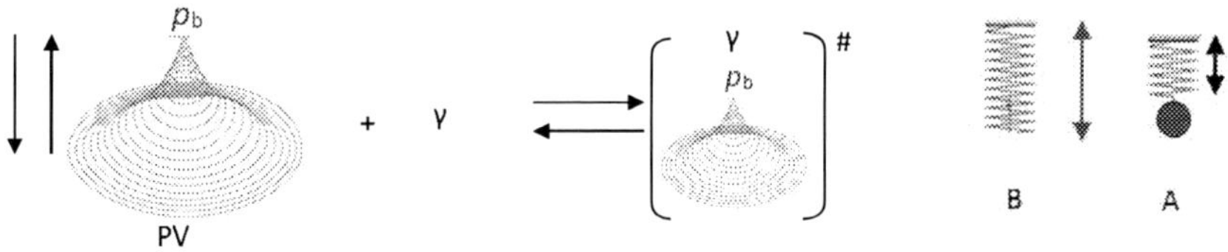

Figure 4. Model of proton oscillations between the physical vacuum (**PV**) and the baryon state (p_b), and the interaction of the proton with the neutrino. On the right, for understanding, a diagram of the "loading" of these neutrino proton oscillations is given. **A** - loaded, **B** - not loaded, states.

Result and Discussion

Molecular Mechanism of Attack by the HSV-1 Virus on Brain Neurons

There was an urgent need to find methods for non-invasive diagnosis and neutralization of the virus attack on the brain *in vivo*, as well as to "repair" the ANC and solve the problem of paralysis.

Traumatic brain wounds are attacked by the herpes virus (HSV-I) [4]. The long lethal period and the difficulty of diagnosing in the early stages of the disease, the complexity and high cost of classical methods for diagnosing the virus, the commonality of external signs with the pathology of cancer (curvature of the muscles of the face, paralysis of the limbs, loss of the shape of brain gliocells) force many researchers to search for alternative ways of rapid diagnosis. At the same time, fast, classical methods of MRT, CT, ECG do not give an answer (there is no reliable diagnosis of the tumor), and the ECG indicates only a violation of electrical signals and nothing more.

In this regard, we have developed a new non-invasive method for the rapid diagnosis of a virus attack on the human brain *in vivo* [1]. The method is based on the analysis of GS from ANC (domains, clusters, coils, coil associates, micellar and sub micellar structures) of a potential donor and a patient. Oscillations of dense and loose conformations of ANCs have very large extinction coefficients, which allows identification of ANCs, but not yet their concentrations. Thus, in probant-70, an attack by the herpes virus of the right part of the brain affected by hematoma was detected due to local destruction of the blood-brain barrier (https://ru.wikipedia.org/wiki/Hematoencephalic _barrier) during surgical resection of "glioblastoma," Figure 5. Therefore, initially attempts were made to understand the mechanism of the attack of the virus on the axon in the neurons of the affected part of the brain. Here, we proceeded from the fact that the attack of the virus led to mechanical damage to tubulins nanotubes and blocking the transmission of the piezoelectric signal from the chromosomes of brain neurons to spinal cord neurons and further to the muscles of the left side of the body (paralysis of the arm, leg, and obturator bladder muscle, as well as time from the time of deformation of the muscles of the left part of the lips of the face). Further, the authors came to the following understanding of the mechanism of virus attack on nanotubes in axons [1, 5], Figure 5.

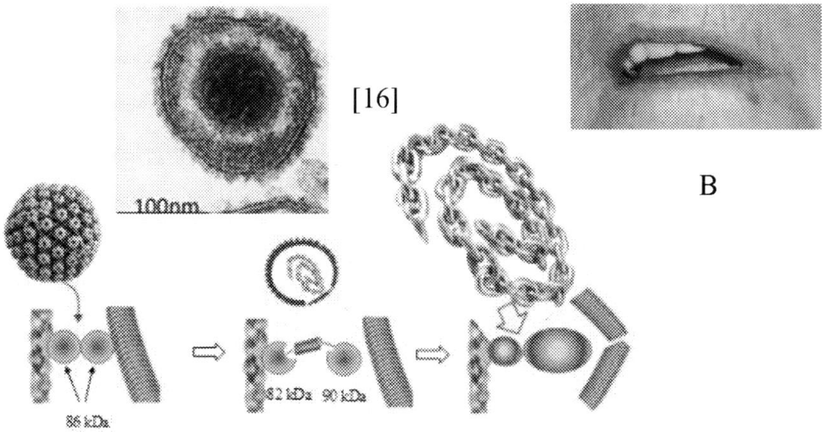

A

Figure 5. **A** - the model of binding of actin and nanotubes of tubulin with the Gas2L1 dimer (cytolinker) and the destructive effect of the virus core (plasmids, ring-shaped DNA, cccDNA, https://de.wikipedia.org/wiki/CccDNA) on the dimer. Subdomain 8.255 Da was indicated by a spiral. Photography was a herpes virus. The mass range of the oscillators in the plasmid was estimated from considerations of its density, close to 1,23 ($m = \rho \cdot V$). **B** - photograph of a part of the probant's face during the HSV-1 attack (https://ru.wikipedia.org/wiki/Bell's palsy).

The virus is in the trigeminal nerve; in the ganglia (https://gaz.wiki/wiki/ru/Gasserian) where it is isolated to the immune system (https://ru.wikipedia.org/wiki/Trinx_nerve#Trinx_nerve_diseases). The virus, from time to time, penetrates through the destruction of the blood-brain barrier to the right side of the brain, where it is easily detected by the GMS method (Figure 9). Due to the difference in masses and charges, the attack of the DNA of the virus genome on the MACF1 cytolinker should lead to strong mechanical stresses in the brain cytoskeleton, loss of stability and gliosis. According to this logic, the virus loosens MACF1 and transforms the coil into a loose conformation with decay into its three subdomains and further stretching of the tubulin nanotube cross-links with actins and their loss of electrical signal transmission functions, i.e., to break the electrical circuit.

Cytoskeletal Repair and Non-Invasive Disruption of HSV-1 in the Brain *In vivo*

The authors have started a search for a fast, non-invasive and mild physical method for repairing the main MACF1 cytolinker *in vivo*. The tool to achieve this goal was the strategy of transferring MACF1 to a dense state, thereby pushing out CccDNA rings and destroying them, Figure 6.

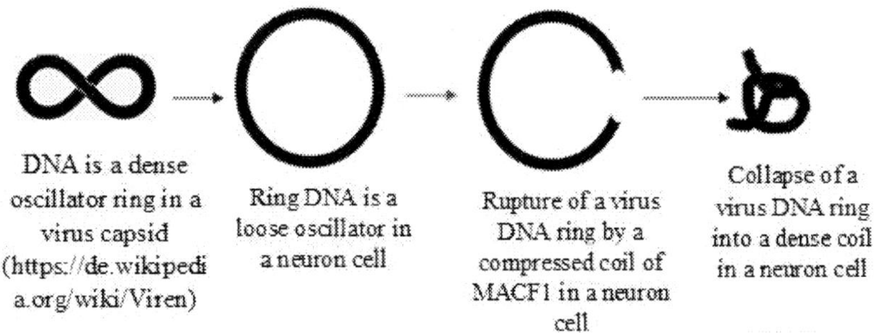

Figure 6. Model of evolution of the DNA ring plasmid (https://en.wikipedia.org/wiki/Plasmid) of the HSV-I virus after infiltrating it into a neuron and pushing it out with a compressed MACF1 cytolinker, destruction and transformation of the DNA molecule into a collapsed coil.

Figure 7 shows the GMS spectrum of the GN of the brain for understanding. The research was focused on the regions of tubulin oscillations in nanotubes and cytolinkers Gas2L1 (growth arrest-specific 2-like, https://en.wikipedia.org/wiki/GAS2L1), MACF1 (https://en.wikipedia. org/wiki/MACF1), which bind nanotubes to albumin [6]. In this report, the authors focused on the work of MACF1, which almost adequately reflected the work of another cytolinker, Gas2L1.

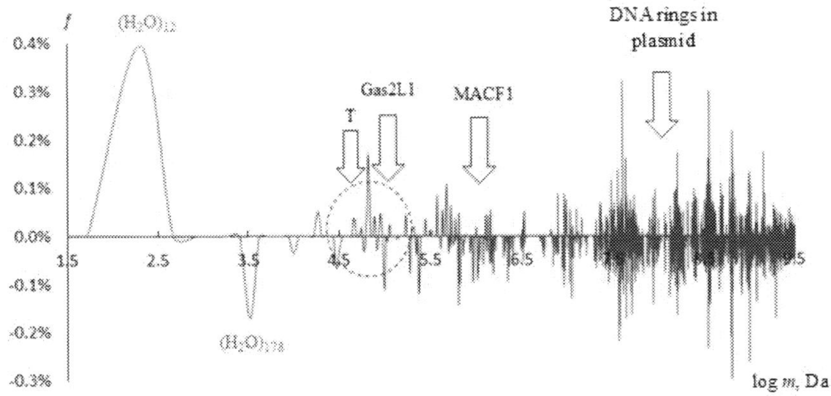

Figure 7. GMS spectrum of the GN brain (right half) of the probant-70.
The vibrational regions of ANC of tubulin (T) and albumin binding coils of Gas2L1, MACF1 and DNA rings in HSV-1 plasmid were indicated. The signals of the base [7] and Chaplin [8] water clusters in the brain cytoskeleton were indicated.

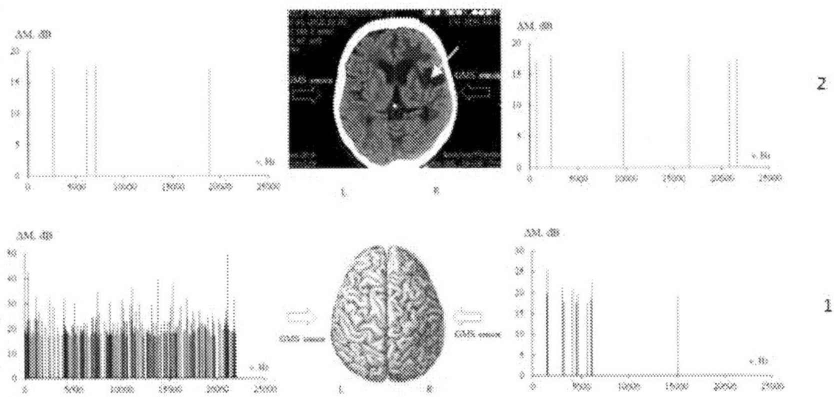

Figure 8. 1 - the structure of digitalized GN in both spheres of the brain (R-right and L - left) of probant-69 in conditions of complete rest (eyes closed), 2 - also, but with forced activation of signals using the left hand (simple raising, spectrum on the right) and the right hand - spectrum on the left. ΔM is the maximum spread in the amplitudes of GN. The photograph of GM CT/SR was taken on November 9, 2019 (the place of early postoperative treatment of glioblastoma is indicated by the oblique arrow (2 isocentric 6 MV-photon-standing fields and 2 single exposure per day from 1.6 Gy to 54.6 Gy and 4 cycles of timodal in 1999 and in 2000).

Figure 8 shows the results of scanning the GN of the probant-70. The probant was erroneously operated on 20 years ago (glioblastoma) and the course of treatment in 2000 "stopped" the growth of the "cancer" (indicated by an oblique arrow). As can be seen, both parts of the brain in the calm state of the patient have similar GN spectra. The scatter amplitudes of the GN (ΔM) are in the normal range for them.

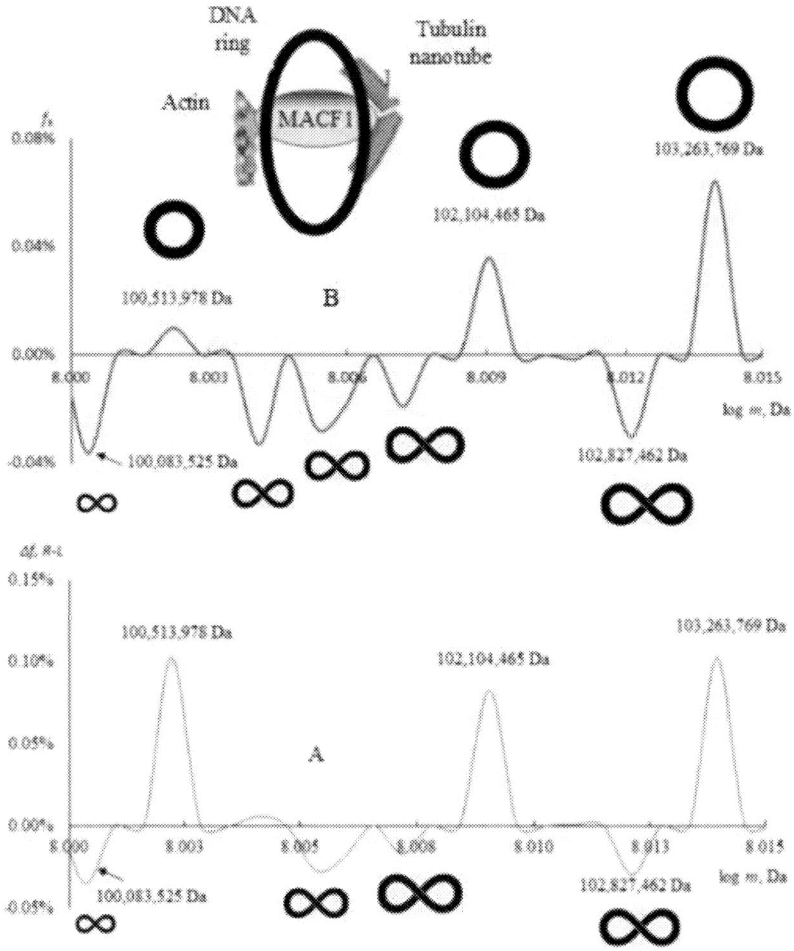

Figure 9. **A** - GMS spectrum of GN difference from the right and the left parts of brain. **B** - GMS spectrum of GN from the right part of the brain. November 30. 2019. A model of the interaction of one DNA ring with a coil of MACF1 was presented on B, above.

In December 2019, cytological examination of cells on the right side, as well as MRT and CT data, gave a negative result for cancer, but the patient had dysmotility and curvature of the lips on the left side of the face, signs of paralysis of the left hand, indicating distortion of electrical signals from the right parts of the brain [9]. Figure 8 shows that the structure of the GN in both parts of the brain strongly depends on the conditions of their forced generation. Under resting conditions, GN from various ANCs are active over the entire spectrum of domains and micelles.

Raising the left hand (GN spectrum on the right) activated the ANC, which were not involved in a calm state, the spectrum was poor in signals, but the spread of their amplitudes increased sharply. Raising the right hand, on the contrary, activated a wide range of signals in the left part of the brain with a very high spread in GN energy (ΔM up to 50). Recall that in the GMS method, ANCs with high motion dynamics (rotation, movement, changes in conformations, configurations, merging of mass concentrations, etc.) are recorded. In this case, the intensity of the signals weakly depends on the ANC concentration and strongly depends on the distance to them [2].

November 30, 2019 probant-70 was hospitalized on suspicion of a relapse of glioblastoma. But before that, the GMS spectra of brain GN were taken, Figure 9. One can see the presence of a number of signals from ANC in the CccDNA region of HSV-2. In the virus capsid, the cccDNA rings were in a compactly packed state (B), which means that they belonged to 5 signals with negative Δf values. 3 signals with positive Δf values related to DNA rings injected with the virus into the cytoskeleton of brain neurons. These were rings in an open, expanded conformation. The GMS spectrum of subtraction of GN of the right part from GN of the left part (A, $\Delta f_{R\text{-}L}$) clarifies the number of DNA collapsed rings (4) in the capsid of the free virus, in the intercellular space, and only 3 species in the axon cytoskeleton.

So, the DNA rings of the virus loosened the cytolinker and destroyed the tubulin nanotubes responsible for the passage of electric current pulses. The axon cytoskeleton experienced a new spectrum of internal mechanical tensions and stopped working. We attempted to influence the conformation of MACF1 in such a way as to return the nanotubes to their initial linear state and push the DNA rings out of the actin-nanotube bundle. For this, the frequency of cytolinker oscillations was calculated according to the first Zubow equation [2]. The cytolinker MACA1 was forced into a collapsed state [10]. This frequency corresponded to 551 Hz. Irradiation of the brain was carried out for 20 minutes, the pressure of the shock waves was no more than 90 ± 5 dB, December 30, 2019 (A) and one month later (B), Figure 10. In this case, a collapsed-expanded equilibrium was achieved in MACF1 coils and the signals in the GMS spectrum practically disappeared.

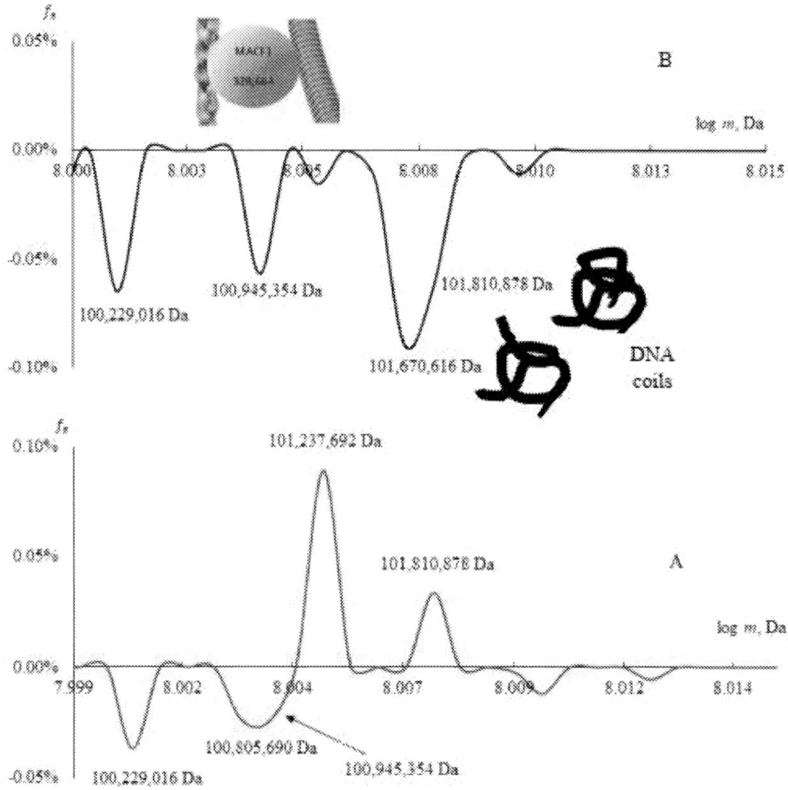

Figure 10. GMS spectra of GN from the right part of brain on January 30, 2020 before irradiation with 551 Hz (**A**) and after irradiation (**B**) for 20 min.

As can be seen from Figure 10, the impact of shock waves on December 30, 2019 led to the destruction of loose ring oscillators of the DNA from the virus, and the repeated impact on January 30, 2020 intensified this process. However, signals from CccDNA in capsids of the free virus still occurred. The next brain irradiation session February 4, 2020 (Figure 11) showed that after 5 days the process of pushing and breaking DNA rings continued (two overlapping signals from coils with comparable masses). So rings with masses of 10,229,016 Da after they were thrown out and clewed lost 145,491 Da. These rings became collapsed coils with masses of 100,083,525 Da. Comparison of DNA masses on February 4, 2020 with their masses on February 6, 2022 (Figure 20) indicates that we are dealing with two genomes of HSV-2 and HSV-1 viruses that are simultaneously in the body. The mechanism of their mixing and distribution dynamics remains unclear.

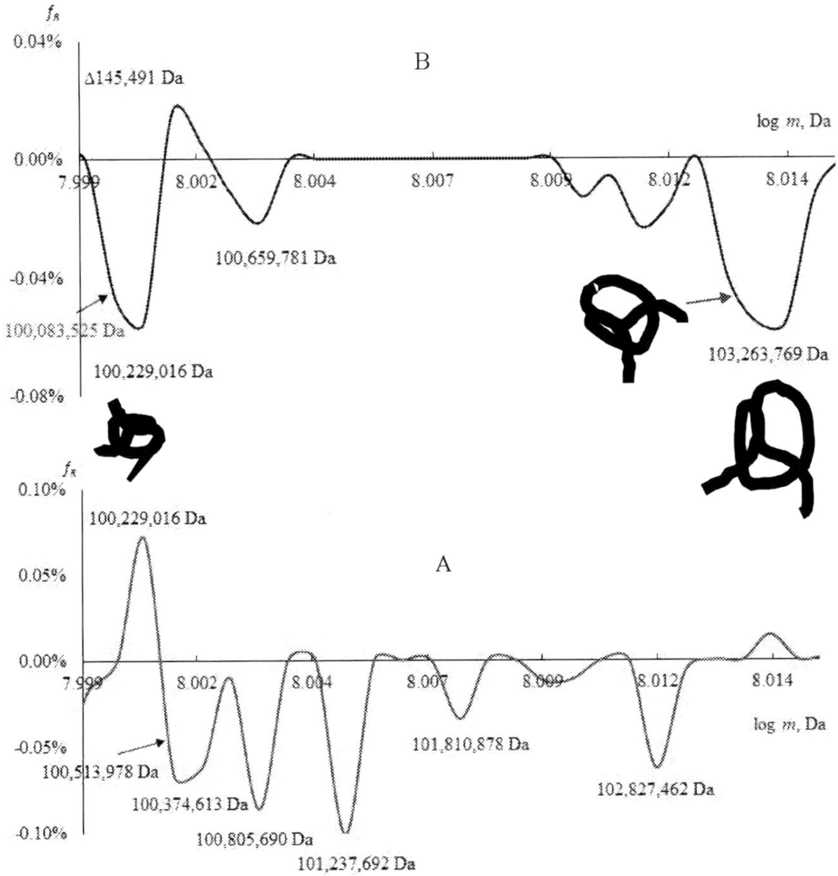

Figure 11. GMS spectra of GN from the right part of brain on February 4, 2020 before irradiation of 551 Hz (**A**) and after irradiation (**B**) for 20 min. 145,491 Da ~ 560 bp.

By this time, the patient's general condition began to noticeably improve, there was a weakening of the signals on the fingers of the left hand and the ability to get off the wheelchair for walking with a cane. It should be noted here that the signals of dense tangles are superimposed on the signals of CccDNA in the capsid of the virus located in the intercellular space of the brain. Therefore, the therapy included a parallel strengthening of the patient's immune system (vitamins).

Figure 12 presented data on the dynamics of conformational changes in MACF1 before repair and after repair of the cytoskeleton of the right side of the brain. It can be seen that when the patient was admitted to the hospital on

November 30, 2019, the MACF1 coils were in a loose state (Figure 9), and after therapy (February 4, 2020) in a dense one (Figure 10). At the same time, at least 4 cytolinker signals have already been detected: two in dense (312,560 and 353,767 Da) and two in loose form (328,664 and 337,052 Da). In the first case, MACF1 lost one subdomain of 16,104 Da, and in the second it attained a subdomain of 16,715 Da. It can be assumed that these subdomains were almost identical and there was a simple redistribution of them between the two types of MACF1coils in the new cytoskeleton. It should also be noted here that the cytoskeleton restoration process did not go through completely, part of MACF1 was still in a loose state (328,664 and 337,052 Da), apparently, weak shock waves do not reach the depths of the brain and the treatment process must be carefully continued.

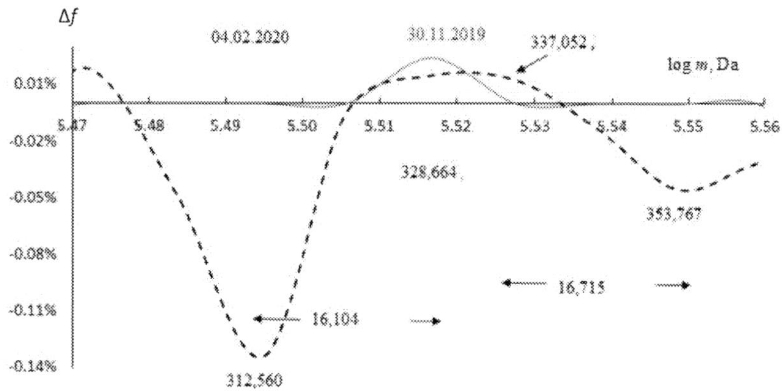

Figure 12. GMS spectra of GN from the right part of brain in the oscillation region of MACF1 coils before irradiation by 551 Hz (November 30, 2019) and after irradiation (February 4, 2020, dashed curve).

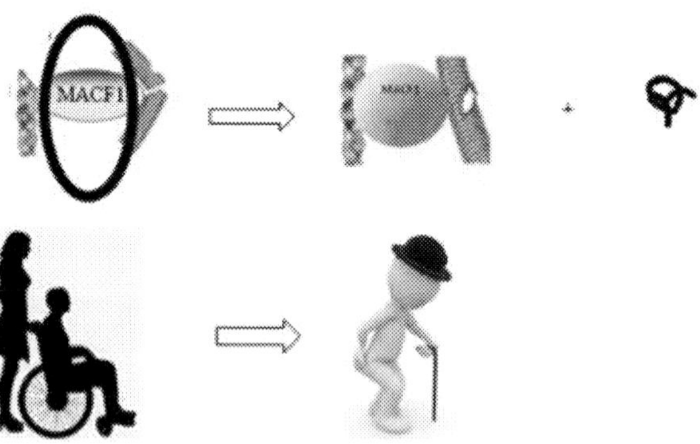

Figure 13. Scheme of repair of the cytoskeleton of the brain.

Thus, the mechanism of repair of the cytoskeleton of the brain can be represented by the following scheme, Figure 13. As followed from this scheme, the process of nanotube recovery was not completed and it still takes time to "fill holes" with kinesins (https://en.wikipedia.org/ wiki/Kinesin).

Sluggish Epilepsy

The therapy of complex irradiation of GN and stimulation of the immune system (vitamins) dramatically improved the condition of the probate, which allowed him to be discharged from the clinic as early as February 2020, i.e., after 3 months and 3 series of therapeutic treatment. However, in 2021, symptoms of indolent epilepsy began to appear and, as a result of a fall, the patient received a new traumatic brain injury (hematoma), Figure 14. After 3 months of treatment, the hematoma disappeared. GMS analysis of the GN from the ANC of the right temple showed no pathologies, but progressive paralysis of the left hand and urinary incontinence were stated (https://ru. wikipedia.org/wiki/ Enuresis).

Therefore, we made attempts to understand these processes from the standpoint of resonant compulsion by an ensemble of brain chromosomal oscillators with a higher potential energy (dominant ensemble of oscillators), oscillations of chromosomes with a lower potential energy (recessive ensemble of oscillators) in the muscle cells of the left hand (Figure 1).

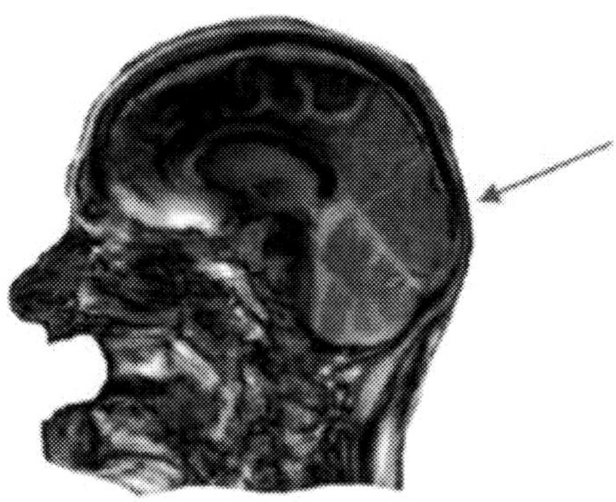

Figure 14. MRT of the probant after falling and hitting the back of the head on the concrete floor on March 23, 2021. Arrow indicates hematoma.

Paresis, Molecular Mechanism and Method of Treatment

Figure 15 shows the GMS spectrum of the muscle of the left hand of the probat-70 after ascertaining progressive paralysis of the left hand (https://ru.wikipedia.org/wiki/Paresis). The hand began to dry up. Attention is drawn to the unusual nature of the signals in the spectrum. Thus, signals of cytoskeletal water clusters are completely absent (broad arrow), however, two strong signals (indicated by asterisks) appeared in the area of loose micellar structures with masses of 9.7 and 87.8 million Dalton, respectively. These signals were also detected in the right side of the brain.

The data in Figure 15 indicate that in the topology of muscle chromosomes, by means of its resonant control of the dominant topology of the brain chromosome, some of the nucleosomes were destroyed with the formation of the free octamers and denatured DNA loops (Figure 16). If the signals from octamer associates are found in the spectra as signals of new and strong oscillators (Figure 15 A), then there are no signals from their DNA strangle loops. This fact can be understood as the formation of unstructured, partially denatured DNA helices and filaments formed from them. According to this model, these signals may reflect the appearance of loose associates of 69 and 622 octamers in the chromosomes of the ANC muscles.

Therapy for restoring long-range order in the muscle through the effect of donor-12 GN on damage in the patient's brain is limited by slow relaxation processes involving large domain and micellar loose structures and, on average, is from 3 to 5% per week.

According to this model, the breakdown of part of the solenoid basic topology of chromosomes, represented, for example, by 52 turns of 12 nucleosomes in each turn, leads to the formation of the coils of proteins from released octamers (156) and loose formations, such as filaments, from DNA helices in denatured form, not giving signals in GMS, Figure 17. These processes, in our opinion, are signs of the onset of the development of Alzheimer's disease (https://en.wikipedia.org/wiki/Alzheimer%27s_disease).

The appearance in the neurons of the brain of coils of proteins and filaments from DNA will become a trigger for the avalanche destruction of the topology of chromosomes and their inactivation as control systems, the progress of syneresis of the brain gel. Therefore, the diagnosis of the beginning of such processes is extremely important, since only at the initial stage of decay is there a real possibility of repair and shift of syneresis in the opposite direction.7.

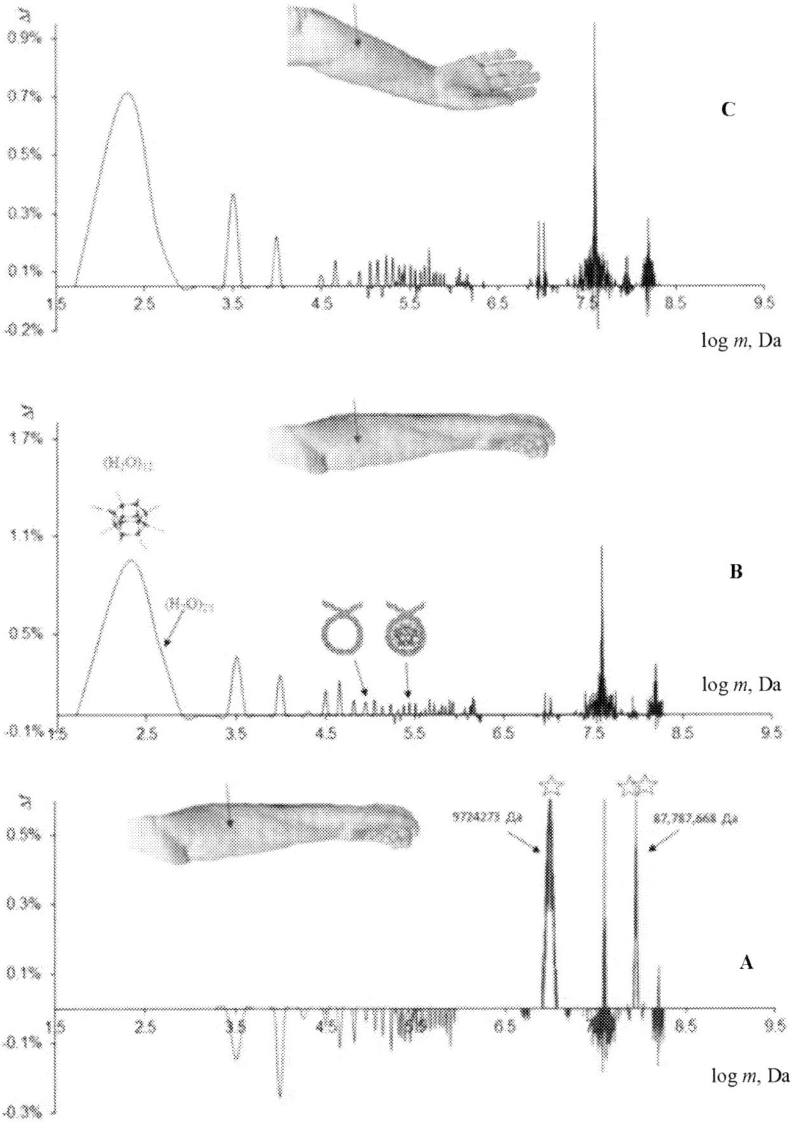

Figure 15. **A** - GMS spectrum of GN from the paralyzed muscle of the left arm of the probant-70 on 26.08.2021. The arrow indicates the location of the GN scan ($N = 657$, $D_c = 19\%$, M_{GMS}=33,162,774, Da). **B** - the same, after treatment with the influence on the right temple of the probant-70 GN of a young donor-12 ($N = 573$, $D_c = 2\%$, M_{GMS} = 19,444,975, Da). **C** - the same, but for the right hand ($N = 583$, $D_c = 2\%$, M_{GMS} = 15,331,016, Da), 26.8.2021.

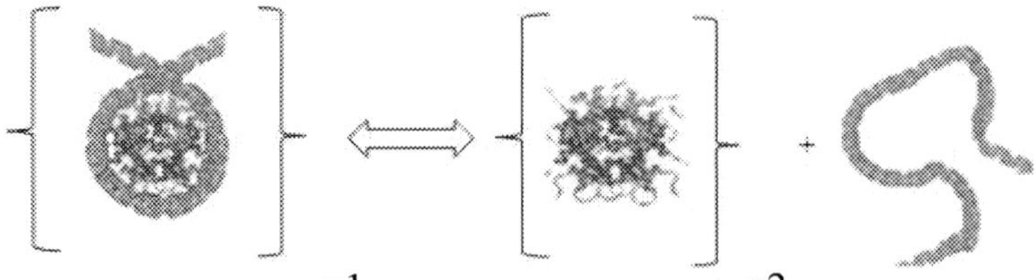

Figure 16. Model of nucleosome disintegration in solenoids of chromosomes of the muscle of the left hand, as a result of compulsion by the dominant oscillator of analogues in the brain during an epileptic seizure. Where, **n1** = 9,724,273/141,145= 69 and **n2** = 87,787,668 /141,145 = 622 (amyloid plaques), Figure 15.

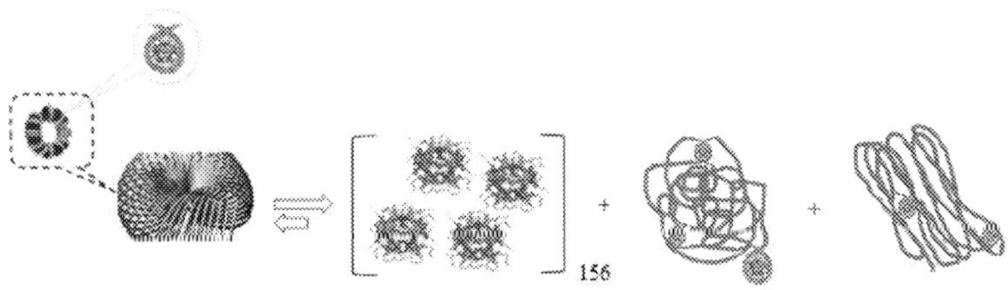

Figure 17. Model of a part of the solenoid construction of the basic topology of chromosomes subjected to decay according to the scheme of Figure 16. An example is given for one turn consisting of 12 nucleosomes (model on the left, top), the number of turns involved in the decay is 52. **A** - a turn of 12 nucleosomes in solenoid **B** and germinal amyloid plaques of 156 octamers **C**, **D** and **E** - coils and filaments of DNA helices.

Therapy

Figure 18 shows the results of brain therapy of probant-70 GN donor-12.

As can be seen from Figure 18, the treatment of the left hand by influencing the main ensemble of nucleosome analogue oscillators in brain neurons had a rapid effect in neutralizing loose octamer coils (Figure 17) in both ensembles of molecular oscillators of the brain and hand (Figure 1), already in the first session. However, in the brain molecular oscillator of octamers (amyloid plaque), there were signals from dense associates, from the decay of 67 nucleosomes (octamers with masses of 9,418,716 Da, 102 Hz) and from 72 and 73 nucleosomes with octamer masses of 10,217,713 Da and 10,307,829 Da, respectively (98 Hz).

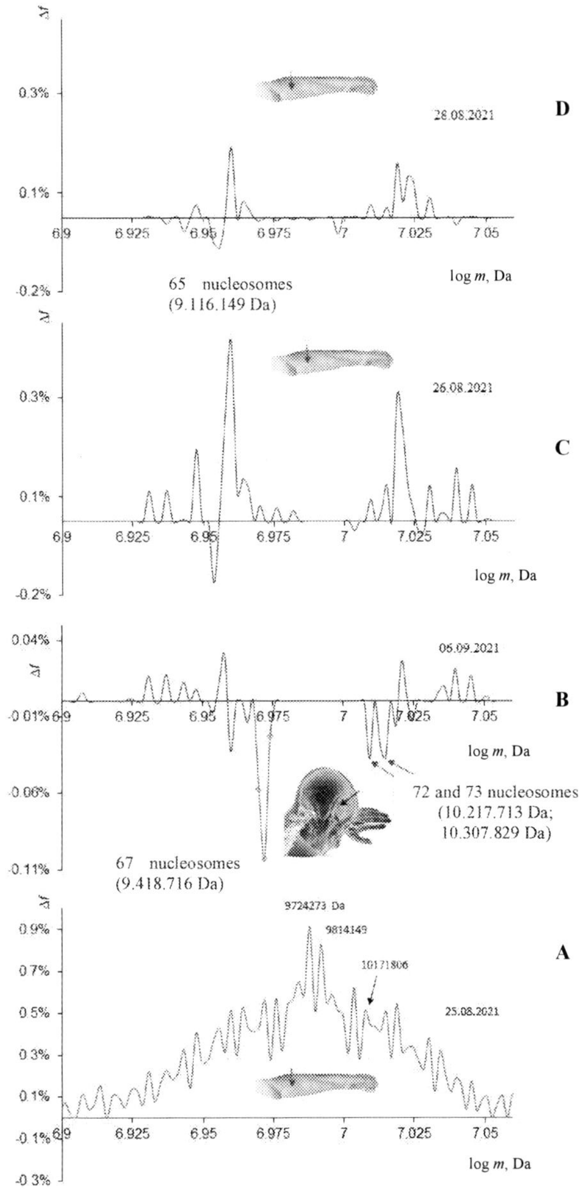

Figure 18. The results of brain therapy of the probant-70 GN donor-12. **A** – GMS spectrum of octamer oscillations (141,145 Da) in nucleosomes of neurons of the left arm muscle (paresis), before irradiation, **B** – GMS spectrum of octamer oscillations in nucleosomes of neurons of the brain of the right part after therapy with GN of donor-12, **C** and **D** – GMS spectra of octamer oscillations in nucleosomes of neurons of the muscle of the left hand after 4 and 5 hours of donor-12 GN therapy (1 h/day).

A similar effect was achieved during the destruction of octamer coils with a peak mass at 87,787,668 Da, Figure 15. As a result, the probant-70 had the ability to bend the left arm at the elbow joint, the hand up to 30°, and a weak reaction of the phalanges of the fingers to the signals of expansion and extension was found, speech improved, clarity of thought, hearing, and stability of gait even without a cane. However, enuresis syndromes remained. Here we believe that the causes of enuresis are complex, namely, problems with systematic insufficient defalization (constipation as a consequence of anti-cancer chemotherapy) and insufficient therapy with donor-12 GN (9.4 and 10.2 million Da, Figure 18 B). Subsequent therapy should have included measures to transform dense octamer associates into loose ones and their restorative implementation into loops of DNA helices (Figures 16 and 17). This, in principle, is possible, Figure 16.

Relapse

The destruction of the blood-brain barrier led to a permanent infiltration of HSV-1 into the right, damaged part of the probation's brain. The signal that the virus penetrated and affected the topology of chromosomes in brain neurons was the re-emergence of Bell's palsy and the appearance of viral lesions on the lips (Figure 5). At this time, a weak signal from the DNA ring of the virus genome (~100 MDa, 31 Hz) in a dense configuration was detected in the GMS, which required the application of an antiviral ointment (Aciclostat) by the probant-70. The virus attack was re-recorded when the probant-70 suddenly fell, which was understood as a relapse of an epileptic seizure. Probant-70 did not lose consciousness, but immediately asked for help. Subsequent scanning of GMS using the GN method of the right hemisphere showed (Figure 19) the appearance of an associate of octamers (amylose plaques, Alzheimer's symptoms) in a loose form with a narrow distribution of masses, which are adequate to those at the maximum in the curve of Figure 18A. The data of Figures 18 and 19 indicated the presence of local zones in the chromosome topology of brain neurons accessible to the virus genome. Finding them requires more research.

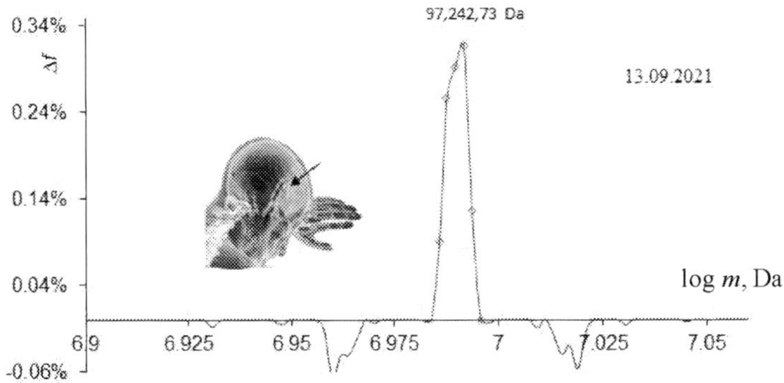

Figure 19. GMS spectrum of octamer oscillations in the nucleosomes of neurons in the right part of the brain after an epileptic seizure and the fall of the probant-70, comments in the text.

Virus

In the GMS spectra, virus signals (Figure 9) are represented by several types, which makes it necessary to understand their morphological constructions at the maximum resolution of the spectrometer. Figure 20 shows the GMS spectra of the brain of the probant-70 after the next treatment.

From the data in Figure 20, the spectra show the effect of donor-12 GN on the rings of the virus genome (A). All oscillators are in a loose configuration, and the difference in masses is (from left to right): 426,327; 278,546; 421,674; 422,588; 423,502, 280,761; 425,021 and 425,935 Da. It can be assumed that their cause is a consequence of the canonical states of the DNA rings in the plasmid. They arise as a result of forced oscillations of the rings in the tight space of the capsid and are accompanied by cycle form breaking and fast restoring. Then, the GMS spectrometer registers the superposition of masses, and after exposure to the GN donor-12, the signals disappear and the DNA rings in the virus genome are destroyed (B).

Figure 21 shows a model of the canonical structural rings of the HSV-1 genome in its capsid, as a simple example. The formation of only 4 canonical structures in the plasmid is shown in the adiabatic equilibrium mode (https://ru.wikipedia.org/wiki/Adiabatic_process). Canonical structures provide reversible processes of rapid decay and recovery, oscillating in a tense state, of only one DNA ring. In this case, a series of new rings and small fragments in a thermodynamically unstable state temporarily follow. The shock wave of the spectrometer registers them in the GMS spectrum as independent units (up to 9 signals). Hence, it is reasonable to believe that external energy impacts on DNA will increase the number of fragments and expand the number of canonical structures.

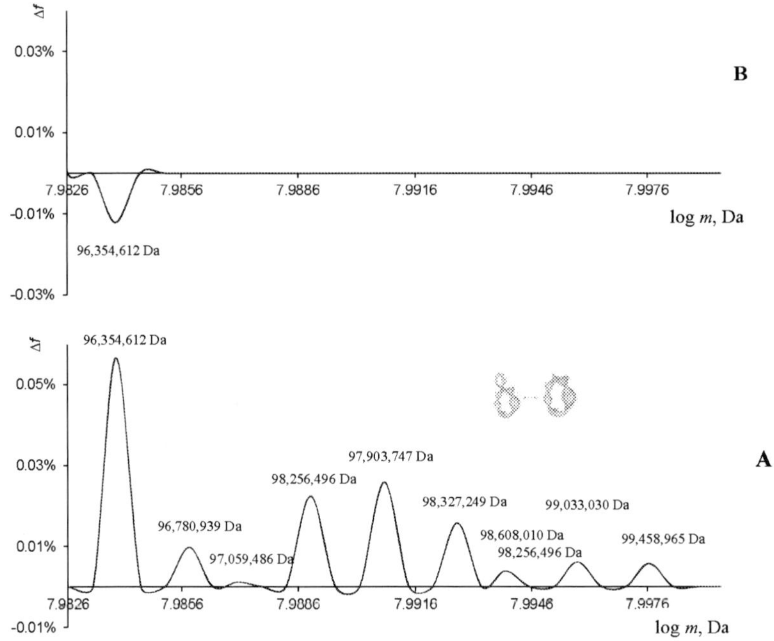

Figure 20. **A** - GMS spectra of the genome of the HSV-1 virus on February 6, 2022, the right hemisphere of the brain of probant-70 and **B** - the same range of DNA oscillations in the genome of this virus after exposure to the HSV-1 donor (granddaughter, 12 years old) and the scheme of reversible decay of oscillating DNA rings of the virus genome.

Nature placed the genome in the capsid in the form of rings due to their low diffusion ability, which prevents the virus from leaving the ring. But the destruction of the ring should increase its diffusion capacity and become an additional source of nucleotides in the body. The destruction of the ring (the formation of "eights") can be expected in the areas of transition from one form of DNA to another. This means that DNA in the genome is heterogeneous in shape (A, B, Z, https://ru.wikipedia.org/wiki/ Deoxyribonucleic_acid) and decay-formation occurs at the sites of maximum tension in the rings during their oscillations. Models of oscillations of a mathematical ring and the tensions arising in it can be found at https://mc.spbstu.ru/userfiles/files/Grad Works/ 2011_bach/zegzhda.pdf.

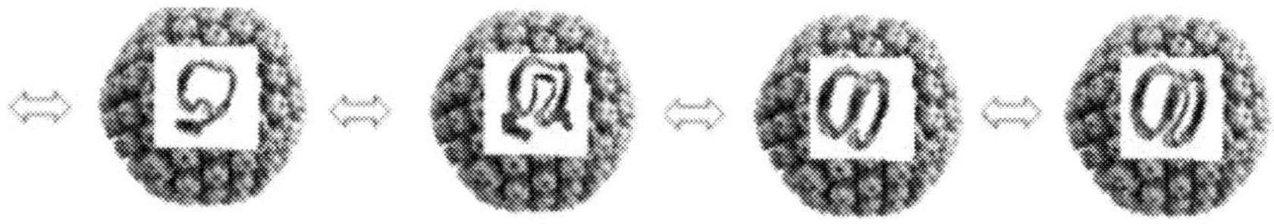

Figure 21. Model of the HSV-1 virus and canonical states of the DNA ring in the plasmid exposed to weak donor-12 GNs. An example is given for only one DNA ring and 4 canonical structures.

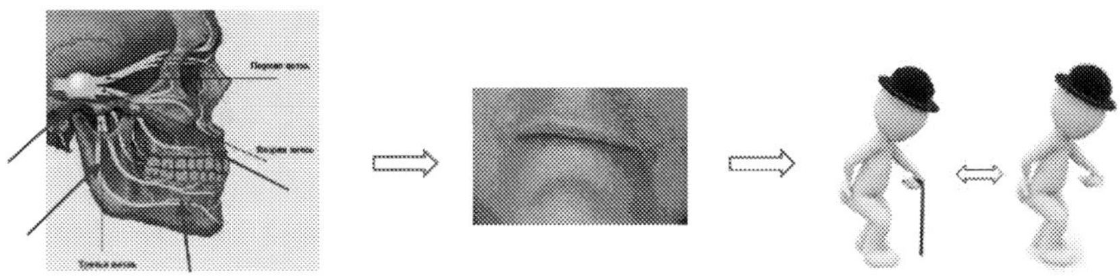

A **B** **C**

Figure 22. **A** - Trigeminal nerve and devirualization sites (indicated by arrows, branches 2 and 3 only). **B** - Result after 2 days, photograph of the patient's lips after non-invasive trigeminal devirualization *in vivo*. **C** - After the start of therapy, Probant began to walk more often even without a cane, but the general weakening of the body, due to hypodynamia of the muscular apparatus, required him to return to it.

So, the external manifestations of a virus attack and LRO monitoring data in the molecular structure of the brain can help the probant-70 prepare for a relapse and prevent its possible severe consequences.

The process of rescue was complicated by the psychological attitude of the probat-70 (not the desire to understand the disease and help the treatment, the banal idea of the hopelessness of the situation and, as a result, laziness). We believe that the healing process, even in this case, can be strengthened by standard methods of physiotherapy, after first convincing the probant of their necessity. On the other hand, frequent MRT and X-ray examinations not only "tortured" the probat-70 with the duration of unsuccessful standard treatment, but also with the lack of clarity of the doctors' positions, which, with a high probability, led to the destruction of the basic topological structures in the chromosomes. The latter requires a deeper study and search for a solution, so it was still difficult to talk about a complete understanding, and even more so about a complete quick recovery of the probate.

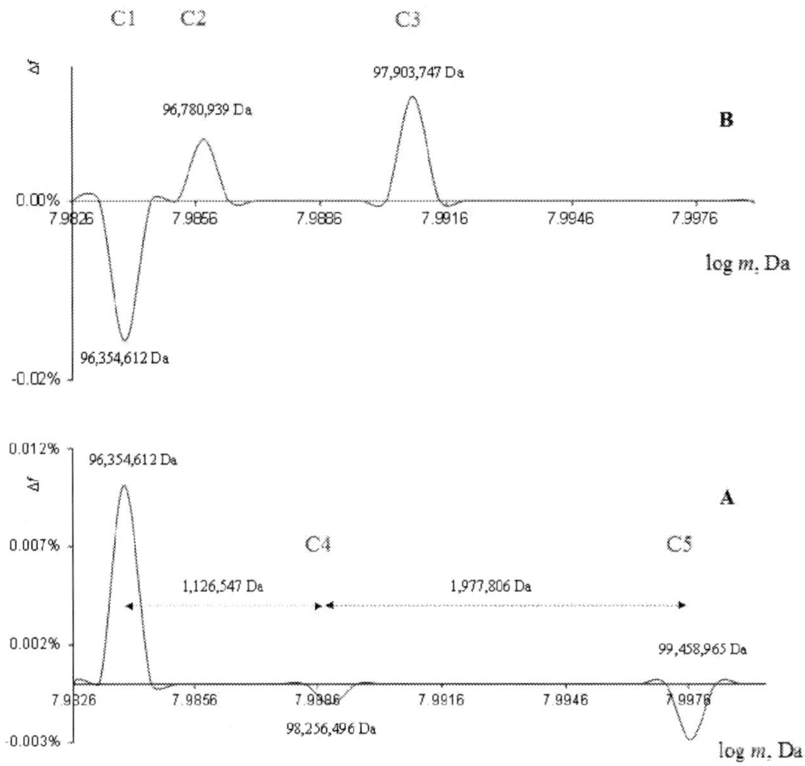

Figure 23. **A** - GMS spectrum, in the region of oscillations of the HSV-2 genome rings (probant-70) and **B** - also for another probant-68 (68 years old) with HSV-1/2; urine of probants (morning).

Thus, brain diseases and the pathologies they cause in other organs can be successfully diagnosed by the non-invasive GMS method in vivo mode, as well as by the advanced capabilities of the method for restoring the basic topology of brain chromosomes. Already after the first therapy in 2021 (Figure 22), the probant began to move more confidently even without a cane. Relapses of the appearance of herpes on the lips became rare, speech and expression of thoughts became clearer, but sporadic.

It should be noted that signals of the virus genome were also registered in other organs (heart, limb muscles) of the probat-70. Further, in order to understand the real number of rings in the virus plasmid, the LRO in the urine of probant-70 with different infection with HSV-1 and HSV-2 viruses was studied, where the products of genome metabolism were expected. Figure 23 shows 2 spectra. One can see the presence of 3 signals (C1, C4 and C5) from oscillating rings in loose form (96,354,612 Da) and 2 in dense form, 98,256,496 and 99,458,965 Da for the HSV-2 virus. The HSV-1 genome is also represented by 3 signals from the rings (C1, C2 and C3), but with somewhat smaller masses: 96,354,612; 96,780,939 and 97,903,747 Da. These data confirm the existence of only 3 DNA rings in the genome of the same type of HSV-1 and HSV-2 viruses (https://en.wikipedia. org/wiki/CccDNA), however, genomes differ in the masses of DNA rings and, possibly, in their conformations.

Alzheimer's Symptomatic

Figure 24 shows photographs of brain damage caused by Alzheimer's disease. It can be seen that the collapse of the brain is associated with the processes of fractionation of all components of the brain into: biopolymers, water, solutions, fats and polysaccharides. These are known from colloidal chemistry processes of gel aging [12] - syneresis (https://ru.wikipedia.org/ wiki/ Syneresis), the driving force of which is cohesive-adhesive separation processes according to the principle: similar to similar. As will be shown below, these processes are reversible, but the restoration of the cytoskeleton will require energy.

The probant-70 had the standard symptoms of Alzheimer's: sporadic loss of memory, hearing, absent-mindedness, slurred speech, poor coordination of movements, and even disruption of the gastrointestinal tract.

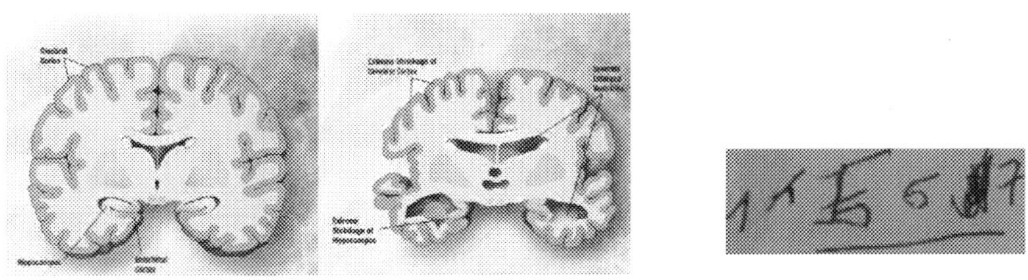

A B C

Figure 24. Photographs of a slice of the brain of a healthy person **A** and **B** prone to Alzheimer's disease (https://ru.wikipedia.org/wiki/Alzheimer's Disease).
C - a sample of recording a phone number by probant-70, 1.3.2022.

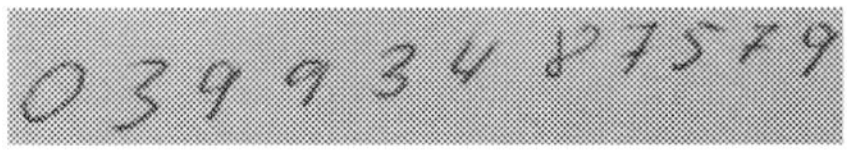

Figure 25. Test in writing a series of numbers with probant-70 after 4 hours of exposure to the affected area of the brain with gravitational noise of the donor (granddaughter, 11 years old). 03.3.2022.

Figure 25 shows the results of the test for writing numbers with probant-70 after 4 hours of exposure (during sleep) to the GN of a granddaughter-donor. Comparison with the previous test (Figure 24) clearly indicates the disappearance of Alzheimer's symptoms. At the same time, coordination in movements improved dramatically, memory and the ability to think logically improved.

The Mechanism of the Appearance of Amylose Plaques in Neurons

Figures 16 and 17 provide insight into the breakdown of solenoid structures of chromosomes and the release of octamer proteins from nucleosomes. It is reasonable to assume that octamer proteins, together with their analogues from other parts of the brain cells, agglomerate into amyloid plaques with masses >0.5 MDa (hAß1-42, [17]), and unfolded DNA with octamer residues into fibrillary structures [13] and helical filaments. [14, 17], Figures 16, 17. Physicians observe this process in optical microscopes, however, the GMS method makes it possible to register octamer agglomeration in the cytoskeletons of brain neurons non-invasively and *in vivo* already at the early stages of nucleosome decay, that is, to monitor the onset of the disease in the early stages of its development.

Alternative mechanisms for the formation of amylose plaques from APP proteins with masses of 110…130 kDa, which are aggregated into oligomeric toxic amyloid-ß-proteins (Aß) and further into fibrillary Aß plaques, have been proposed [17]. However, the very origin of APP proteins remains unclear.

Restoration of the Molecular Structure of the Cytoskeleton of Neurons

Since the process of syneresis can be reversible, the authors attempted to restore the cytoskeleton of neurons. The attempt was based on the well-known

Chladni phenomenon (https://ru.wikipedia.org/wiki/ Figures_Chladni). To do this, samples of the right hemisphere of the donor without pathologies (granddaughter, 12 years old) were taken and the cytoskeleton of neurons in the right part of the brain of probant-70 was exposed to them (Figures 18 and 20). The result was expected. The macromolecular structure of the cytoskeleton of neurons in the brain of probant-70 was restored. Probant-70 already after 2...3 days (the time of relaxation processes for macromolecules) noticed a progress. Speech and coordination, memory began to recover, and after 3 months he entered the rhythm of life, but, as it turned out, the procedure must be repeated every 4-6 months. During this time, the cytoskeleton of neurons remained stable. Instability is associated with virus attacks on the trigeminal nerve. Therefore, it was concluded that it is necessary to reduce the level of viruses in the whole body through the use of a complex of pharmaceuticals (https:// flexikon.doccheck.com/de/Bell-L%C3%A4hmung).

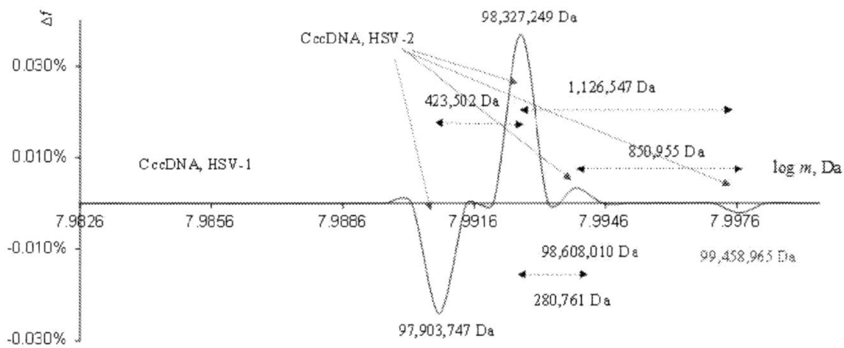

Figure 26. GMS spectrum, in the region of oscillations of the HSV-1 and HSV-2 genome rings (probant-70). 2.3.2022.

So, patient-70 was prescribed acyclovir (200 mg x every 4 hours a day, for a week, https://ru.wikipedia.org/wiki/wiki/Acyclovir). Already after the first day in his urine, the signals of the HSV-1 genome disappeared, but the signals of the HSV-2 genome appeared (Figure 26). The symptoms of Bell's palsy disappeared and there were signs of suppression of paresis (weak movements of the fingers of the left hand). Since the likelihood of recurrence is still high, it was decided to continue chemotherapy and physiotherapy, as well as the impact of donor GN on the injury site on the right side of the brain.

Storage of Chromosome Topologies (SCT)

The analysis of the course of the disease indicated the urgent need to create an individual data repository on the basic topology of chromosomes for each citizen in case of damage (accidents, wars, sports, aging and disease). These data should be compiled for each local brain function at the age of 12...15 years and updated every 10...20 years. Such a repository will allow not to turn to donors with a different brain morphology and basic chromosome topology, but to use their own data, which, in our opinion, will lead to synergy in the processes of brain recovery and treatment.

Conclusion

The GMS method allows you to quickly monitor the GN from the ANC of the brain in real time.

ANC in the cytoskeleton of the brain are formed under the influence of the gravitational noise of the Universe.

Chromosomes of neurons, in the locations of brain functions, remotely and resonantly interact with analogous chromosomes in neurons of other organs of the body, as a powerful dominant oscillator, forcing their analogs to corresponding topological changes.

Pathologies are associated primarily with a violation of the harmonic oscillations of the chromosomes of the brain and chromosomes in the cells of other organs as a single oscillator.

A method has been found for soft repair of the brain cytoskeleton in the mode of non-invasive physical impact of weak shock waves on the cytoskeletal ligaments.

Soft non-invasive influence on the long-range order of ANC in the brain *in vivo* is the future of medicine.

The HSV-1 virus easily penetrates through lesions in the blood-brain barrier and attacks neurons, and is able to affect the basic topology of their chromosomes.

Frequent exposure to MRT and X-rays leads to a disruption in the basic topology of chromosomes that resonates with counterparts in other organs of the body, which initiates various forms of epilepsy.

Irradiation of the damaged brain of a GN donor patient makes it possible to restore the destroyed topology of brain chromosomes and stop epileptic processes.

Non-invasive devirulization of the trigeminal nerve with GMS technology tools makes it possible to block the entry of HSV-1 into the damaged part of the brain.

The GMS method allows monitoring the impact of the herpes virus on neuronal brain chromosomes and their topological local forms responsible for motor functions.

The genome of HSV-1 and HSV-2 is represented by 3 DNA rings that are in dynamic equilibrium in the capsid, which can be represented as canonical structures, with products of their rapid decay and rapid formation.

The symptomatology of epileptic pathology, in viral infections, is the result of the attack of the virus genome on tubulin structures, leading to the destruction of nanotubes and sporadic blocking of the electrical signal between neurons.

Alzheimer's disease is the result of the destruction of the solenoid structures of nucleosomes in the topology of the chromosomes of brain neurons.

The GMS method will make it possible to create a backup storage of data on the topology of chromosomes in case of damage to the brain cytoskeleton.

References

[1] Zubow K., Zubow A., Zubow V. A. New Fast Non Invasive Diagnostic of Human Brain at Molecular Level: Brain Treatment. *Horizons in Neuroscience Research.* Eds. Andres Costa & Eugenio Villalba. Nova Publisher Inc. 2020, vol. 39, https://novapublishers.com/shop/horizons-in-neuroscience-research-volume-39/.

[2] Zubow K., Zubow A. V., Zubow V. A. *The Way to the ETIs. Applied gravitational mass spectroscopy.* Nova Sci. Publ. NY, 2014. https://www.novapublishers.com/catalog/product_info.php?products_id=42668&osCsid=5bd85d42dc273360fd48126de7be9daf.

[3] Zubow K., Zubow A., Zubow V. A. Nucleosome States and Sub Ensemble of Histones in Brain form Memory. Chromosomes - a powerful accumulator of potential energy. Horizons in Neuroscience Research. Eds. Andres Costa & Eugenio Villalba. Nova Publisher Inc. 2022. *Horizons in Neuroscience Research.* Volume 43, in print.

[4] Lindemann A. *Herpes simplex Virus Typ 1 Latenz in humanen Hirnnervganglien als virale Pathogenese der akut unilateralen Vestibulopathie* [*Herpes simplex virus type 1 latency in human cranial nerve ganglia as a viral pathogenesis of acute unilateral*

vestibulopathy]. Dissertation, 2019, Medizinischen Fakultät der Ludwig-Maximilians-Universität München [Medical faculty of the Ludwig-Maximilians-University Munich.]. https://edoc.ub.uni-muenchen.de/24172/2/ Lindemann_Anja.pdf.

[5] Zubow K., Zubow A., Zubow V. A. A method for non-invasive repair of the brain cytoskeleton after an HSV-I attack. Virus deactivation mechanism. *Horizons in Neuroscience Research.* Eds. Andres Costa & Eugenio Villalba. Nova Publisher Inc. 2020, vol.40, pp. 225-240. https://novapublishers.com/shop/horizons-in-neuro science-research-volume-40/.

[6] Dieudonnée van de Willigel, Jessica JA Hummell, Celine Alkemade at all. Cytolinker Gas2L1 regulates axon morphology through microtubule-modulated actin stabilization. *EMBO reports* 20:e47732|2019, pp. 1-20. doi 10.15252/embr. 201947732.

[7] Bogdanov E. V. Manturova G. M. Equicluster model of water. *Biomedical Electronics*, 2000, No. 7, pp. 19-28.

[8] Prof. Chaplin in http://www.lsbu.ac.uk/water/index.html.

[9] Shingo Murakami, MD; Mutsuhiko Mizobuchi, MD; Yuki Nakashiro at al. Bell Palsy and Herpes Simplex Virus: Identification of Viral DNA in Endoneurial Fluid and Muscle. *Annals of Internal Medicine*; 1996, vol. 124(1_Part_1), pp. 27-30. doi: 10.7326/0003-4819-124-1_Part_1-199601010-00005.

[10] Zubow K., Zubow A., Zubow V. A. Properties of Atomic Nuclei Ensembles (Molecular Clusters and Domains) as a New Form of Matter. *Horizons in World Physics.* Ed. Albert Reimer. NY, Nova Publish. Inc. 2020, vol. 302, pp. 119-141. https://novapublishers.com/shop/horizons-in-world-physics-volume-302/.

[11] Annika Lenz, Lars Ojamäe. On the stability of dence versus cage-shaped water clusters: Quantum-chemical investigations of zero-point energies, free energies, basis-set effects and IR spectra of $(H_2O)_{12}$ and $(H_2O)_{20}$. *Chem. Phys. Letters*. 2006, v. 418, pp. 361-367.

[12] Frolov Yu. G. Course of colloid chemistry. Surface phenomena and dispersed systems. — M.: *Chemistry*, 1988. 464 p.

[13] Xiaoyan Hua, Scott L. Crickb, Guojun Buc, Carl Friedend, Rohit V. Pappub, and Jin-Moo Leea. Amyloid seeds formed by cellular uptake, concentration, and aggregation of the amyloid-beta peptide. *PNAS*, December 1, 2009, vol, 106, no. 48, pp. 20324–20329. www.pnas.org/cgi/doi/10.1073/pnas.0911281106.

[14] Sperling RA, Mormino EC, Schultz AP, Betensky RA, Papp KV, Amariglio RE, Hanseeuw BJ, Buckley R, Chhatwal J, Hedden T, Marshall GA, Quiroz YT, Donovan NJ, Jackson J, Gatchel JR, Rabin JS, Jacobs H, Yang HS, Properzi M, Kirn DR, Rentz DM and Johnson KA (2019) The impact of amyloid-beta and tau on prospective cognitive decline in older individuals. *Ann Neurol* 2:181-193.

[15] Trojanowski JQ and Lee VM (1994) Paired helical filament tau in Alzheimer's disease. The kinase connection. *Am. J Pathol* 144:449-453.

[16] Mettenleiter, T.C. Budding events in herpesvirus morphogenesis. *Virus Res,* 2004. Vol. 106, no.2, pp. 167-80.

[17] Sarah Schemmert. *In vivo Charakterisierung Amyloid-β-Oligomer eliminierender D-enantiomerer Peptide zur Therapie der Alzheimer'schen Demenz*. Dissertation.

Januar 2018. Mathematisch-Naturwissenschaftlichen Fakultät der Heinrich-Heine-Universität Düsseldorf. *FRG* [*In vivo characterization of amyloid-β-oligomer eliminating D-enantiomeric peptides for the treatment of Alzheimer's dementia*. Dissertation. January 2018. Faculty of Mathematics and Natural Sciences at the Heinrich Heine University in Düsseldorf. FRG]. https://docserv.uni-duesseldorf.de/servlets/ DerivateServlet/Derivate-48515/Dissertation_Sarah%20 Schemmert.pdf.

Chapter 2

The Role of the Thalamus in the Nociception

Alfonso Alfaro-Rodríguez[1], Ana Micov[2], Samuel Reyes-Long[1], Herlinda Bonilla-Jaime[3], Circe Monserrat Vázquez-Bonilla[4], Ana Lilia Dotor-Llerena[1], Cindy Bandala[1,5] and José Luis Cortes-Altamirano[1,6,*]

[1]División de Neurociencias, Instituto Nacional de Rehabilitación, "Luis Guillermo Ibarra Ibarra," Ciudad de México, México
[2]Department of Pharmacology, Faculty of Pharmacy, University of Belgrade, Serbia
[3]Departamento de Biología de la Reproducción, Universidad Autónoma Metropolitana-Iztapalapa, Ciudad de México, México
[4]Facultad de Medicina, Universidad Nacional Autónoma de México, Ciudad de México, México
[5] Escuela Superior de Medicina, Instituto Politecnico Nacional, Ciudad de México, México
[6] Departamento de Quiropráctica, Universidad Estatal del Valle de Ecatepec, Estado de México, México

Abstract

Long it has been recognized the thalamus as the entry gate to the brain for the sensory input transmission from the periphery. In the relay of the nociceptive input to a painful sensation a combination of processes in the periphery, spinal cord and brain are involved, but not completely understood. The thalamus has a very rich nuclear organization; more than

* Corresponding Author: jlcortesaltamirano@gmail.com.

In: Horizons in Neuroscience Research. Volume 48
Editors: Andres Costa and Eugenio Villalba
ISBN: 979-8-88697-230-6
© 2022 Nova Science Publishers, Inc.

20 nuclei have been identified, and it can be classified from an evolutionary perspective, from the interconnectivity of the fibers and from the cytoarchitectonic and anatomic-functional organization. The thalamic nuclei of the medial line conform two independent endogenous systems that exert some control over the nociceptive input: the medial dorsal nucleus that participates in the descendent facilitation of the development of mechanical allodynia, and the ventral medial that specifically mediates the descendent inhibition of thermal hyperalgesia. More recently, the periventricular nucleus, located in the medial line, has been recognized to have modulatory effects in the nociceptive pathway. In this way the thalamus along with other areas of the cerebral cortex play a crucial role in the integration of the sensitive information. The interconnectivity of the cortico-thalamic projections prompts a complex network of communication that paired with the several neurotransmitters result in the integration of the painful response. In the present chapter, we will discuss the distal components along with the sensitive receptors and the interconnectivity relevant to the nociception focusing on the modulatory role of the thalamus.

Keywords: thalamus, nociception, pain, neurotrasmitters, neurophysiology

Introduction

The thalamus is a vital structure lying deep within the brain and possesses a number of important roles, such as sensory and motor function, attention and memory, plus, is a key relay station for the transmission of nociceptive information to the cerebral cortex (Lenz et al., 2000). Several classifications of the thalamic nuclei have been proposed ranging from an evolutionary point of view (Elliot, 1969), to characteristics of connectivity of fibers and functions (Afifi y Bergman, 1999), and cytoarchitectonic and anatomic-functional criteria (Hirai y Jones, 1989; Morel et al., 1997). The complex relationship between the thalamic nuclei and the cerebral cortex is underlined by the synapses between these two great structures and the neurophysiological properties of them (Che et al., 2006; Park et al., 2017).

The thalamus has long been considered as a simple relay station for sensory information from the periphery to the cortex. However, the view of 'just' transferring sensory signals from subcortical nuclei to the cortex, has been replaced with the conception that thalamic neurons play a central role in the selection, amplification, and prioritization process that determines which type of information should be available to the cortex at any given time

(Sherman, 2005, Sherman and Guillery, 1998). Being the so-called 'gate-keeper' of the cortex, thalamic neurons regulate the flow of rapidly changing sensory signals, thus allowing the cortex to adjust to the constantly evolving behavioral and environmental demands (Sherman, 2005). To regulate the number of sensory signals that reach the cortex, thalamic neurons must themselves be subjected to a variety of modulatory inputs that originate in cortical, hypothalamic, brainstem, spinal and intrathalamic nuclei (Sherman and Guillery, 1996; McCormic, 1992).

On the other hand, nociception is the integration of harmful sensory information from the environment produced by a tissue injury that is transmitted to the Central Nervous System (CNS) by nociceptors, which are a group of sensory receptors whose main characteristic is the capacity to differentiate between harmful stimuli from those that are innocuous, among the former is pain, which is the perception of an agonizing sensation of variable magnitude.

The thalamus plays a crucial role in the integration of the ascending pain signals on their way to the cerebral cortex through the lateral and medial thalamic nociceptive pathways. The lateral thalamic pathway mediates the sensory-discriminative (referring to the intensity, location, and duration of pain) component of pain, while the medial thalamic pathway encodes affective-motivational (referring to the unpleasantness of pain and motivation to escape the pain) pain aspects. The thalamus is also part of a complex neural network involved in pain modulation (Melzack, 1999).

Thalamus Nociceptive Pathways

In Thalamus the nociceptive information is integrated, it is the relay structure of the afferent information to the cerebral cortex, plus it is responsible for the processing of said information and has a strong impact on cortical functions. In the last decade the participation of specific pathways for the cortical recognition of pain has been recognized (Treede RD, 1999), therefore, we can consider that the sensation of pain has a representation in the cerebral cortex. Nociceptive information is transmitted from the spinal cord to the thalamus (spinothalamic pathway) and to the cerebral cortex (thalamocortical), through five ascending pathways (Table 1).

The participation of the thalamus in the nociceptive pathways is currently under constant scrutiny, its importance in pain processing is amply recognized. The fact that the ascending pathways end in different regions of the thalamus and the role of nociceptive mediation are under constant investigation, however, it has already been shown that the spinothalamic pathway integrates not only nociceptive, but also tactile and thermal information, and as it ascends through the brainstem it sends information to the reticular formation (Lenz, 1998). Thus, the thalamus serves as a relay station for ascending nociceptive pathways and descending cortical circuits (Apkarian, 2007; Kuner and Kuner, 2021).

Table 1. Ascending nociceptive pathways from the thalamus

Nociceptive Pathways	Description
Spinothalamic bundle a) Spinothalamic side b) Spinothalamic previous	Ascending pathway, made up of axons from specific neurons of Rexed laminae I and V-VII of the posterior horn. Ascending towards the white matter, ending in the thalamus. Its electrical stimulation produces pain a) Lateral spinothalamic: Located in the lateral cord, transmits nociceptive and thermal information b) Anterior spinothalamic: Small, located in the anterior cord, transmits non-discriminatory information (crude)
Spinoreticular bundle	Ascending pathway, made up of axons from laminae VI and VII of Rexed. From the anterolateral quadrant of the spinal cord and descends to both the reticular formation and the thalamus. Bilateral, not crossed. Many of these axons do not cross the midline. Region responsible for wakefulness and warning of injury.
Spinomesencephalic bundle	Ascending pathway, made up of axons from Rexed laminae I and V of the anteroexternal quadrant of the spinal cord to the reticular formation and to the gray matter with a pathway from the spinoparabrachial bundle, also projects to the parabrachial nuclei and in turn these parabrachial nuclei project to the amygdaloid nucleus composed mainly of the limbic system, that is, the system involved in emotions. Therefore, it has been established that this beam contributes to the affective component of pain. Some axons go to the dorsal part of the external funiculus. Also called the descending pain inhibition system by termination in the periaqueductal gray matter and raphe nuclei of the midbrain, which are thought to give rise to fibers that modulate nociceptive transmission.
Cervicotalamic bundle	Ascending pathway, arises in the external white matter of the two upper cervical segments of the spinal cord via nociceptive neurons in the external cervical nucleus of laminae III and IV of Rexed. They cross the midline and ascend in the medial lemniscus to the ventroposterior and posteromedial nuclei of the thalamus.
Spinohypothalamic bundle	Ascending pathway, made up of axons from neurons in laminae I, V, and VIII of Rexed. They go to the supraspinal autonomic control centers. They are considered to activate neuroendocrine and cardiovascular responses.

(Rolf-Detlef, 2002; Kandel et al., 2012; Perea-Bartolomé et al., 2004).

Ascending Nociceptive Projections

The classic ascending nociceptive pathway consists of a three-neuron chain that transmits pain signals from the periphery to the cerebral cortex, with two stations in the dorsal spinal cord and thalamus/brainstem. The thalamus is one of the central areas most consistently activated by painful stimuli. It receives nociceptive inputs from ascending nociceptive pathways directly via the spinothalamic and trigeminothalamic tracts and indirectly via the spinobulbar tract (Figure 1). The spinothalamic tract conveys both noxious and non-noxious signals to the lateral (mostly) and medial (partially) thalamus (Dostrovsky and Craig, 2013; Bastuji et al., 2016; Groh et al., 2018). The spinobulbar tract conveys mainly noxious signals to the medial thalamus via an additional synaptic relay within the brainstem homeostatic regions, such as the reticular formation, periaqueductal grey matter (PAG), and the parabrachial nucleus. The dorsal column-medial lemniscal pathway, usually associated with non-nociceptive afferents, could also conduct nociceptive signals from the viscera to the thalamus (Dostrovsky and Craig, 2013).

Cells Origin of Ascending Nociceptive Projections

The cell bodies of second-order neurons are located in three distinct regions of the spinal gray matter: laminae I, IV-V, and VII-VIII. The main nociceptive projection neurons originate from laminae I (in primates, almost half of the spinothalamic cells are located in this lamina) and V. Second-order neurons can be functionally classified into nociceptive-specific (responding exclusively to noxious stimuli) and wide-dynamic range (responding to noxious and innocuous stimuli) neurons. A prototypical lamina I neuron is a nociceptive-specific neuron with a small receptive field that projects largely to the lateral thalamus, whereas a lamina V neuron is a wide-dynamic range neuron with a large receptive field, projecting largely to the medial thalamus. In the absence of nociceptive input, lamina I projection neurons are quiescent and display no spontaneous activity (Keller et al., 2007), thus showing some kind of preference for encoding noxious input under normal conditions (Chisholm et al., 2021). The axons of the spinothalamic neurons show a topographic organization and a dorsoventral segregation, with superficial lamina cell axons being more dorsally located than deeper lamina cell axons (Apkarian, 2007).

Terminations of Ascending Nociceptive Projections

It is not entirely clear which thalamic nuclei are functionally driven directly via ascending nociceptive pathways. Anatomical and functional specificity, as well as taxonomic differences between species, make identifying the thalamic nuclei involved in nociception even more complicated. Based on anterograde tracing experiments in primates and silver-staining degeneration subsequent to cordotomy in humans, the spinothalamic terminations in six distinct nuclei are determined (using nomenclature common to the primate brain; Dostrovsky and Craig, 2013):

- The posterior part of the ventral medial nucleus (VMpo)
- The ventral posterior nuclei, i.e., ventroposterior lateral (VPL), ventroposterior medial (VPM), and ventroposterior inferior (VPI) nuclei
- The ventral lateral nucleus (VL)
- The central lateral nucleus (CL)
- The parafascicular nucleus (Pf)
- The ventral caudal part of the medial dorsal nucleus (MDvc).

Many controversies are woven about the existence and role of VMpo in pain processing. Reputable sources state that VMpo serves as a primary projection target for lamina I spinothalamic cells in primates, whereas it is rudimentary or non-existent in non-primates (Dostrovsky and Craig, 2013; Craig, 2014). The role of the ventrobasal nuclei, which are still considered the principal thalamic somatosensory nuclei, is more widely accepted. The VPL is the most important nucleus of the ventrobasal complex, encoding tactile, proprioceptive, and nociceptive signals in the firing rates (low firing rates at innocuous stimuli and high firing rates at noxious stimuli) (Treede, 2002; Groh et al., 2018). Nearly all neurons from the ventrobasal complex are of the wide-dynamic range type, while VMpo neurons are almost exclusively nociceptive-specific.

According to the nuclei involved, the thalamic nociceptive pathways are divided into a lateral and a medial part. The lateral thalamic nociceptive pathway (VPL, VPM, VPI, and VMpo) was supposed to subserve the sensory-discriminative aspects of pain, and the medial thalamic nociceptive pathway (CL, Pf, and MDvc) the affective-motivational aspects. Given that nociceptive-specific neurons make up the majority of neurons in the medial thalamic nuclei, the medial thalamic pathway is thought to be more pain-specific (Dostrovsky and Craig, 2013; Whitt et al., 2013). There is growing evidence that the medial thalamic pathway contributes to the discriminative aspects of nociception as well as to the modulation of nociceptive signals (Apkarian et al., 2011).

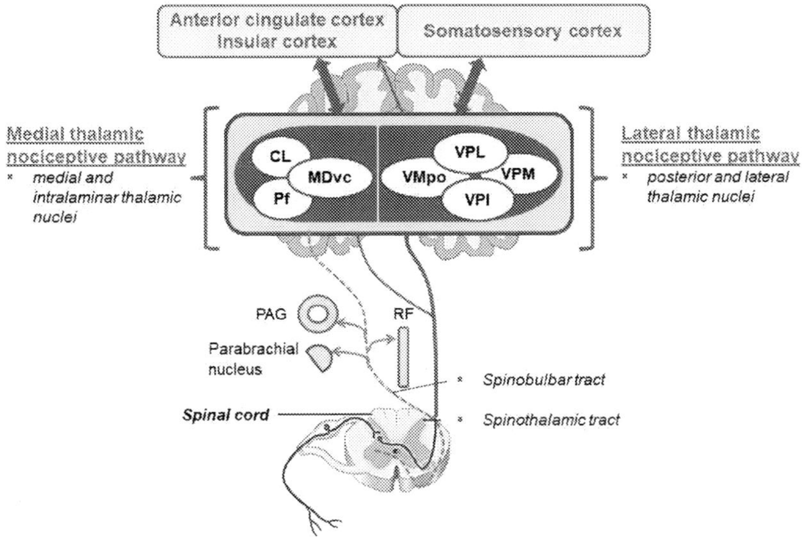

Figure 1. Scheme depicting the lateral and medial thalamic nociceptive pathways with corresponding input and output connections. Due to clarity, the trigeminothalamic tract is omitted. VMpo, posterior part of the ventral medial nucleus; VPL, ventroposterior lateral nucleus; VPM, ventroposterior medial nucleus; VPI, ventroposterior inferior nucleus; VL, ventral lateral nucleus; CL, central lateral nucleus; Pf, parafascicular nucleus; MDvc, ventral caudal part of the medial dorsal nucleus; PAG, periaqueductal grey matter; and RF, reticular formation.

The thalamic neurons, both projection neurons and GABAergic interneurons, have two functional modes: relay (constant firing rate) and oscillatory (bursting firing rate) mode. The thalamic neurons transmit afferent signals to the cortex in relay mode under normal circumstances (Krahe and Gabbiani, 2004).

Ventromedial Thalamic Function in Nociceptive Response

The Ventral Posterior Complex (VPC) is a region of the thalamus where sensitive information coming from ascending somatic sensory pathways converges. The VPC is a well-organized region, it is formed by the Ventral Posterior Lateral nucleus (VPL) and the Ventral Posterior Medial Nucleus (VPM) (Smith, 2008), in the following sections we will describe the afferences and efferences that these two nuclei have, the main neurotransmitters present, as well as their involvement in the nociceptive response.

The thalamus comprises three major cell types: the relay cells, which project their axons to the cerebral cortex or the striatum; interneurons, which have their axons and synapsis in the same nuclei; and the reticular neurons, which send their axons to the dorsal thalamus. The VPL receives sensory information from the Dorsal Column-Medial Lemniscal System and nociceptive information from second-order neuron from the Anterolateral System, however, maintaining the organization that defines the VPC, the neurons from these two systems do not combine but instead contact different classes of relay neurons. Then, third-order neurons from the VPL synapse with the primary somatosensory cortex (S1) particularly in the areas 1 and 3b. The VPL receives nociceptive information from the whole-body except the face, and it has been determined that it mediates the sensory discriminative component of pain: the intensity, location, and quality of the noxious stimuli (Purves et al., 2012).

On the other hand, the VPM receives sensitive information from the nociceptor of the face, which synapse to the trigeminal complex and the ascends throughout the Trigeminothalamic Tract, arriving then, to the VPM, which in turns projects third-order neurons to the area 3a of the S1 (Kandel et al., 2012).

Glutamate and GABA are the two transmitters released at most synapses in the dorsal thalamus, plus, the thalamus is importantly innervated by dopamine, which according to Sánchez-González et al., (2005) influences the activity of cortical, striatal, and amygdaloid regions to which the thalamus is connected. However, the authors report that the lowest densities are present in the primary sensory relay nuclei, which includes the VPL and VPM. In a further report, García-Cabezas et al. (2007) also report the presence of dopamine axons in the thalamus of the macaque, with few innervations to the VPC. In contrast, there are more monoamines projections to the thalamus, as was reported by Westlund et al., (1990), They reported that the VPL of primates receives an important amount of serotoninergic innervation, plus by means of HPLC they found a norepinephrine concentration four times that of serotonin in the rat VPL nucleus.

Changes in the Ventral Posterior Complex of the Thalamus under pathological conditions. Given that the VPL and VPM are the relay structures of the nociceptive process between the peripheral nervous system (PNS) and the CNS, several lines of research show that they regulate or participate in several pathologies that have pain as a common symptom.

Neuropathic pain is a clinical sign present in many diseases, and it can even be a pathology by itself, when resulting from nerve injury is often resistant to pharmacotherapy. Two principal manifestations of neuropathic pain, thermal hyperalgesia, and mechanical allodynia are mediated through different mechanisms and separate neuronal pathways, C fibers have limited effects on mechanical allodynia, whereas Aδ fibers transmit innocuous mechanical and thermal information. Neuropathic pain is also the major and the most disabling symptom even under analgesic therapy.

Patel et al., (2018) in a model of spinal nerve ligated Sprague-Dawley rats, described how descending noradrenergic inhibition of spinal excitability impacts sensory coding in the VPL of the thalamus. The authors propose that for those patients with small and/or large fiber neuropathy, where deafferentation of spinal neurons is likely, a significant component of ongoing pain may be driven by ectopically firing spinal neurons. Iwata et al., (2011) sought to characterize the changes in neuronal activity in the VPL in a rat model of peripheral neuropathic pain, the authors found that peripheral neuropathic pain is associated with significant changes in the firing of VPL neurons with receptive fields in the contralateral injured hind paw. In a more recent report, Chao et al., (2021) recruited forty-one patients with pathology-proven small fiber neuropathy with reduced skin innervation, their results indicate that the precentral gyrus was the most involved region in the structural influences of SFN on the brain. Specifically, the connectivity between the precentral gyrus and the somatosensory VPL and motor VLa and VLp nuclei in the thalamus was reduced, and the connectivity reduction between the precentral gyrus and these thalamic nuclei was associated with burning, tingling, mechanical allodynia, or numbness. The authors conclude that the reduction in white matter connectivity between the VPL and the precentral gyrus implicates alterations in sensorimotor integration after chronic neuropathic pain and supports the selection of the primary motor cortex as a target for noninvasive stimulation to alleviate chronic neuropathic pain.

Regarding the VPM, Okada et al., (2019) hypothesized that activation of neurons by noxious stimulation of orofacial tissues projecting to VPM after trigeminal nerve injury depends, in part, on the modality of the applied. Then, they quantified the change in the distribution pattern of VPM projection neurons in trigeminal spinal subnucleus caudalis (Vc) activated by capsaicin injection or mechanical stimulation to the upper lip after chronic constriction injury of the infraorbital nerve in rats. The researchers suggest that capsaicin may have recruited mechanically insensitive C fibers and heat-insensitive Ad fibers in Vc-VPM pathway, plus, that ascending nociceptive pathways from Vc to VPM are activated differentially in a stimulus modality-specific manner. However, Montes et al., (2005) presented a clinical case in which clinically typical central thalamic pain developed in the absence of any demonstrable lesion of the VPM. Our data rather indicate that, although the VPC does not represent the exclusive sensory thalamic relay for thermal nociceptive inputs, lesions in this area sparing the VPM are sufficient to produce central pain. It is likely, however, that other patients may present pain after thalamic lesions that do affect the VPM, underscoring the proteiform mechanisms of central pain.

Zhato et al., (2006) found that peripheral nerve injury (CCI) results in long-distance changes in responsiveness to peripheral stimulation in third-order pain processing neurons of the VPL of the thalamus that receive inputs from the injured contralateral sciatic nerve in animals that display lowered behavioral nociceptive thresholds. Our new data also document the abnormal expression of the Nav1.3 voltage-gated sodium channel transcripts in the VPL during this time of neuronal hyperresponsiveness and reduced nociceptive thresholds. Our results demonstrate for the first time, that changes in sodium channel expression within the thalamus are associated with abnormal sensory processing and chronic neuropathic pain after CCI.

Current therapies focused on the Ventral Posterior Complex of the Thalamus. In order to manage chronic pain in consequence of damage to the different regions of thalamus, including ventral posterior complex, pharmacological and nonpharmacological therapies have been proposed. Several studies have been carried where the administration of drugs individually or in combinations with different routes of administration has been employed: oral, intramuscular, and intravenous. This drug included cannabinoids (Wolf et al., 2020), opioid analgesics (Trang et al., 2015), anticonvulsants (Hebestrei et al., 2017), antidepressants (Widerström-Noga et al., 2015) intravenous infusions of anesthetic drugs (Chen-Tung Yen et al., 2013). Other non-pharmacological interventions encompass physical therapy (Cunningham et al., 2019), electroacupuncture (Shen et al., 2021), cognitive-behavioral therapy and other psychological therapies (Cunningham et al., 2019; Khera et al., 2021), laser stimuli and intracerebral electrodes (Bastuji et al., 2016), neurostimulation methods like reoccurring electrical stimulation (Dydyk and Munakomi, 2022), transcutaneous electrical nerve stimulation (Davis et al., 2000), repetitive transcranial magnetic stimulation (Rokyta et al.,

2012; Jeanmonod et al., 2012; Lin et al., 2018), motor cortex stimulation (Tsubokawa et al., 1991), deep brain stimulation (Rokyta et al., 2012; Boccard et al., 2015), radiation therapy and radiosurgery (Hayashi et al., 2007; Lovo et al., 2018), stellate ganglion block (Liao et al., 2017) and as a last resort, neurosurgical procedures such as mesencephalic tractotomy (Shieff et al., 1987; Shieff et al., 1990) and Gamma Knife thalamotomy (Franzini et al., 2021). Regarding the pain caused by neoplasms in the thalamus, resection of the tumor improves this symptom (Cao et al., 2015). However, most of the clinical studies where the efficacy of the aforementioned therapeutic alternatives has been shown, are not exclusive to the management of pain due to specific damage in the ventral posterior complex of the thalamus, neither thalamus specific.

In this sense, examples of the etiology of pain secondary to thalamic injury could be due to a brain tumor or a cerebrovascular event (Vartiainen et al., 2016), where different regions of the thalamus are damaged directly or indirectly in consequence of biochemical and mechanical cell damage. The inflammation and oxidative response that the hemorrhage or lack of irrigation causes in most of the regions of this anatomical point provokes neuropathic chronic pain disorders and thalamic pain syndrome (Dydyk and Munakomi, 2022). The tumor growth and intracranial pressure that causes cell death, necrosis and/or apoptosis, generates molecules related to the etiology of acute and chronic pain (Hadidchi et al., 2019).

Descending Cortical Input Projections

Corticothalamic projections arise in almost every area of the cerebral cortex. Although both the lateral and medial thalamus receive the terminations of corticothalamic fibers, the medial thalamus is especially affected. For example, the primary somatosensory cortex projects backwards to the posteriomedial nucleus (Mease et al., 2016; Groh et al., 2018), whereas the prefrontal cortex sends excitatory projections to the mediodorsal thalamus (Mitchell, 2015). Cortical projections to the medial thalamus together with projections from the thalamus to the cortex form the corticothalamocortical loop. The contribution of such corticothalamocortical loops to pain processing remains unknown (Kuner and Kuner, 2021). It is possible that some of the thalamic nuclei with nociceptive responses are activated polysynaptically by the cortical or subcortical structures and by the ascending nociceptive pathways (Groh et al., 2018).

Neurochemical Communication within Thalamic Input Nociceptive Pathways

Nociceptive signals are transmitted to the thalamus by glutamatergic neurons in the spinothalamic, trigeminothalamic, dorsal column-medial lemniscal, and spinoreticulothalamic pathways. Corticothalamic communication is also acquired by glutamatergic neurotransmission. Spinobulbar projections are more neurotransmitter-abundant as they include cholinergic, serotonergic, and noradrenergic neurons. Within the thalamic pathways (especially within the thalamic reticular nucleus), inhibitory GABAergic interneurons play an important role in the modulation of nociceptive signals (Apkarian, 2007; Dostrovsky and Craig, 2013).

Thalamic Output Nociceptive Pathways

The thalamus integrates and processes nociceptive signals arising from multiple ascending pathways before sending information to the various parts of the cortex and subcortical structures. According to human brain imaging research, the primary (S1) and secondary (S2) somatosensory corticies, the anterior cingulate cortex, the insular cortex, and the prefrontal cortex are the cortical regions most commonly activated by noxious stimuli. Noxious stimuli also affect certain subcortical areas like the PAG, hypothalamus, amygdala, hippocampus, and cerebellum.

Thalamocortical Nociceptive Pathways

The second-order neuron forms a synapse with the third-order neuron, thus, forming the thalamocortical nociceptive pathways. These pathways follow a somatotopic arrangement, meaning that certain regions of the body are represented in specific cortical (subcortical) areas, with thalamic nuclei serving as relay stations. The lateral thalamic nuclei convey information mainly to the somatosensory cortex, supporting discriminative pain assessment. The medial thalamic nuclei innervate primarily limbic cortices (the anterior cingulate cortex and insular cortex), supporting affective-motivational pain aspects (Apkarian, 2007; Groh et al., 2018).

In primates, primary and secondary somatosensory cortices receive noxious somatosensory input from the ventrobasal complex. Some of the well-recognized thalamocortical pairs are VPL-S1 and VPI-S2 (Apkarian, 2007; Dostrovsky and Craig, 2013). The limbic cortices are mainly activated via medial thalamic nuclei (MDvc and Pf send projections to the anterior cingulate cortex and the insular cortex). Medial thalamic nuclei also innervate the hypothalamus and amygdala, emphasizing the involvement of the medial thalamus in the affective-motivational component of pain and autonomic control as well. Limbic cortices also receive nociceptive input from the lateral thalamic nuclei: VMpo primarily projects to the posterior insular cortex (further to the amygdala), while the ventral parts of the ventroposterior nucleus and VPI innervate the anterior cingulate cortex and the insular cortex (Craig and Dostrovsky, 2013).

Encoding Nociceptive Signals

Noxious and innocuous signals converge progressively as signals travel to the central circuits. In line with this observation, nociceptive-specific neurons are in the minority in the spinal cord and are even rarer in thalamic nuclei (Kenshalo et al., 1980; Patel and Dickenson, 2016). Furthermore, the pronounced convergence of nociceptive pathways with other sensory pathways within the same nucleus is observed. How the brain discriminates between nociceptive and innocuous signals remains poorly understood. A suggested explanation is that the lateral thalamus encodes multimodal information (tactile, proprioceptive, nociceptive) in the firing rate mode, with low firing rates at non-noxious and high firing rates at noxious intensities (Kenshalo et al., 1980; Treede, 2002; Groh et al., 2018). By using firing rate threshold, the cortex also discriminates between noxious and non-noxious stimuli. The medial thalamic pathway seems to be more pain-specific (Whitt et al., 2013), so pain intensity coding could be a unique feature of the lateral thalamic nociceptive pathway.

Neurochemical Communication within Thalamic Output Nociceptive Pathways

Thalamic output to the cortex is mediated by glutamatergic neurotransmission and consequently by the activation of NMDA and non-NMDA receptors.

CGRP neurons have been shown to provide thalamo-amygdalar communication, which may also be important in generating emotional responses to painful stimuli (Apkarian, 2007).

Maladaptation of the Thalamic Nociceptive Pathways in Chronic Pain

Because of the many unresolved concerns, chronic pain remains a challenge for basic scientists and physicians. Chronic pain is characterized by substantial neuroplastic changes and reorganization in many brain regions. Neuroplasticity implies functional and structural changes with varying intensities depending on the type of chronic pain. The thalamus undergoes neuroplastic remodeling, especially under neuropathic pain conditions. Various changes that intervene in the thalamic regions have been identified through electrophysiological, immunohistochemistry, and functional imaging studies. Some of them are discussed below (Groh et al., 2018; Kuner and Kuner, 2021).

Abnormal Neuronal Excitability

Chronic pain is associated with altered pattern and/or frequency of discharges of the thalamic neurons, which in patients suffering from chronic pain fire in a bursting pattern (i.e., oscillatory mode). However, it is not clear if such a firing is a result of and/or the cause of chronic pain (Krahe and Gabbiani, 2004; Groh et al., 2018). Bursting firing activity is common in the medial thalamus, but it is also observed in the lateral thalamus. The mechanisms responsible for the altered thalamic firing have not been elucidated yet. Thalamic T-type calcium channels are most probably involved in the generation of burst firing and oscillatory behavior in thalamocortical dysrhythmia (Liao et al., 2011). Altered neural–astrocyte coupling has also been suggested to be responsible for altered thalamocortical activity under neuropathic pain states (Alshelh et al., 2016).

Increased expression of sodium channels (Nav1.3) in the ventral posterolateral nucleus of the thalamus was determined after peripheral nerve injury (Zhao et al., 2006). Increased expression of CaV3.1 T-type Ca2+-channels could also promote sensitization of thalamic neurons after peripheral nerve injury (Choi et al., 2016). As a result, these channels could be attractive targets for neuropathic pain analgesic development.

Changes in Thalamic Blood Flow

Thalamic hypoperfusion has been observed in patients suffering from various neuropathic pain conditions (Nakabeppu et al., 2001) and fibromyalgia (Williams and Gracely, 2006). The reduced thalamic blood flow might be the cause of the altered thalamic response in patients with neuropathic pain.

Molecular Neuroplasticity

Following peripheral and/or spinal cord injuries, molecular neuroplasticity (altered neurotransmitter release/response and/or altered ion channels/ receptors expression) is evidenced in many supraspinal structures, including the thalamus. Increased glutamatergic neurotransmission and interaction with NMDA/AMPA receptors induces depolarization of the thalamic neurons in the ventroposterolateral nucleus (Bordi and Quartaroli, 2000). It has been suggested that enhanced glutamatergic transmission in the ascending pain pathways is due to overexpression of Homer proteins, which causes increased expression of NMDA and metabotropic glutamatergic receptors within thalamic nuclei (Obara et al., 2013). Serotonergic neurotransmission is reduced in the ventrobasal complex, which in turn reduces the descending inhibitory input to the spinal cord (Goettl et al., 2002). The loss of inhibitory activity of GABAergic interneurons also contributes to molecular neuroplasticity in thalamic nociceptive pathways under chronic pain (Zhang et al., 2017). Furthermore, μ-opioid receptor-mediated G-protein activity was reduced in the thalamus after peripheral nerve injury, indicating an apparent desensitization in receptors from this region (Hoot et al., 2011) and an additional mechanism of molecular neuroplasticity.

Changes in Glial Activation

Microglial cells in the thalamus have been suggested to be involved in neuropathic pain development. Neuroplastic changes after chronic constriction injury upregulate certain neuroimmune modulator in the thalamus, which induces microglial activation. These findings suggest that the reactivation of microglia cells and secretion of inflammatory cytokines in the thalamus by peripheral nerve injuries facilitate the excitation of pain thalamic neurons under peripheral (Zhao et al., 2007) and central (Nagasaka et al., 2017) neuropathic pain conditions.

Supraspinal Structures on the Pain Process

The thalamus is the primary relay nucleus that receives ascending projections from the spinal cord and is thought to process the pain sensation component. It is one of the supraspinal structures that have been extensively investigated because it receives projections from ascending pathways. Such as spinal lamina 1 neurons that project extensively to the ventrobasal complex (ventral posterolateral + ventral posteromedial) and to the posterior group of thalamic nuclei (Dado et al., 1994).

On the other hand, we know that the nociceptive neurons of the ventrobasal complex project especially to the primary somatosensory cortex and this pathway constitutes the lateral pain system that plays an important role in stimulus discrimination (Craig, 2003). Another important aspect to address is the affective-motivational aspect of pain that is mediated by the medial pain pathway, which includes the intralaminar thalamic nuclci and thc posterior aspect of the ventromedial thalamic nuclei that projects to the somatosensory cortex and limbic structures (Desbois, 2001). On the other hand, fibers from the paracentral nucleus connect to cortical structures such as the lateral orbital, lateral agranular and dorsomedial prefrontal areas that play an important role in cognitive functions, aggressive behavior and emotional states. Neurons originating in lamina VII/VIII project to the medullary reticular formation, ventrolateral periaqueductal and intralaminar thalamic nuclei (Sewards, 2003).

There is an extensive projection from the intralaminar nuclei to the cortex, including the anterior cingulate cortex that favors the motivational aspects of pain. These brain structures, including the thalamus, are parts of a neural network involved in pain modulation that requires further research to understand the complexity of pain perception (Friedman, 1986).

Interestingly, some midline nuclei have been verified to function as novel "nociceptive discriminators" and form two distinct endogenous systems that control noxious responses: the mediodorsal nucleus of the thalamus that participates in the descending facilitation underlying the development of mechanical allodynia and the ventromedial nuclei of the thalamus that specifically mediates descending inhibition of thermal hyperalgesia in rats (You et al., 2013).

There is extensive evidence describing the important contribution of the thalamus to the hyperalgesic responses (increased painful response to noxious stimuli) associated with peripheral lesions. Studies in rats have shown that following hind paw inflammation or peripheral nerve injury, ventrobasal thalamic neurons (ventral posterolateral plus ventral posteromedial) exhibited lower thresholds and peripherally enhanced evoked responses (Whissell et al., 2016; Vertes, 2008).

C-fos markers in thalamus in relation to changes in neuronal activity in response to pain. Electrophysiological and functional imaging studies show functional changes occurring in the thalamus under neuropathic pain conditions. The contribution of the thalamus in neuropathic pain is also supported by other studies, such as immunohistochemical studies. The expression of a gene, c-fos, is considered an early marker of long-term functional changes in neuronal activity. After noxious stimulation, induction of c-fos expression has been observed in several thalamic nuclei, e.g., midline nuclei, intralaminar nuclei, paraventricular nucleus and VPL (Erdos et al. 2003). The level of c-fos was increased in supraspinal regions, including the thalamus, frontal cortex and periaqueductal gray matter four days after sciatic nerve ligation. Reorganization of thalamic neurons occurred within an average of 5 to 6 hours after sciatic nerve ligation presenting changes in receptive fields eliciting responses to noxious stimuli and the strength of cross-correlation of activation of thalamic neurons (Erdos et al. 2003). On the other hand, peripheral nerve injury was observed in addition to biochemical abnormalities in the thalamus, such as reduced serotonin (5-HT) release in the contralateral ventrobasal complex that may reduce inhibitory input to spinal cord projections and thalamic relay neurons (Goettl et al. 2002; Okada et al. 2019). Ultimately, this led to decreased antinociception or even facilitation of neurons that enhance pain perception.

Studies have shown that NMDA receptors are involved in somatosensory and nociceptive transmission in the thalamus (Tarrés-Gatius et al. 2020). NMDA receptors in VPL are important in the development and maintenance of hyperalgesia in rats.

Blockade of NMDA receptors in the thalamus reduced nociceptive transmission in neuropathic and normal rats. Although NMDA receptor subunits have been found in the medial thalamus their role in mediating nociception in the structure has not been proven (Bordi et al. 2000; Shaw et al. 2020) so further research is required.

Role of the Neurotramsmitters in Thalamic Nociceptive Response

Gamma Aminobutiric Acid (GABA) activation results in inhibitory response, which is mediated through three different receptor subtypes, named GABAA, GABAB and GABAC (Steiger and Russek, 2004; Wafford, 2005; Calver et al., 2003; Kaupmann et al., 1997; Kuner et al., 1999; Chebib, 2004). Nociceptive input is believed to be modulated in the thalamus by intrinsic inhibitory mechanisms. Since GABA mediates most inhibitory actions in the thalamus, the distribution of the three currently known receptor subtypes, may regulate the processing of nociceptive information (Neto et al., 2006).

The dorsal thalamus and ventral thalamus are the main components that connect intimately with the cerebral cortex. The reticular thalamic nucleus (RT) and the zona incerta (ZI) are the most important nuclei in the ventral thalamus. Both nuclei are GABAergic, and neurons in the ventral thalamus project primarily to the dorsal thalamus to modulate thalamic information flow (Yen et al., 1985; Power et al., 1999).

Studies suggest that in some thalamic nuclei, opioid-induced antinociception might be mediated by the GABAergic system (Jia et al., 2004). In the medial thalamus, most neurons were excited by noxious stimuli and this neuronal excitation was reduced by GABA and by THIP (4,5,6,7-tetrahydroisothiazolo-[5,4-c]pyridine-3-ol), a GABAA agonist. Behavioral tests using the rat tail-immersion assay showed that the injection of GABA or GABAA agonist in the thalamus induced an antinociceptive effect, suggesting that GABAA receptors located in the parafascicular nucleus might be responsible for this antinociceptive response (Reyes-Vazquez et al., 1986). On the other hand, GABA receptors in the nucleus have been shown to modulate trigeminovascular nociceptive transmission in thalamic relay neurons in the ventroposteromedial nucleus that are activated by a trigeminovascular nociceptive stimulus in association with migraine (Andreou et al., 2010)

Recently in the posterior nucleus of thalamus, a key sensorimotor structure, Park et al., (2017) found that presynaptic GABAB receptors are present on both GABAergic and glutamatergic terminals, but only those on GABAergic terminals are tonically active. The authors also observed that release from GABAergic terminals, but not glutamatergic terminals, is suppressed by cholinergic activation and that a subpopulation of GABAergic terminals is regulated by cannabinoids. These results suggest that in posterior nucleus of thalamus exist multiple regulatory mechanisms concurrently, where a maladaptive plasticity in this inhibition leads to severe pathologies, including chronic pain (Masri et al., 2009) and migraine (Burstein et al., 2010). These results agree with what was reported by Ipponi et al., (1999) where they mention an increase in endogenous levels of GABA in the medial thalamus which induced an antinociceptive behavior that was evaluated by noxious mechanical, chemical and thermal stimulation. This antinociception was reversed by a selective GABAB receptor antagonist, suggesting that the antinociceptive effect of tiagabine on the thalamus was mediated by GABAB receptors.

Studies in ventral posterior nuclei have shown that the expression levels of GABAB(1b) mRNA were altered in response to a prolonged noxious input arising from a monoarthritic ankle in the rat (Ferreira-Gomes et al., 2004). On the other hand, Xiao et al., (2005) reports that GABA(A) receptor may be involved in mediating the 5-HT-induced antinociception in ventral posterior nuclei possibly through a disinhibition mechanism.

In case of Glutamate, is the principal excitatory neurotransmitter in the brain. Evidence from the last several decades indicates that the excitatory amino acid glutamate plays a significant role in nociceptive processing. Glutamate and glutamate receptors are located in areas of the brain, spinal cord and periphery that are involved in pain sensation and transmission. Glutamate acts at several types of receptors, including ionotropic (directly coupled to ion channels) and metabotropic (directly coupled to intracellular second messengers). There are three families of ionotropic receptors with intrinsic cation permeable channels N-methyl-D-aspartate (NMDA), alpha-amino-3-hydroxy-5-methyl-4-isoxazolepropionic acid (AMPA) and kainite acid and there are three groups of metabotropic, G protein-coupled glutamate receptors (mGluR) that modify neuronal and glial excitability through G protein subunits acting on membrane ion channels and second messengers such as diacylglycerol and cAMP (Meldrum, 2000).

The actions of glutamate in the brain seem to be more complex. Activation of glutamate receptors in thalamus seems to be pronociceptive (Eaton and Salt, 1990). However, Zhang et al., (1997) observed that the microinjection of neurotransmitter glutamate into ventral posterior nuclei had antinociceptive effect. Salt et al., (2014) made in vivo study with multi-barrel iontophoretic electrodes from single neurons in the thalamus of rats. They found that thalamic responses are mediated primarily via mGlu1 receptors, the inactivation of somatosensory cortex resulted in a reduction of thalamic nociceptive responses. These results underline the importance of mGlu1 receptors in the processing of sensory information in the thalamus, particularly with respect to nociceptive responses. Furthermore, the involvement of mGlu1 receptors may reflect the activity of descending cortico-thalamic afferents.

On the other hand, the Serotonin is a molecule with diverse effects in the central nervous system as well as in the periphery. It can bind to postsynaptic serotonin receptors (5-HT receptors) or serotonin autoreceptors on the presynaptic membrane. The 5-HT receptors are divided into seven subfamilies (5-HT1-7) and 15 receptor subtypes. Serotonin is present at high density in thalamic nucleus, and the presence of 5-HT1A and 5-HT7 receptors in the thalamus involved in nociceptive processes has been reported (Noseda et al., 2017; Cortes Altamirano et al., 2020).

Drugs that inhibit serotonin transporter are frequently used to treat pain syndromes, e.g., neuropathy or fibromyalgia, where mechanical allodynia is present. The ventral posterior nuclei of thalamus and the hypothalamus are major supraspinal projection regions for spinal neurons that transmit nociceptive information and are innervated by monoaminergic fibers. A study determined that peripheral neuropathy induce changes in extracellular monoamines in the rat thalamus. Neuropathic rats had significantly decreased 5-HT content in thalamus, this study found changes in monoamine release in supraspinal structures in neuropathic rats, suggesting a release of serotonin from the ventral posterior nuclei of the thalamus modulate the neuropathic pain (Goett et al., 2002).

The role of each receptor and its association with pain conditions are not known with any certainty, and experimental studies with both agonists and antagonists have shown that serotonin acts as an important neuromodulator with both nociceptive and antinociceptive effects. The specific effect depends on the type of receptor, amount of substance, and anatomical region where the action takes place. For example, the 5-HT1A receptor in the CNS of rat model studies is associated with pain inhibition (antinociception) within the spine, while peripheral 5-HT can be responsible for the increase in the inflammatory response, thus exerting a nociceptive effect (Fillingim et al., 2008).

The serotonin has long been implicated in migraine pathophysiology (Hegerl and Juckel, 1993; Sucuteri, 1972). The serotonergic innervation in ventroposterior medial of thalamus is originating mainly in the rostral raphe (Westlund et al., 1990; Nothias et al., 1988; Consolazione, 1984), and that depending on the amount of serotonin release in the thalamus its effect, it could be facilitatory (at low concentration) or inhibitory (at high concentration) (Eaton SA, Salt, 1989). Shields and Goadsby, (2006) reported serotonin receptors modulate trigeminovascular responses in ventral posterior nuclei of thalamus using in vivo model of trigeminovascular nociception, they observed a potentially novel action for the serotonin 5-HT1B/1D receptor agonists, which are so effective in acute migraine in the thalamus. The serotonergic innervation of thalamic trigeminovascular neurons provide an anatomical substrate for a predominantly inhibitory effect of serotonin on trigeminovascular information transmission between the thalamus and cortex (Shields and Goadsby, 2006).

Finally, Cortes Altamirano et al., (2020) evaluated the nociceptive effect of Levetiracetam (LEV) on the expression of 5-HT1A and 5-HT7 receptors in the thalamus of rat. The results confirmed the expression of the 5-HT1A and 5-HT7 receptors in the thalamus and its role in pain modulation.

Conclusion

With all the information and evidence displayed above we can conclude that the thalamus is the main gateway for the transmission of sensory information from the periphery to the cortex. The studies described in the present chapter showed that the thalamus is an important structure that mediates the different components of pain: discriminative sensory components and affective-motivational components. The thalamus also participates in descending inhibition in order to modulate nociceptive inputs to the dorsal horn of the spinal cord.

Changes in biochemistry, immediate early gene expression, thalamic blood flow and response properties of thalamic neurons have been found in neuropathic pain models. These data indicate that the thalamus has an important role to play in modulating nociception in normal and neuropathic pain syndrome.

References

Alshelh Z, Pietro FD, Youssef AM, Reeves JM, Macey RM, Vickers ER, Peck CC, Murray GM, Henderson LA. Chronic Neuropathic Pain: It's about the Rhythm. *J Neurosci.* 2016;36(3):1008-18. doi: 10.1523/JNEUROSCI.2768-15.2016.

Andreou AP, Shields KG, Goadsby PJ. GABA and valproate modulate trigeminovascular nociceptive transmission in the thalamus. *Neurobiol Dis.* 2010;37(2):314-23. doi: 10.1016/j.nbd.2009.10.007.

Apkarian A. Nociceptive Processing in the Thalamus. In: Schmidt R, Willis W (eds) *Encyclopedia of Pain.* Springer, Berlin, Heidelberg. 2007. doi.org/10.1007/978-3-540-29805-2_2765.

Apkarian VA, Hashmi JA, Baliki MN. Pain and the brain: specificity and plasticity of the brain in clinical chronic pain. *Pain.* 2011 Mar;152(3 Suppl):S49-S64. doi: 10.1016/j.pain.2010.11.010.

Bastuji H, Frot M, Mazza S, Perchet C, Magnin M, Garcia-Larrea L., Thalamic Responses to Nociceptive-Specific Input in Humans: Functional Dichotomies and Thalamo-Cortical Connectivity. *Cereb Cortex.* 2016 Jun;26(6):2663-76.

Bastuji H, Frot M, Mazza S, Perchet C, Magnin M, Garcia-Larrea L. Thalamic Responses to Nociceptive-Specific Input in Humans: Functional Dichotomies and Thalamo-Cortical Connectivity. *Cereb Cortex.* 2016;26(6):2663-76. doi: 10.1093/cercor/bhv106.

Boccard SGJ, Pereira EAC and Aziz TZ. Deep brain stimulation for chronic pain. *J Clin Neurosci.* 2015 Oct;22(10):1537-43.

Bordi F, Quartaroli M. Modulation of nociceptive transmission by NMDA/glycine site receptor in the ventroposterolateral nucleus of the thalamus. *Pain.* 2000;84(2-3):213-24. doi: 10.1016/s0304-3959(99)00205-5.

Bordi F, Quartaroli M. Modulation of nociceptive transmission by NMDA/glycine site receptor in the ventroposterolateral nucleus of the thalamus. *Pain.* 2000;84(2- 3):213-24.

Burstein R, Jakubowski M, Garcia-Nicas E, Kainz V, Bajwa Z, Hargreaves R, Becerra L, Borsook D. Thalamic sensitization transforms localized pain into widespread allodynia. *Ann Neurol.* 2010; 68: 81–91. doi:10.1002/ana.21994.

Calver AR, Michalovich, D, Testa T, Robbins M J, Jaillard C, Hill J, Szekeres P G, Charles KJ, Jourdain S, Holbrook JD, Boyfield I, Patel N, Medhurst AD, Pangaloset MN. Molecular cloning and characterisation of a novel GABAB-related G-protein coupled receptor. *Brain Res. Mol. Brain Res.* 2003 20;110(2):305-17. doi: 10.1016/ s0169-328x(02)00662-9.

Cao, L., Li, C., Zhang, Y., & Gui, S. Surgical resection of unilateral thalamic tumors in adults: approaches and outcomes. *BMC Neurology*. 201515(1):1-13.

Chao CC, Tseng MT, Lin YH, Hsieh PC, Lin CH, Huang SL, Hsieh ST, Chiang MC. Brain imaging signature of neuropathic pain phenotypes in small-fiber neuropathy: Altered thalamic connectome and its associations with skin nerve degeneration. *Pain.* 2021 May 1;162(5):1387-99.

Che B, Ab A, A HA. The role of the thalamus in modulating pain. *Malaysian Journal of Medical Sciences*, Vol. 13, No. 2, July 2006 (11-18). Chebib, 2004

Chebib M. GABAC receptor ion channels. *Clin. Exp. Pharmacol. Physiol.* 2004; 31, 800–804.

Chisholm KI, Lo Re L, Polgár E, Gutierrez-Mecinas M, Todd AJ, McMahon SB. Encoding of cutaneous stimuli by lamina I projection neurons. *Pain.* 2021;162(9):2405-2417. doi: 10.1097/j.pain.0000000000002226.

Choi S, Yu E, Hwang E, Llinás RR. Pathophysiological implication of CaV3.1 T-type Ca2+ channels in trigeminal neuropathic pain. *Proc Natl Acad Sci USA.* 2016 Feb 23;113(8):2270-5. doi: 10.1073/pnas.1600418113.

Consolazione A, Priestley JV, Cuello AC. Serotonin-containing projections to the thalamus in the rat revealed by a horseradish peroxidase and peroxidase antiperoxidase double-staining technique. *Brain Res.* 1984; 26;322(2):233-43. doi: 10.1016/0006-8993(84) 90113-6.

Cortes-Altamirano JL, Reyes-Long S, Bonilla-Jaime H, Clavijo-Cornejo D, Vargas J, Bandala C, Alfaro-Rodriguez A. Acute administration of levetiracetam in tonic pain model modulates gene expression of 5HT 1A and 5HT 7 receptors in the thalamus of rats (Rattus norvergicus). *Mol Biol Rep*. 2020;47(5):3389-3396. doi: 10.1007/ s11033-020-05419-1

Craig AD. A new view of pain as a homeostatic emotion. *Trends Neurosci.* 2003;26(6):303-07.

Craig AD. Topographically Organized Projection to Posterior Insular Cortex from the Posterior Portion of the Ventral Medial Nucleus (VMpo) in the Long-tailed Macaque Monkey. *J Comp Neurol*. 2014; 522(1): 36–63. doi: 10.1002/cne.23425.

Cunningham NR, Kashirkar-Zuck S and Coghill RC. Brain mechanisms impacted by psychological therapies for pain: identifying targets for optimization of treatment effects. *Pain Rep*. 2019 Aug 7;4(4):e767.

Dado RJ, Katter JT, Giesler GJ, Jr Spinothalamic and spinohypothalamic tract neurons in the cervical enlargement of rats. I. Locations of antidromically identified axons in the thalamus and hypothalamus. *J Neurophysiol.* 1994;71(3):959-80.

Dahlstrom A, Fuxe K. Evidence for the existence of monoamine-containing neurons in the central nervous system. *Acta Physiologica Scandinavica*. 1964; 62, 1–55.

Davis KD, Kwan CL, Crawley AP, and Mikulis DJ. Electrical Nerve Stimulation Can Be Used as a Tool in fMRI Studies of Pain- and Tingling-Evoked Activations. 2000. *Pain Research and Management*, 5(1), 81–86.

Desbois C, Villanueva L. The organization of lateral ventromedial thalamic connections in the rat: a link for the distribution of nociceptive signals to widespread cortical regions. *Neuroscience.* 2001;102(4):885-98.

Dostrovsky JO, Craig AD. Ascending Projection Systems. In: McMahon S, Koltzenburg M, Irene Tracey I, Turk DC (eds) *Wall & Melzack's Textbook of Pain*, 6th ed, Elsevier Saunders. Philadelphia, 2013, pp. 182-197.

Dydyk AM, Munakomi S. *Thalamic Pain Syndrome*. [Updated 2022 Feb 9]. In: StatPearls [Internet]. Treasure Island (FL): StatPearls Publishing; 2022.

Eaton SA, Salt TE. Modulatory effects of serotonin on excitatory amino acid responses and sensory synaptic transmission in the ventrobasal thalamus. *Neuroscience*. 1989;33(2): 285-92. doi: 10.1016/0306-4522(89)90208-x.

Erdos B, Lacza Z, Tóth IE, Szelke E, Mersich T, Komjáti K, Palkovits M, Sándor P, Mechanisms of pain-induced local cerebral blood flow changes in the rat sensory cortex and thalamus. *Brain Res.* 2003;960(1-2):219-27.

Ferreira-Gomes J, Neto FL, Castro-Lopes JM. Differential expression of GABAB(1b) receptor mRNA in the thalamus of normal and monoarthritic animals. *Biochem Pharmacol*. 2004;68(8):1603-11. doi: 10.1016/j.bcp.2004.07.018.

Fillingim RB, King CD, Ribeiro-Dasilva MC, Rahim-Williams B, Riley JL. III Sex, gender, and pain: A review of recent clinical and experimental findings. *J. Pain*. 2009;10:447–485. doi: 10.1016/j.jpain.2008.12.001

Franzini A, Attuati L, Zaed I, Moosa S, Stravato A, Navarria P, Picozzi P, Gamma Knife central lateral thalamotomy for the treatment of neuropathic pain. *J Neurosurg*. 2020 Jul 24;1-9.

Friedman DP, Murray EA. Thalamic connectivity of the second somatosensory area and neighboring somatosensory fields of the lateral sulcus of the macaque. *J Comp Neurol.* 1986;252(3):348-73.

García-Cabezas MÁ, Rico B, Sánchez-González MÁ, Cavada C. Distribution of the dopamine innervation in the macaque and human thalamus. *Neuroimage*. 2007 Feb 1;34(3):965-84.

Goettl VM, Huang Y, Hackshaw KV, Stephens Jr RL. Reduced basal release of serotonin from the ventrobasal thalamus of the rat in a model of neuropathic pain. *Pain.* 2002 Sep;99(1-2):359-66. doi: 10.1016/s0304-3959(02)00209-9.

Greene DJ, Marek S, Gordon EM, Siegel JS, Gratton C, Laumann TO, Gilmore AW, Berg JJ, Nguyen AL, Dierker D, Van AN, Ortega M, Newbold DJ, Hampton JM, Nielsen AN, McDermott KB, Roland JL, Norris SA, Nelson SM, Snyder AZ, Schlaggar BL, Petersen SE, Dosenbach NUF. Integrative and Network-Specific Connectivity of the Basal Ganglia and Thalamus Defined in Individuals. *Neuron.* 2020;105(4):742-758.e6. doi: 10.1016/j.neuron.2019.11.012.

Groh A, Krieger P, Mease RA, Henderson L. Acute and Chronic Pain Processing in the Thalamocortical System of Humans and Animal Models. *Neuroscience*. 2018;387:58-71. doi: 10.1016/j.neuroscience.2017.09.042.

Hadidchi S, Surento W, Lerner A, Liu CSJ, Gibbs WN, Kim PE, Shiroishi MS. Headache and Brain Tumor. *Neuroimaging Clinics of North America.* 2019. 1-10.

Hayashi M, Chernov MF, Taira T, Ochiai T, Nakaya K, Tamura N, Goto S, Yomo S, Kouyama N, Katayama Y, Kawakami Y, Izawa m, Muragaki Y, Nakamura R, Iseki H, Hori T, Takakura K, Outcome after pituitary radiosurgery for thalamic pain syndrome. *Int J Radiat Oncol Biol Phys*. 2007 Nov 1;69(3):852-7.

Hebestrei JM and May A. Topiramate modulates trigeminal pain processing in thalamo-cortical networks in humans after single dose administration. *PLoS One*. 2017 Oct 9;12(10):e0184406.

Hegerl U, Juckel G. Intensity dependence of auditory evoked potentials as an indicator of central serotonergic neurotransmission: a new hypothesis. *Biol Psychiatry*. 1993; 33:173–187. doi: 10.1016/0006-3223(93)90137-3.

Hoot MR, Sim-Selley LJ, Selley DE, Scoggins KL, Dewey WL. Chronic neuropathic pain in mice reduces μ-opioid receptor-mediated G-protein activity in the thalamus. *Brain Res*. 2011;1406:1-7. doi: 10.1016/j.brainres.2011.06.023.

Ipponi A, Lamberti C, Medica A, Bartolini A, Malmberg-Aiello P. Tiagabine antinociception in rodents depends on GABA(B) receptor activation: Parallel antinociception testing and medial thalamus *GABA microdialysis.* 1999; 5:368(2-3):205-11. doi: 10.1016/s0014-2999(99)00034-5.

Iwata M, LeBlanc BW, Kadasi LM, Zerah ML, Cosgrove RG, Saab CY. High-frequency stimulation in the ventral posterolateral thalamus reverses electrophysiologic changes and hyperalgesia in a rat model of peripheral neuropathic pain. *Pain*. 2011 Nov 1;152(11):2505-13.

Jeanmonod D, Werner B, Morel A, Michels L, Zadicario E, Schiff G, Martin E, Transcranial magnetic resonance imaging-guided focused ultrasound: noninvasive central lateral thalamotomy for chronic neuropathic pain. *Neurosurg Focus*. 2012;32(1):E1.

Jia H, Xie YF, Xiao DQ, Tang JS. Involvement of GABAergic modulation of the nucleus submedius (Sm) morphine-induced antinociception. *Pain*. 2004;108(1-2):28-35. doi: 10.1016/j.pain.2003.11.012.

Kandel ER, Schwartz JH, Jessel TM, Siegelbaum SA, Hudspeth AJ. 2012. *Principles of Neural Science*. 5th Edition. New York: McGraw-Hill Professional.

Kaupmann K, Huggel K, Heid J, Flor PJ, Bischoff S, Mickel SJ, McMaster G, Angst C, Bittiger H, Froestl W, Bettler B. Expression cloning of GABA(B) receptors uncovers similarity to metabotropic glutamate receptors. *Nature* 1997; 20;386(6622):239-46. doi: 10.1038/386239a0.

Keller AF, Beggs S, Salter MW, De Koninck Y. Transformation of the output of spinal lamina I neurons after nerve injury and microglia stimulation underlying neuropathic pain. *Mol Pain*. 2007;3:27. doi: 10.1186/1744-8069-3-27.

Kenshalo Jr DR, Giesler Jr GJ, Leonard RB, Willis WD. Responses of neurons in primate ventral posterior lateral nucleus to noxious stimuli. *J Neurophysiol*. 1980 Jun;43(6): 1594-614. doi: 10.1152/jn.1980.43.6.1594.

Khera T, Rangasamy V. Cognition and Pain: A Review. *Front Psychol*. 2021 May 21;12:673962. doi: 10.3389/fpsyg.2021.673962.

Krahe R, Gabbiani F. Burst firing in sensory systems. *Nat Rev Neurosci*. 2004;5(1):13-23. doi: 10.1038/nrn1296.

Kuner R, Kohr G, Grunewald S, Eisenhardt G, Bach A, Kornau HC. Role of heterodimer formation in GABAB receptor function. *Science*. 1999; 1;283(5398):74-7. doi: 10.1126/science.283.5398.74.

Kuner R, Kuner T. Cellular Circuits in the Brain and Their Modulation in Acute and Chronic Pain. *Physiol Rev*. 2021 Jan 1;101(1):213-258. doi: 10.1152/physrev. 00040. 2019.

Liao C, Yang M, Liu P, Zhong W and Zhang W. Thalamic pain alleviated by stellate ganglion block: A case report. *Medicine* (Baltimore). 2017 Feb;96(5):e6058.

Liao YF, Tsai ML, Chen CC, Yen CT. Involvement of the Cav3.2 T-type calcium channel in thalamic neuron discharge patterns. *Mol Pain*. 2011 Jun 4;7:43. doi: 10.1186/ 1744-8069-7-43.

Lin H, Li, W, Ni J and Wang Y. Clinical study of repetitive transcranial magnetic stimulation of the motor cortex for thalamic pain. *Medicine* (Baltimore). 2018 Jul;97(27):e11235.

Lovo EE, Torre B, Campos F, Caceros V, Reyes WA, Barahona KC, Cruz C, Arias J, Alho E, Contreras WO, Stereotactic Gamma Ray Radiosurgery to the Centromedian and Parafascicular Complex of the Thalamus for Trigeminal Neuralgia and Other Complex Pain Syndromes. *Cureus*. 2019 Dec 19;11(12):e6421. doi: 10.7759/cureus.6421.

Masri R, Quiton RL, Lucas JM, Murray PD, Thompson SM, Keller A. Zona incerta: a role in central pain. *J Neurophysiol*.2009; 102: 181–191. doi:10.1152/jn.00152.2009.

Mease RA, Sumser A, Sakmann B, Groh A. Cortical Dependence of Whisker Responses in Posterior Medial Thalamus In Vivo. *Cereb Cortex*. 2016 Aug;26(8):3534-43. doi: 10.1093/cercor/bhw144.

Meldrum B S. Glutamate as a neurotransmitter in the brain: review of physiology and pathology *J Nutr*. 2000;130(4S Suppl):1007S-15S. doi: 10.1093/jn/130.4.1007S.

Melzack R. From the gate to the neuromatrix. *Pain*. 1999;Suppl 6:S121-S126. doi: 10.1016/S0304-3959(99)00145-1.

Mitchell A. The mediodorsal thalamus as a higher order thalamic relay nucleus important for learning and decision-making. *Neurosci Biobehav Rev*. 2015 Jul;54:76-88. doi: 10.1016/j.neubiorev.2015.03.001.

Montes C, Magnin M, Maarrawi J, Frot M, Convers P, Mauguière F, Garcia-Larrea L. Thalamic thermo-algesic transmission: ventral posterior (VP) complex versus VMpo in the light of a thalamic infarct with central pain. *Pain*. 2005 Jan 1;113(1-2):223-32.

Nagasaka K, Takashima I, Matsuda K, Higo N. Late-onset hypersensitivity after a lesion in the ventral posterolateral nucleus of the thalamus: A macaque model of central post-stroke pain. *Sci Rep*. 2017;7(1):10316. doi: 10.1038/s41598-017-10679-2.

Nakabeppu Y, Nakajo M, Gushiken T, Tsuchimochi S, Tani A, Kanmura Y. Decreased perfusion of the bilateral thalami in patients with chronic pain detected by Tc-99m-ECD SPECT with statistical parametric mapping. *Ann Nucl Med*. 2001 Oct;15(5): 459-63. doi: 10.1007/BF02988354.

Neto FL, Ferreira-Gomes J, Castro-Lopes JM. Distribution of GABA receptors in the thalamus and their involvement in nociception. *Adv Pharmacol*. 2006;54:29-51. doi: 10.1016/s1054-3589(06)54002-5.

Noseda R, Borsook D, Burstein Rami. Neuropeptides and neurotransmitters that modulate thalamo- cortical pathways relevant to migraine headache. *Headache*. 2017;57(2): 97–111. doi:10.1111/head.13083.

Nothias F, Onteniente B, Roudier F, Peschanksi M. Immunocytochemical study of serotoninergic and noradrenergic innervation of the ventrobasal complex of the rat thalamus. *Neurosci Lett*. 1988; 95:59–63. doi: 10.1016/0304-3940(88)90632-5.

Obara I, Goulding SP, Hu JH, Klugmann M, Worley PF, Szumlinski KK. Nerve injury-induced changes in Homer/glutamate receptor signaling contribute to the development and maintenance of neuropathic pain. *Pain*. 2013;154(10):1932-1945. doi: 10.1016/j.pain.2013.03.035.

Okada M, Fukuyama K, Ueda Y. Lurasidone inhibits NMDA receptor antagonist-induced functional abnormality of thalamocortical glutamatergic transmission via 5-HT7 receptor blockade. *Br J Pharmacol*. 2019 Oct;176(20):4002-4018.

Okada S, Katagiri A, Saito H, Lee J, Ohara K, Iinuma T, Bereiter DA, Iwata K. Differential activation of ascending noxious pathways associated with trigeminal nerve injury. *Pain*. 2019 Jun 1;160(6):1342-60.

Park A, Ying L, Radi M, Asaf K. Presynaptic and extrasynaptic regulation of posterior nucleus of thalamus. *J Neurophysiol*. 2017;118(1): 507–519. doi: 10.1152/jn.00862.2016.

Patel R, Dickenson AH. Neuronal hyperexcitability in the ventral posterior thalamus of neuropathic rats: modality selective effects of pregabalin. *J Neurophysiol*. 2016;116(1):159-70.

Patel R, Qu C, Xie JY, Porreca F, Dickenson AH. Selective deficiencies in descending inhibitory modulation in neuropathic rats: implications for enhancing noradrenergic tone. *Pain*. 2018 Sep;159(9):1887.

Power BD, Kolmac CI, Mitrofanis J. Evidence for a large projection from the zona incerta to the dorsal thalamus. *J Comp Neurol* 1999;404:554e65.

Purves D, Augustine GJ, Fitzpatrick D, Hall WC, LaMantia AS, White LE. 2012. *Neuroscience*. 5th Edition Sinauer Associates.

Reyes-Vazquez C, Enna SJ, Dafny N. The parafasciculus thalami as a site for mediating the antinociceptive response to GABAergic drugs. *Brain Res*. 1986; 24:383(1-2):177-84. doi: 10.1016/0006-8993(86)90018-1.

Rokyta R and Fricová J. Neurostimulation methods in the treatment of chronic pain. *Physiol Res*. 2012;61(Suppl 2):S23-31. doi: 10.33549/physiolres.932392.

Salt TE, Jones HE, Copeland CS, Sillito AM. Function of mGlu1 receptors in the modulation of nociceptive processing in the thalamus. *Neuropharmacology*. 2014;79 (100):405-11.

Sánchez-González MÁ, García-Cabezas MÁ, Rico B, Cavada C. The primate thalamus is a key target for brain dopamine. *Journal of Neuroscience*. 2005 Jun 29;25(26):6076-83.

Sewards TV, Sewards MA. Representations of motivational drives in mesial cortex, medial thalamus, hypothalamus and midbrain. *Brain Res Bull*. 2003;61(1):25-49.

Shaw AD, Muthukumaraswamy SD, Saxena N, Sumner RL, Adams NE, Moran RJ, Singh KD. Generative modelling of the thalamo-cortical circuit mechanisms underlying the neurophysiological effects of ketamine. *Neuroimage*. 2020 Nov 1;221:117189.

Shen Z, Zhang H, Wu Z, He Q, Liu J, Xu Y, Yao S, He X, Chen Y, Liang Y, Liu B, Jiang Y, Fang J, Du J, Zhu X, Wu M, We Y, Sun J, Xu C, Fang J, Shao X, Electroacupuncture Alleviates Chronic Pain-Induced Anxiety Disorders by Regulating the rACC-Thalamus Circuitry. *Front Neurosci*. 2021 Jan 11;14:615395.

Shieff C and Nashold BS Jr. Stereotactic mesencephalotomy. *Neurosurg Clin N Am*. 1990 Oct;1(4):825-39.

Shields KG, Goadsby PJ. Serotonin receptors modulate trigeminovascular responses in ventroposteromedial nucleus of thalamus: a migraine target? *Neurobiology of disease*. 2006;23(3):491-501. doi: 10.1016/j.nbd.2006.04.003.

Sicuteri F. Headache as possible expression of deficiency of brain 5-hydroxytryptamine (central denervation supersensitivity). *Headache*. 1972; 12:69–72. doi: 10.1111/j.1526-4610.1972.hed1202069.x.

Smith Y. 2008. *The thalamus in: Neuroscience in medicine. Conn, P. M. 6th Edition* Springer Science & Business Media.

Steiger JL, Russek SJ. GABAA receptors: Building the bridge between subunit mRNAs, their promoters, and cognate transcription factors. *Pharmacol Ther*. 2004;01(3):259-81. doi: 10.1016/j.pharmthera.2003.12.002.

Tarrés-Gatius M, Miquel-Rio L, Campa L, Artigas F, Castañé A. Involvement of NMDA receptors containing the GluN2C subunit in the psychotomimetic and antidepressant-like effects of ketamine. *Transl Psychiatry*. 2020 Dec 10;10(1):427.

Trang T, Al-Hasan, R, Salvemini D., Salter MW, Gutstein H, Cahill CM, Pain and Poppies: The Good, the Bad, and the Ugly of Opioid Analgesics. *J Neurosci*. 2015 Oct 14;35(41):13879-88.

Treede RD. Spinothalamic and thalamocortical nociceptive pathways. *J Pain.* 2002;3(2): 109-12; doi: 10.1054/jpai.2002.122951.

Tsubokawa T, Katayama Y, Yamamoto T, Hirayama T and Koyama S. Treatment of thalamic pain by chronic motor cortex stimulation. *Pacing Clin Electrophysiol.* 1991 Jan;14(1):131-4.

Tu Y, Fu Z, Mao C, Falahpour M, Gollub RL, Park J, Wilson G, Napadow V, Gerber J, Chan ST, Edwards RR, Kaptchuk TJ, Liu T, Calhoun V, Rosen B, Kong J. Distinct thalamocortical network dynamics are associated with the pathophysiology of chronic low back pain. *Nat Commun*. 2020;11(1):3948. doi: 10.1038/s41467-020-17788-z.

Vartiainen N, Perchet C, Magnin M, Creac'h C, Convers P, Nighoghossian N, Mauguière F, Peyron R, Garcia-Larrea L, Thalamic pain: anatomical and physiological indices of prediction, *Brain*. 2016. 139 (3):708–722.

Vertes RP, Hoover WB (2008) Projections of the paraventricular and paratenial nuclei of the dorsal midline thalamus in the rat. *J Comp Neurol* 508 :212-237. 10.1002/cne. 21679.

Wafford KA. GABAA receptor subtypes: Any clues to the mechanism of benzodiazepine dependence? *Curr. Opin. Pharmacol*. 2005; 5(1):47-52. doi: 10.1016/j.coph.2004. 08.006.

Westlund KN, Sorkin LS, Ferrington DG, Carlton SM, Willcockson HH, Willis WD. Serotoninergic and noradrenergic projections to the ventral posterolateral nucleus of the monkey thalamus. *Journal of Comparative Neurology*. 1990 May 8;295(2):197-207.

Whissell PD, Tohyama S, Martin LJ (2016) The use of DREADDs to deconstruct behavior. *Front Genet* 7 :70. 10.3389/fgene.2016.00070.

Whitt JL, Radi Masri R, Pulimood NS, Keller A. Pathological activity in mediodorsal thalamus of rats with spinal cord injury pain. *J Neurosci.* 2013;33(9):3915-26. doi: 0.1523/JNEUROSCI.2639-12.2013.

Widerström-Noga E, Cruz-Almeida Y, Felix ER and Pattany PM. Somatosensory phenotype is associated with thalamic metabolites and pain intensity after spinal cord injury. *Pain*. 2015 Jan;156(1):166-174.

Williams DA, Gracely RH. Biology and therapy of fibromyalgia. Functional magnetic resonance imaging findings in fibromyalgia. *Arthritis Res Ther*. 2006;8(6):224. doi: 10.1186/ar2094.

Wolf J, Urits I, Orhurhu V, Peck J, Orhurhu MS, Giacomazzi S, Smoots D, Piermarini C, Manchikanti L, Kaye AD, Kaye RJ, Viswanath O, The Role of the Cannabinoid System in Pain Control: Basic and Clinical Implications. *Curr Pain Headache Rep*. 2020 Jun 6;24(7):35.

Xiao DQ, Zhu JX, Tang JS, Jia H. GABAergic modulation mediates antinociception produced by serotonin applied into thalamic nucleus submedius of the rat. *Brain Res*. 2005;1057(1-2):161-7. doi: 10.1016/j.brainres.2005.07.053.

Yen CT and Lu PL. Thalamus and pain. *Acta Anaesthesiol Taiwan*. 2013 Jun;51(2):73-80.

Yen CT, Conley M, Hendry SH, Jones EG. The morphology of physiologically identified GABAergic neurons in the somatic sensory part of the thalamic reticular nucleus in the cat. *J Neurosci.* 1985; 5(8):2254-68. doi: 10.1523/JNEUROSCI.05-08-02254. 1985.

You HJ, Lei J, Niu N, Yang L, Fan XL, Tjølsen A, Li Q (2013) Specific thalamic nuclei function as novel 'nociceptive discriminators' in the endogenous control of nociception in rats. *Neuroscience* 232 :53-63. 10.1016/j.neuroscience.2012.12.021.

Zhang C, Chen RX, Zhang Y, Wang J, Liu FY, Cai J, Liao FF, Xu FQ, Yi M, Wan Y. Reduced GABAergic transmission in the ventrobasal thalamus contributes to thermal hyperalgesia in chronic inflammatory pain. *Sci Rep.* 2017;7:41439. doi: 10.1038/ srep 41439.

Zhang XF, Hu XT, White FaJ, Wolf ME. Increased responsiveness of ventral tegmental area dopamine neurons to glutamate after repeated administration of cocaine or amphetamine is transient and selectively involves AMPA receptors. *J Pharmacol Exp Ther.* 1997;281(2):699-706.

Zhao P, Waxman SG, Hains BC. Modulation of thalamic nociceptive processing after spinal cord injury through remote activation of thalamic microglia by cysteine cysteine chemokine ligand 21. *J Neurosci.* 2007;27(33):8893-902. doi: 10.1523/JNEUROSCI. 2209-07.2007.

Zhao P, Waxman SG, Hains BC. Sodium channel expression in the ventral posterolateral nucleus of the thalamus after peripheral nerve injury. *Mol Pain.* 2006;2:27. doi: 10.1186/1744-8069-2-27.

Chapter 3

Physical Exercise Improves Cognition and Memory: A Short Review

G. Sridevi*, **PhD**
Department of Physiology, SRM Dental College and Hospital, Saveetha University, Chennai, India

Abstract

Physical exercise is a bodily movement caused by skeletal muscles with the expenditure of energy. It helps a person to stay energetic throughout the day. It activates the physiological systems of the body by acting on the heart and lungs, reduces stress and anxiety, and causes improvements in mood as well. This review exclusively concentrates on the influence of physical exercise on improvements in cognition and memory. Literature reports support the association that exercise activates brain plasticity by stimulation of growth factors that develop new connections between brain cells. Many researchers found evidence that hippocampal neurogenesis starts to diminish with aging, and this could be partially opposed by exercise in mouse models. Human studies also added support to this association that aerobic and neuromotor exercises increased memory performance in elderly subjects with improvements in short-term memory and long-term memory.

Keywords: physical exercise, fitness, brain cognition, memory

* Corresponding Author's Email: sridevig.sdc@saveetha.com.

In: Horizons in Neuroscience Research. Volume 48
Editors: Andres Costa and Eugenio Villalba
ISBN: 979-8-88697-230-6
© 2022 Nova Science Publishers, Inc.

Introduction

Physical exercise plays an important role in maintenance of healthy wellbeing of an individual. Physical exercise is considered to be any bodily movement caused by skeletal muscles with the expenditure of energy. It makes a person stay energetic and fit throughout the day. It activates the physiological systems of the body, increases the force of contraction of heart, improves the respiratory cycles, reduces stress and anxiety, improves mood and boosts happiness, improves self-confidence, etc. It reduces the risk of developing heart disease, hypertension, obesity, raised blood glucose levels, osteoporosis, coronary artery disease, depression and even colon cancer.

A well-balanced exercise program can promote general health of the body, increases endurance and slows down the effects of aging. The benefit of exercise is not only limited to physical well- being and health. It also enhances emotional well-being as well. Regular physical activity acts to endorse the health, postpones and prevents predominant musculoskeletal disorders like mechanical low back pain, arthritis, spinal deformities, neck and shoulder pain and muscular disorders.

Types of Exercise

Well-Balanced Exercise Program

Endurance Exercises

Physical exercises that repeat a sequence of muscle contractions for many repetitions are considered as endurance exercises [1]. Endurance exercises like brisk walking and dancing improve cardiovascular fitness and respiratory health and enhance the movement of the circulatory system. This type of endurance training can be performed easily in ways such as climbing flights of stairs.

Strength Training Exercises

Strength training exercises are workouts that involve the work of muscles by applying a resistance against the action of that particular muscle. The resistance offered to the muscle must be of appropriate strength to make the target muscle fatigue at about 8-12 repetitions of exercise. Strength training workouts involve lifting weights or the use of resistance bands. This type of exercise can increase muscle strength and improve the performance of everyday activities like carrying groceries or lifting heavy goods [2].

Balance Exercises

Balance training involves exercises that strengthen the muscles to keep the body in an upright position. They improve postural stability and balance. This type of exercise can be intense enough in maintaining the postural balance as in yogic poses. Examples of such exercises are standing on one leg or a yogic posture and doing tai chi [3].

Stretching Exercises

Stretching is type of physical exercise where a specific muscle or tendon is maximally flexed or stretched. This type of exercise improves the elasticity of muscles and improves muscle tone. This exercise increases the flexibility of muscles and joints. Even many day-to-day activities like bending down is an example of stretching exercises [4].

Physical Benefits of Exercise

To Maintain Body Weight

A balanced workout of about of 150 minutes a week of aerobic activity with moderate intensity for 5 days a week would maintain an ideal body weight. Previous reports suggested strong scientific evidence that physical activity maintains body weight over time. The adequate amount of exercise required by each body varies from person to person. Also, a high amount of physical activity with a well-adjusted diet plan reduces the amount of calories and helps to reduce overweight [4].

Strengthens the Bones and Muscles

Physical exercise ensures good protection of the bones, joints, and muscles of the body. Keeping bones, joints, and muscles active in a good healthy workout ensures a good day-to-day activity and keeps a person physically active. Previous literature reports revealed that aerobic exercises confined to muscle-strengthening and bone-strengthening of moderately intense level can reduce *the loss of bone density* that occurs with age. Also, physically active people *have a lower risk of hip fracture* compared to physically inactive people. It also improves stability of a person and reduces the risk of falling and fall-related injuries. Physical exercises help to reduce the inflammatory processes of arthritis and other rheumatic conditions. *Buildup of strong healthy muscle.* Muscle endurance and strengthening exercises like lifting weights can increase or maintain muscle mass and strength. This proves its benefit in elderly people who experience reduced muscle mass and muscle strength with the progression of age [4].

Increase the Longevity of Life

Scientific reports revealed that physical activity reduces the risk of early death caused due to heart disease and some cancers. It ensures a lower risk of mortality to 33% compared to physically inactive people only with a small exercise regimen for about 150 minutes a week. Vigorous-intensity activity also reduces the risk of premature death [4].

Exercise and Brain

Physical exercise not only activates the muscles and joints, but also influences the brain. Exercise acts on the brain in various aspects. It improves the physiological circulation of blood with increased heart rate and improves the oxygenation of brain tissues. It releases many hormones that provide a nutrition-based environment for brain growth.

Exercise activates brain plasticity by stimulating the growth of new connections between brain cells with important cortical areas of the brain. Recent research demonstrated that exercise increases the development and release of new growth factors in the brain that ensure good new neuronal connectivity inside the brain. Aerobic exercise is of great benefit to the body and brain. It acts not only to improve the brain connections but also repairs damaged brain cells. A daily morning exercise before going to work increases the spike of brain activity and prepares us for the mental stresses that we are about to face for the rest of the day. It increases the retention of new information and prepares us to better react to complex situations at office work [5, 6].

Previous literature states evidence to link the effect of physical exercise to the brain. The Physical Activity Guidelines for Americans, given by the U.S. Department of Health and Human Services in the year 2018, stated the guidelines of physical activity in four classes of age. 1. Preschool-Aged Children in the age group of 3-5 years were physically active throughout the day and they seem to have good growth and development, enhanced mental capacity and social interaction. 2. Adolescent children in age group of 6-17 years had a minimum of 60 min per day to an aerobic exercise with moderate and a vigorous physical activity at least 3 days per week. These children also seem to have good mental ability and cognition. Adults are ones who do not move more and sit throughout the day and they would perform only 150-300 min of aerobic exercise with moderate-intensity for 75-150 min at least 2 days a week and they start developing cognitive deficits and memory loss. 4. Old Adults - they do less muscular activity and physical exercise, which poses them to develop degenerative conditions like dementia, Alzheimer's disease, Parkinson's disease, etc. The last two groups of people who are vulnerable to such neurophysiological disorders must do much aerobic and muscle-strengthening activities to maintain a healthy brain function [7, 8].

Previous reports suggested the link between physical activity and brain functions. It suggested that brain function is activated by delivering of regulatory molecules into the blood because these substances are packaged into endocytic vesicles and they finally deliver their cargoes to the brain through the brain capillary endothelial cells. It is also stated that exercise stimulates release of exosomes and tiny vesicles into the blood circulation [9].

Animal Studies on Physical Exercise Linked to Cognition

Previous studies reported that animal studies had showed that physical exercise has a generous action on health and also increases the plasticity of the nervous system. Supporting new evidence indicates that physical exercise exerts its action on cognition of the brain by affecting molecular events that relate to energy metabolism and synaptic plasticity. The report also found that the molecular machinery of physical exercise that stimulates the brain is brain-derived neurotrophic factor which acts at the higher interface of metabolism and plasticity [10].

The effects of motor exercise on cognition were mainly studied in rodents by use of specific training on wheels and locomotor activity analyses. Studies on healthy rats have demonstrated that an increase in intense motor activity gradually increases the proliferation rates of neurons and glia cells and angiogenesis in the hippocampus and neocortex and cerebellum. This motor activity produces changes in neurotransmitter levels of serotonin, noradrenalin, and acetylcholine and promotes the release of brain-derived neurotrophic factor and the insulin-like growth factor-1 [11].

Reports suggested that animals performing motor exercise showed significant improvements in spatial abilities and cognitive domains such as executive functions. This gives supporting evidence that motor exercise improves cognitive functions. Voluntary exercise doubled the number of surviving newborn cells in amounts similar to enrichment condition. A study on adult mice exposed to conditions, like enriched and standard housing along with voluntary and forced exercise, observed that physical exercise doubled the number of surviving newborn cells [10, 12]. A few reports by Kronenberg et al., 2006 [13] also suggested that structural and functional changes like gliogenesis, synaptogenesis, neurogenesis, angiogenesis and significant alteration in neurotransmission systems and increasing in neurotrophic factors were more evident in older animals, particularly in animal models of neurodegenerative diseases [11].

Another report reveals that the levels of performance in behavioral tasks like spatial tasks causes different facets of spatial cognitive functions [11]. Some reports on animal models reveal the fact that motor activity improves cognitive performance through epigenetic mechanisms and influences the expression of genes involved in neuroplasticity. The important molecular processes that underlie such epigenetic mechanisms involve DNA methylation, histone modifications and expression of microRNA. The process of DNA methylation produces repressive effects of memory-suppressor genes to serve the expression of neuroplasticity-promoting genes and memory consolidation genes. And the histone acetylation is a requisite for consolidation of long-term memory [14]. Another recent study reported that 4 weeks of motor exercise in animal models significantly evidenced an increasing activity of enzymes which are involved in histone acetylation or deacetylation and these epigenetic mechanisms determine the expression of BDNF [15].

Some reports suggested that the hippocampus is an area of the brain that is sensitive to the benefits of PA and is also particularly vulnerable to age-related decay. It is already known that the hippocampus is involved in learning and memory processes [16].

It was also proposed that voluntary exercise greatly enhanced neurogenesis in dentate gyrus of adult mouse. It is previously stated that hippocampal neurogenesis starts diminishing with aging and this can be partially opposed after exercise. Thus, exercise-enhanced hippocampal neurogenesis is more evident in learning in aged mice [17]. This enhanced hippocampal neurogenesis is attributed to better microcirculation and increased growth factors. A report suggested three mechanisms that pose the beneficial effects of exercises to be actions of orexin-A/hypocretin-1, hypothalamic orexinergic neurons communication with hippocampus and hippocampal neurogenesis and functions.

Another study reported the influence of exercise on hippocampal structure and function, with assessment of parameters like spatial memory and pattern separation, evaluation of brain structure and plasticity, production of neurotrophic factors, and the vasculature of the brain. Studies supported the evidence of hippocampal neurogenesis in rodent models exposed to more physical activity. More converging evidence proved that exercise benefits include higher brain functions and improved cognition in mammals with a reduced risk for Alzheimer's disease (AD) and improved life span in humans [18].

Previous literature reported the benefits of exercise on neurogenesis as an extension to mouse models of degenerative diseases such as Alzheimer's Disease and Down Syndrome. Also, the studies added the therapeutic benefit of physical exercise with better improvement in cognitive function during cognitive impairment and dementia [19].

Another literature revealed that running (RUN) increases the development and formation of new neurons in the hippocampus, improves the neuronal spine density, increases the synaptic plasticity and neurotrophin levels, and enhances spatial memory function in mice compared with sedentary animals. Furthermore, housing rodents in identical-sized cages with either social or isolated conditions observed that the enriched environment without a running wheel does not enhance neurogenesis and increase neurotrophin levels [20].

Evidence on Physical Exercise Linked to Cognition and Memory in Human Studies

Neuroplasticity is a mechanism that occurs following physical exercise that is evidenced even in humans. Many study trials demonstrated that in adults, physical exercise determines structural changes in the brain like increased gray matter volume in frontal and hippocampal regions and greatly reduces damage to the gray matter [16].

Also, physical exercise facilitates the release of neurotrophic factors like peripheral BDNF which is related to cognitive functioning [21]. It increases the cerebral blood flow, improves cerebrovascular health and improves the actions of glucose and lipid metabolism that nourish the brain [11].

Another report evidenced this relationship by cross-sectional and epidemiological studies indicating that physical exercise improves cognitive functions in young and older adults [22]. This could be achieved by increasing the memory abilities, attentional processes and executive-control processes [23, 24].

Many studies demonstrated that physical exercise could prevent cognitive decline which is greatly linked to aging. This reduces the risk of developing dementia and reduces the level of deterioration in executive functions of the brain [25].

A few recent studies have found new relationships by examining imaging studies on the hippocampus in older humans and observed that aerobic fitness produced differences in the volume and brain structure that were related to cognitive performance as a function of aerobic fitness. A study by Erickson et al., worked with 165 healthy older adults aged between 59 to 81 years with good cognition and cardiorespiratory fitness who were exposed to maximal graded exercise test, and their hippocampal volume was assessed using functional magnetic resonance imaging (fMRI) and a performance of spatial memory task. The report revealed that higher fitness was associated with higher volume of hippocampus bilaterally, and this observation was greatly associated with better spatial memory performance [26].

Another study by Pereira et al., 2007 [27], measured the cerebral blood volume in adult humans around the mean age of 33 years by exposing them to 12 weeks of aerobic exercise training. The results revealed that exercise selectively influenced the dentate gyrus and produced profound changes in the cerebral blood volume with efficient cardiorespiratory fitness. These structural changes were influenced by improved cognitive performance by Rey Auditory Verbal Learning Test after the aerobic exercise training. And like mouse models, this data also suggests that in the hippocampal area, the dentate gyrus is uniquely susceptible to physical exercise indicated by exercise-related behavior causing neurogenesis in the brain.

Historical perspectives have also evidenced this association between physical exercise and cognitive functioning of the brain. Another scientist, Spirduso, also investigated the association of exercise with cognition in older subjects and reported that aerobic exercise was beneficial to the initiation and execution of action, particularly reaction time [28].

Another systematic literature search with six electronic databases and 5957 records found that physical exercise in the form of resistance training and resistance exercises produced evidential brain changes, particularly in the frontal lobe, with good improvements in executive function. Also, this resistance training resulted in lower white matter atrophy and lower volumes of white matter lesion. Thus, the report evidenced the cautious use of the physical exercise training on brain studies [29].

Reports also suggested that episodes of physical exercise led to higher concentrations of peripheral blood lactate and these levels were more linked to the improvements in executive functions [30]. Also, the production of lactate in the muscles is likely to be utilized for cognitive processes because it can cross the blood-brain barrier with the availability of monocarboxylate transporters. These raised concentrations of peripheral lactate might trigger the release of serum BDNF [31].

Physical Exercise Enhances Memory

Evidence was reported by researchers that exercise regimens involving aerobic and neuromotor exercises led to increase in the memory performance in elderly subjects in executive functions for short-term memory and incidental memory for long-term memory consolidation. A study compared the effects of aerobic exercise and neuromotor exercise in nearly 40 subjects for 36 sessions with a workout of 50 minutes, 3 days a week for period of 12 weeks and the intensity of activity was measured by Borg scale. The results expressed that significant improvements were identified after the exercise intervention period in both groups for parameters on nomination and incidental memory [32].

Another study investigated the aerobic physical fitness program towards ventilatory threshold and improvements in cognitive functions during a 6-month exercise program in 46 healthy inactive men aged 60-75 years. They were assessed for blood viscosity and physical and memory evaluation after using a cycle ergometer, 60 minutes every day for 3 times per week. The study revealed that there were significant improvements in memory, decreased blood viscosity and higher aerobic capacity in the aerobic physical fitness program [33].

Also, many studies revealed that physical exercise promoted delayed brain aging and degenerative pathologies in conditions like Alzheimer's Disease, diabetes, and multiple sclerosis, evidencing that physical exercise improves cognitive processes and memory and creates a sense of wellbeing Studies also evidenced the effects of various types of exercise on motor- and non-motor- clinical features of Parkinson's Disease and reported positive results and even proved in animal models with improved cell proliferation and migration of neural progenitors and hinders age-related deterioration with improvements in the vascularization of substantia nigra [33].

Conclusion

In the present day, life expectancy is increasing throughout the world and it is of much importance to maintain a better independent life with a sense of wellbeing. This can be achieved with proper physical fitness in the form of physical exercise that can also enrich the mental status of a person. Physical exercise promotes positive biological and psychological effects that influence the brain and promote good cognitive functioning and can also counteract the pathological process of aging. Although the beneficial effects of physical exercise are evident, care must be ensured to choose the appropriate exercise regimen for maximum benefits.

References

[1] *Benefits, need and importance of daily exercise.* Available from: https://www.researchgate.net/publication/306118434_Benefits_need_and_importance_of_daily_exercise [accessed Jun 04 2021].

[2] https://www.heart.org/en/healthy-living/fitness/fitness-basics/endurance-exercise-aerobic#:~:text=Also%20called%20aerobic%20exercise%2C%20endurance,and%20improves%20your%20overall%20fitness.

[3] https://www.mydr.com.au/sports-fitness/strength-training-exercises/.

[4] Weerapong P., Hume P. A., Kolt G. S., (2004). "Stretching: Mechanisms and Benefits for Sports Performance and Injury Prevention." *Physical Therapy Reviews*. 9 (4): 189-206. doi: https://10.1179/108331904225007078. S2CID 71435119.

[5] https://www.webmd.com/fitness-exercise/a-z/balance-training#:~:text=Balance%20training%20involves%20doing%20exercises,some%20very%20challenging%20yoga%20poses.

[6] https://www.brainhq.com/brain-resources/everyday-brain-fitness/physical-exercise/.

[7] *Physical Activity Guidelines for Americans.* 2nd ed. U.S. Department of Health and Human Services; Washington, DC, USA: 2018. [(accessed on 1 June 2019)]. Available online: https://health.gov/paguidelines/second-edition/ [Google Scholar].

[8] Piercy K. L., Troiano R. P., Ballard R. M., Carlson S. A., Fulton J. E., Galuska D. A., George S. M., Olson R. D. The Physical Activity Guidelines for Americans. *JAMA*. 2018;320:2020-2028. doi: https://10.1001/jama.2018.14854.

[9] Whitham M., Parker B. L., Friedrichsen M., Hingst J. R., Hjorth M., Hughes W. E., Egan C. L., Cron L., Watt K. I., Kuchel R. P., et al., Extracellular Vesicles Provide a Means for Tissue Crosstalk during Exercise. *Cell Metab.* 2018;27:237-251.e4. doi: https://10.1016/j.cmet.2017.12.001.

[10] van Praag H., Shubert T., Zhao C., Gage F. H. (2005). Exercise enhances learning and hippocampal neurogenesis in aged mice. *J. Neurosci.* 25, 8680-8685. https://10.1523/JNEUROSCI.1731-05.2005.

[11] Mandolesi L., Gelfo F., Serra L., Montuori S., Polverino A., Curcio G., Sorrentino G., (2017). Environmental factors promoting neural plasticity: insights from animal and human studies. *Neural Plast.* 2017, 1-10. https://10.1155/2017/7219461.

[12] Langdon K. D., Corbett D. (2012). Improved working memory following novel combinations of physical and cognitive activity. *Neurorehabil. Neural Repair* 26, 523-532. https://10.1177/1545968311425919.

[13] Kronenberg G., Bick-Sander A., Bunk E., Wolf C., Ehninger D., Kempermann G. (2006). Physical exercise prevents age-related decline in precursor cell activity in the mouse dentate gyrus. *Neurobiol. Aging* 27, 1505-1513. https://10.1016/j.neurobiolaging.2005.09.016.

[14] van Kesteren MT, Ruiter DJ, Fernandez G, Henson RN. 2012. How schema and novelty augment memory formation. *Trends Neurosci* 35: 211–219

[15] Maejima H., Kanemura N., Kokubun T., Murata K., Takayanagi K. (2018). Exercise enhances cognitive function and neurotrophin expression in the hippocampus accompanied by changes in epigenetic programming in senescence-accelerated mice. *Neurosci. Lett.* 665, 67–73. 10.1016/j.neulet.2017.11.023

[16] Colcombe S. J., Erickson K. I., Scalf P. E., Kim J. S., Prakash R., McAuley E., Elavsky S., Marquez D. X., Hu L., Kramer A. F., (2006). Aerobic exercise training increases brain volume in aging humans. *J. Gerontol. A Biol. Sci. Med. Sci.* 61, 1166-1170. https://10.1093/gerona/61.11.1166.

[17] Heine VM, Maslam S, Joels M, Lucassen PJ (2004) Prominent decline of newborn cell proliferation, differentiation, and apoptosis in the aging dentate gyrus, in absence of an age-related hypothalamus-pituitary-adrenal axis activation. *Neurobiol Aging* 25: 361–375

[18] Chaddock-Heyman L., Erickson K. I., Holtrop J. L., Voss M. W., Pontifex M. B., Raine L. B., Hillman C. H., Kramer A. F., (2014). Aerobic fitness is associated with greater white matter integrity in children. *Front. Hum. Neurosci.* 8:584. https://10.3389/fnhum.2014.00584.

[19] Rodrigues L., Dutra M.F., Ilha J., Biasibetti R., Quincozes-Santos A., Leite M.C., Marcuzzo S., Achaval M., Goncalves C.A. Treadmill training restores spatial cognitive deficits and neurochemical alterations in the hippocampus of rats submitted to an intracerebroventricular administration of streptozotocin. *J. Neural Transm.* 2010;117:1295–1305.

[20] Kobilo T, Yuan C, van Praag H. Endurance factors improve hippocampal neurogenesis and spatial memory in mice. *Learn Mem.* 2011b;18:103–107

[21] Hötting K., Röder B. (2013). Beneficial effects of physical exercise on neuroplasticity and cognition. *Neurosci. Biobehav. Rev.* 37, 2243–2257. 10.1016/ j.neubiorev.2013.04.

[22] Lista I., Sorrentino G. (2010). Biological mechanisms of physical activity in preventing cognitive decline. *Cell. Mol. Neurobiol.* 30, 493–503. 10.1007/s10571-009-9488-x Baylor A. M., Spirduso W. W. Systematic aerobic exercise and components of reaction time in older women. *J Gerontol.* 1988;43:121–126

[23] Kramer A. F., Hahn S., Cohen N. J., Banich M. T., McAuley E., Harrison C. R., et al.. (1999). Ageing, fitness and neurocognitive function. *Nature* 400, 418–419. 10.1038/22682

[24] Colcombe S., Kramer A. F. (2003). Fitness effects on the cognitive function of older adults. *Psychol. Sci.* 14, 125–130. 10.1111/1467-9280.t01-1-01430 [

[25] Herold F., Törpel A., Schega L., Müller N. G. Functional and/or structural brain changes in response to resistance exercises and resistance training lead to cognitive improvements – a systematic review. *Eur Rev Aging Phys Act* 16, 10 (2019). https://doi.org/10.1186/s11556-019-0217-2

[26] Erickson KI, Prakash RS, Voss MW, et al. Aerobic fitness is associated with hippocampal volume in elderly humans. *Hippocampus.* 2009;19(10):1030-1039. doi:10.1002/hipo.20547

[27] Pereira A. C., Huddleston D. E., Brickman A. M., Sosunov A. A., Hen R., McKhann G. M., Sloan R., Gage F. H., Brown T. R., Small S. A. An in vivo correlate of exercise-induced neurogenesis in the adult dentate gyrus. *Proc Natl Acad Sci U S A.* 2007;104:5638–5643.

[28] Tsukamoto H., Suga T., Takenaka S., Tanaka D., Takeuchi T., Hamaoka T., Isaka T., Ogoh S., Hashimoto T. Repeated high-intensity interval exercise shortens the positive effect on executive function during post-exercise recovery in healthy young males. *Physiol Behav.* 2016;160:26–34

[29] Riske L., Thomas R. K., Baker G. B., Dursun S. M. Lactate in the brain: an update on its relevance to brain energy, neurons, glia and panic disorder. *Ther Adv Psychopharmacol.* 2017;7:85–9. https://doi.org/10.1177/2045125316675579

[30] Thuanne da Silva Santos, Saulo Vasconcelos Rocha, Lélia Renata Carneiro Vasconcelos. The effect of physical exercise on the memory of elderly - an intervention study. Motriz. *Revista de Educação Física* 2019: 25(4)

[31] Antunes H. K., De Mello M. T., Santos-Galduróz R. F., Galduróz J. C. F., Aquino Lemos V., Tufik S. and Bueno O. F. A. Effects of a physical fitness program on memory and blood viscosity in sedentary elderly men. *Brazilian Journal of Medical and Biological Research* (2015) 48(9): 805-812.

[32] Carlo Maria Di Liegro, Gabriella Schiera, Patrizia Proia and Italia Di Liegro. Physical Activity and Brain Health. *Genes* 2019, 10, 720; doi:10.3390/genes 10090 720

[33] Cohen A. D.; Tillerson J. L.; Smith A. D., Schallert T., Zigmond M. J. Neuroprotective effects of prior limb use in 6-hydroxydopamine-treated rats: Possible role of GDNF. *J. Neurochem.* 2003, 85, 299–305.

Chapter 4

Astrocytes Migration and Their Molecular Role in the Recuperation of Damaged Nervous Tissue

Haneesha Vishwa Sai, Ryan Brice and Li Yao*
Department of Biological Sciences, Wichita State University,
Wichita, Kansas, USA

Abstract

Astrocytes are abundant glial cells that exhibit highly diversified physiological roles in healthy and diseased nervous systems. They also play significant roles in various cell processes of the central nervous system (CNS) that actively participate in neuronal regulation for functional regeneration and repair of brain or spinal cord injuries. Astrocytes are specialized to assist in the reduction of damaged tissue surrounding the injury site and simultaneously stitch back the disrupted blood brain barrier (BBB) in support of neural tissue and maintenance of brain homeostasis. Astrocytes use a popular cell-to-cell communication mechanism to respond to various signaling molecules. A glial scar is the result of astrocytes' migration to the target site and their extensive proliferation to prevent further damage to cells. During reactive astrogliosis, astrocytes tend to upregulate and downregulate the expression of various proteins required for cell migration and repair, like glial fibrillary acidic protein (GFAP), $\alpha_v\beta_3$, integrin, fibronectin, aquaporin (AQP)-4, Rho GTPases, syndecan-4 proteoglycan, connexin (Cx) 43, Cx30, and hemichannels (HCs), which are critical for migration. Astrocytes thrive at injury sites during brain or spinal cord injuries and

* Corresponding Author's Email: li.yao@wichita.edu.

In: Horizons in Neuroscience Research. Volume 48
Editors: Andres Costa and Eugenio Villalba
ISBN: 979-8-88697-230-6
© 2022 Nova Science Publishers, Inc.

assist the process of neuronal survival. In this review, we will discuss the origin, development, functionality, physiology, and pathology of astrocytes, further expanding on the significant roles that migration plays in the repair of damaged nervous tissue. Astrocyte migration is critical for performing several functions during both physiological and pathological conditions.

Keywords: astrocytes, migration, neural injury, neural regeneration, recuperation

Introduction

Astrocytes are one of most abundant and diversified glial cells that perform several functions in the neural tissue of the central nervous system (CNS). As shown through previous studies, astrocytes correlate with various physiological functions, including, but not limited to, the provision of nutrients, regulation of extracellular ionic concentration, synaptogenesis, control of penetrability of the blood-brain barrier (BBB), and initiation of multiple pathological processes in the brain [1]. Based on their morphology, anatomy and spatial orientation, astrocytes are categorized into two main subtypes: protoplasmic and fibrous [2]. Protoplasmic astrocytes are more spread out and portray extensively branched short processes. Fibrous astrocytes show radial distribution of long but less-branched processes. Some astrocytes portray a mixed morphology, like an intermediate appearance of fibrous and protoplasmic astrocytes, which are situated in gray and white matter regions. The glial fibrillary acidic protein (GFAP) and S-100 beta (a cytosolic Ca^{2+}-binding protein) are some of the markers used more frequently. GFAP is a specific intermediate filament protein in astrocytes and is essential for expression of the normal functioning of fibrous astrocytes in regulation of CNS white matter and integrity of the BBB [3].

During CNS development, neurons are formed prior to the formation of glial cells through radial glia that serve as a scaffold to support cell migration and also as a substrate of neural stem cells (NSCs) for both neural and glial cells [4]. Previous studies have shown that the developing spinal cord has revealed astro-glial-specific transcription factors that create a gliogenic switch where NSCs transition from neurogenesis to gliogenesis during development in the ventricular zone (VZ). Nuclear factor I-A (NFIA) is one such transcription factor, which is significant for embryonic gliogenesis, including astrocytogenesis [5]. Gliogenesis is possible with the involvement of factors such as Notch signaling, transcriptional repressor N-CoR, methylase Dnmt1, and histone methylation [6].

Differentiating astrocytes migrate to reach their final functioning site during development, whereas astrocytes in the adult brain are more latent under regular physiological conditions [7]. The arrangement of astrocytes in the brain are distinct as tiling domains and do not intertwine their processes [8, 9]. This occurrence is thought to be due to contact inhibition during postnatal development and is often lost during neurodegenerative disorders or after brain injury (BI) or spinal cord injury (SCI) [9].

Astrocytes and other glial cells show a rapid response to the events of BI or SCI and participate in repair and recovery at the injury site. During the initial stages of injury, disrupted axons have been shown to inhibit molecules from the myelin sheath of the oligodendrocytes. The myelin ligands and neuronal receptors interconnect and lower the regenerative capacity of the damaged neuronal processes [10].

Reactive astrogliosis is a process that alters the morphological and molecular structures of cells post injury [9]. This is provoked by various molecules from the blood, inflammatory cells, secretions from injured cells such as adenosine triphosphate (ATP), endothelin-1, pro-inflammatory cytokines such as tumor necrosis factor (TNF) and interleukin (IL)1y, interferon (IFN)y, and IL-6 [11–14]. Astrocytes near the injury site are altered to the reactive state from the latent state and suffer from cellular hypertrophy, thereby further changing into a fibroblast-like morphology and enhancing the expression of varied proteins such as GFAP, vimentin, nestin, and inducible nitric oxide synthase (iNOS) [15]–[17].

Reactive astrocytes are distinguished through cellular hypertrophy, extensions of processes and enhanced expression of GFAP, nestin, and other such intermediate filaments [18]. After severe injury, astrocytes undergo hypertrophy of their cell body and processes, and migrate to the site of injury to proliferate extensively. These changes alter the astrocyte arrangement, and the amplified astrocytes overlap to form a glial scar that functions to isolate the injured tissue to prevent exposure of the healthy surrounding neurons to unsafe molecules [19]. To successfully contain the injury site, astrocytes change their polarity accordingly and migrate; upon reaching the affected site, they uptake the extracellular signals such as glutamate, free iron, cytokines, ATP, and adenosine diphosphate (ADP) [20]. Reactive gliosis exhibits two roles, an advantageous one where it serves as a barrier to protect the CNS from extended damage, and another disadvantageous one where it impedes axonal regeneration and neuronal survival [9, 21]. During formation of the glial scar (within 24 hours of injury), astrocytes extensively secrete and deposit chondroitin sulfate proteoglycans (CSPGs) into the extracellular matrix (ECM), in tandem with myelin inhibitor molecules, to create unfavorable conditions for axonal regeneration [22].

Astrocyte Origin, Development, and Heterogeneity

Astrocytes are known to emerge from neural progenitor cells called radial glia, which are obtained from neuroepithelium. They originate through the process of asymmetric division [23]. At the initial stage of nervous system development during the neuronogenic period, the uneven division of radial glia creates immature neurons or neuron-restricted intermediate progenitors [24]. Two main stages in the development of the nervous system are neurogenesis and gliogenesis. Neurogenesis precedes gliogenesis using pro-neurogenic factors like neurogenin-1. The beginning of neurogenesis is regulated by NFIA, which is a transcription factor that works in alliance with sox 9 via Notch signaling or the transcriptional repressor N-CoR. These pathways intersect with the Janus kinase (JAK)/signal transducer and activator of transcription (STAT) signaling cascade where STAT3 is co-activated with the p300/CBP complex, which links to the astroglia gene promoter and results in the expression of genes specific to astrocytes, such as GFAP [25–27]. It is important to suppress this signaling cascade, which is responsible for gliogenesis, in order to promote neurogenesis using neurogenin-1 and other pro-neural factors such as Ngn2, NeuorD1, and Mash1, which bind with p300/CBP, thus terminating gliogenesis. Similarly, several factors of cytokines from the IL-6 family, such as the ciliary neurotrophic factor (CNTF), leukemia inhibitor factor (LIF), and cardiotrophin (CT)-1, which use signal-transducing co-receptors LIFRβ and gp130 to activate the JAK/STAT signaling cascade, thus regulating the process of gliogenesis [28]. This shows that the subpopulations of radial glia (neuronogenic, gliogenic, and multipurpose) coordinate to work together [29].

In the subventricular zone (SVZ) where asymmetrical division of radial glia is observed, the intermedial glial cells produced progress to form immature astrocytes. They further migrate in multiple layers of the cortical region and proliferate extensively. In the cortical layer I, or marginal zone (embryonic and neonatal cortex), neural progenitors that form neurons, oligodendrocytes, and astrocytes have been observed to populate ventral and dorsal telencephalic VZs. Astrocytes found in cortical layers I–IV emerge from progenitors of the marginal zone and cause different morphological changes of deeper and superficial astroglia [30, 31]. Embryonic astrogliogenesis is just one way of populating astrocytes in the CNS. In rodents, the majority of astrocytes are formed during the second and third postnatal weeks; in humans, the same gliogenesis also spreads into adulthood, contributing to the overall glial population. During postnatal astrogenesis, the symmetrical division of differentiated astrocytes in the CNS is responsible for more than 50 percent of astrocytes in the overall population [32]. Astrocytes are also produced from radial glia that lose their apical processes and change their morphology to transform into protoplasmic astrocytes, thus leading to the 10–15 percent mature astroglia population. Some astrocytes that are directly derived from radial glia turn into undifferentiated stem cells [33, 34]. There are two main phases of astrogliogenesis: one is during embryogenesis via intermediate glial progenitors, through asymmetrical division of radial glia in which the glial progenitors migrate, multiply, and transform into astrocytes; the other is in the postnatal stage of astrogliogenesis, where the radial glia undergo direct transformation into astrocytes and symmetrical division of the differentiated astrocytes [35].

Astrocyte Activity Post-Acute Brain Injury

Brain injury may cause infarction or selective neuronal death based on the intensity and period of the event. Infarction is characterized by the accidental casualty of glia and neurons. Neurons maintain close interaction with astrocytes for their survival. Hence, at any injured site where astrocytes fail to thrive, it is implied that neuronal survival at that location will be questionable, but if there are astrocytes surviving, then this is a promising condition of synaptic remodeling and neurite outgrowth to recoup and compensate for the lost cells. Astrocytes are more resistant to multiple affronts, including ischemia, than neurons; however, sometimes protoplasmic astrocytes are more sensitive to the effects of brain insults than fibrous astrocytes, thus proving the variance of resistance among different subtypes of astrocytes [36].

Astrocytes play crucial roles in supporting neuronal growth and survival during acute brain injuries. These include glutamate uptake, glutamate release, metabolic intermediates release, oxygen free radicals scavenging, extra-cellular K^+ and H^+ buffering, gap junction (GJ) coupling, BBB and brain edema influences, second injury and recovery effects, inflammatory response and gliosis, and axonal regeneration barriers [37]. During serious conditions like ischemia, hypoglycemia, and trauma, the glutamate toxicity mechanism leads to neuronal death [38]. Removal of glutamate from the ECM is achieved by Na^+-dependent transporters confined to astrocytes [39]. Many studies have described the important role of these glutamate astrocyte transporters, termed GLAST and GLT-1, in regulating the toxic levels of extracellular glutamate concentration [40]. Glutamate uptake needs movement against the concentration gradient, which requires high energy; the intracellular glutamate concentration ranges from 1 to 10 MM, and the extracellular glutamate concentration usually ranges below 10 MM, in glia and neurons [41]. To overcome the concentration gradient, the influx of each glutamate ion of 3 Na^+ ions and 1 H^+ ion is carried out by efflux of the 1K^+ ion. The energy spent to perform this action is estimated to be a large part of total brain ATP turnover. The main advantage of glutamate uptake by astrocytes is shifting the high energy expenditure by neurons in the process. Other glutamate transporters possess the ability to move substrates either inward or outward, referred to as uptake reversal [42].

At the stages of ATP depletion due to severe ischemia, the membranes supported by ATP collapse and terminate the uptake process, in turn initiating the efflux of glutamate by versal of the uptake [43]. Astrocytes release glutamine, which is a precursor for synthesis of neurotransmitter glutamate [44–46]. Surrounding the uptake of astrocytes, glutamate is released by neurons at the synapses and, by using the glutamine synthetase enzyme, convert it into glutamine [47]. The astrocytes further release glutamine for neuronal uptake and metabolize it into glutamate to be packaged in synaptic vesicles [48].

Inhibition of the glutamine synthetase enzymatic function through pharmacological drugs leads to the mitigation of glutamine levels in the brain, which decreases the K^+ level, in turn evoking glutamate release and reducing the effects of ischemia [49]. Ischemic BI is mainly caused by reactive oxygen species (ROS) [50]. Glutathione is a primary antioxidant compound in the brain, the absence of which increases the chances of ischemic injury [51]. In comparison with neurons, astrocytes consist of higher concentrations of glutathione along with other enzymes in glutathione metabolism [52]. In the same way, the flow of glucose via the pentose phosphate pathway in astrocytes is two times that produced by neurons, indicating the greater capability of astrocytes in scavenging ROS compared to neurons. This oxidant-scavenging mechanism in astrocytes supports neuronal survival [53]. During ischemia, elevated extracellular K^+ concentrations may cause cell swelling, the release of glutamate, and anoxic depolarizations. Astrocytes portray two mechanisms (active and passive) to limit these increased extracellular K^+ concentrations [54]. The electrical coupling in glial cells enhances the passive movement of K^+ ions from extracellular space into the cytoplasm of astrocytes. This increases the intracellular K^+ concentration that is redistributed among coupled cells via the K^+ current all through the glial syncytium, resulting in spatial buffering [55]. Gap junctions of astrocytes allow for the intracellular transfer of ions and other molecules, such as $Ca2^+$ and inositol triphosphate [56].

The efficiency of astrocyte coupling is regulated by several neuro-transmitters, cytokines, and many other bioactive substances [57]. Certain conditions like the increase in intracellular Ca^{2+}, reduced pH, and fewer oxygen free radicals prevent coupling during ischemia [58]. However, multiple subsets of gap junctions do remain available even during brain insults [59]. Post-cerebral ischemia and brain edema impair local and surrounding blood flow by damaging long-fiber channels. Brain edema is categorized as both vasogenic, because of the transcapillary movement of water and other solutes across the BBB, and also cytotoxic, because of the osmotic swelling of cellular elements [60].

Astrocyte processes cover up most of the abluminal capillary surface and form some part of the physical BBB [61]. Astrocytes induce the creation of compact intercellular junctions between capillary endothelial cells and modulate the expression along with the function of endothelial cell transporters, thereby contributing to the function of the BBB [62]. During any kind of secondary BI, astrocytes at the site of injury initiate the exhibition of two major actions: hypertrophy and extensive proliferation, or astrogliosis [63]. Macrophages and microglia migrate to the injury site to guard against this response, Reactive astrocytes elevate the expression of structural proteins such as GFAP and vimentin [64]. After the ischemia expression of many proteins such as copper-zinc superoxide dismutase, glutathione peroxidase, and metallothionein, all are upregulated, thereby increasing their capacity to decrease ROS [65]. An evolved conservatory function of reactive astrogliosis is to seclude the region of injury post BI. Because the brain consists of fewer fibroblasts compared to other tissues in the body, astrocytes construct a "barricade" around the lesion site, called anisomeric gliosis. The glial scar formed as a result of this could be an obstacle for regenerating axons [66]. Reactive astrocytes are identified by the enhanced expression of GFAP, and this adds to the barrier property of the glial scar for axonal extension. GFAP anti-sense DNA shows the expression of laminin, which allows neurite growth in this condition [66, 67]. Matrix metalloproteases (MMPs) and their inhibitors are components produced by reactive astrocytes that design the remodeling of ECM components and affect the glial scar architecture formed at the injury site. In this way, the reactive astrocytes promote the recovery of BBB [68].

Role of Astrocytes Post-Spinal Cord Injury

During the functional recovery stage post-spinal cord injury, it has been observed that astrocytic responses are important for neural tissue repair and regeneration [69]. The reactive astrocytes developed gradually migrate to the site of injury, resulting in glial scar formation, which was initially thought to be harmful for the pathophysiology of SCI; however, the functioning of these cells before glial scar formation has proven to be beneficial for tissue repair and recuperation of motor-functioning abilities [69]. To understand the role of the STAT3 molecule, it was particularly reduced in reactive astrocytes of genetically modified mice through a nestin gene promoter/enhancer, which resulted in decreased migration to the epicenter of the injury site, thereby leading to a broader region of injury, damaged contraction of incoming inflammatory cells, and constrained overall functional recovery [69, 70]. In the same mice, when the suppressor of the cytokine signaling-3 protein (SOCS3) was weakened in reactive astrocytes, contrasting results were observed, such as accelerated migration of astrocytes to the inflammatory cells, constriction of the lesion region, and sudden elevation in the functional recovery [71]. In the chronic phase of SCI, the same reactive astrocytes may cause physical and chemical barriers for axonal regeneration [71]. It was observed that the reactive astrocytes selectively upregulated NES, CTNNB1, AXIN2, PLAUR, MMP2, and MMP13 marker genes, and that the scar-forming astrocytes upregulated CDH2, SOX9, XYLT1, CHST11, CSGALNACTL1, ACAN, PCAN, SLIT2 marker genes [72]. The reversible nature of the reactive astrogliosis process has been proven via transplantation of reactive astrocytes into injured spinal cord, where they formed astrocytic scars, and when they were transplanted into naïve spinal cord, they morphologically returned to naïve astrocytes [72]. Similarly, the marker genes of scar-forming reactive astrocytes were highly upregulated when the cells were transplanted into injured spinal cord, while the marker genes of reactive astrocytes were repressed when planted in naïve spinal cord. Based on the results obtained, the reversible nature of reactive astrocytes when placed under certain varied conditions has been proven [72].

Table 1. Molecules and genes of astrocytes involved in SCI and BI

Molecule(s)	Function	Reference
Glial fibrillary acidic protein (GFAP)	Is expressed in subpopulation of astrocytes in CNS	[3, 18, 22, 73]
Vimentin	Is expressed in immature astrocytes (protoplasmic and fibrous astrocyte subpopulations); is highly expressed in reactive astrocytes	[16, 17, 74, 75]
N-cadherin	Assists in transformation of reactive astrocytes to scar-forming	[72]
Signal transducer and activator of transcription-3 (STAT3)	Assists in migration of reactive astrocytes towards injury epicenter; increases contraction of infiltrating inflammatory cells; promotes functional recovery (regulator of reactive astrogliosis)	[69, 70]
Suppressor of cytokine signaling-3 protein (SOCS3)	Provides negative feedback molecule of STAT3	[70, 71]
Interleukin-6 (IL-6)	Upstream effectors of STAT3 pathway; aggregates invading inflammatory cells	[71]
Anti-integrin beta1 antibody (anti-beta1 Ab) (antibody to collagen-binding integrin)	Prevents scar formation due to no expression of N-cadherin and GFAP	[72]
Chondroitin sulfate proteoglycan genes (CSPGs): XYLT1, CHST11, CSGALNACTL1, ACAN, PCAN	Abundantly inhibit extracellular axonal regeneration; exhibit gene expression in astrocytic scar area post-SCI	[76–78]
Slit2	Guides axons limiting/repulsive gene	[76, 79]
CDH2, SOX9	Are marker genes for scar-forming astrocytes	[72]
NES, CTNNB1, AXIN2, PLAUR, MMP2, MMP13	Act as marker genes for reactive astrocytes	[72]
Integrins: $a_1ß_1$, $a_2ß_1$, $a_{10}ß_1$, $a_{11}ß_1$	Play a significant role as ECM receptors in cell-Coll1 interaction	[80]
Collagen-1	Induces scar formation upon interaction with reactive astrocytes	[72]
ECM genes: COLLA1, COLLA2	COLL-1 genes that are highly expressed in affected spinal cord	[72, 80]
N-cadherin nAb, N-cadherin-neutralizing body	Prohibit transformation of RAs into SAs	[72]

Astrocytes turn reactive after SCI conditions and benefit by assisting in the repair function; however, when they turn into scar-forming astrocytes, they might be detrimental to the SCI repair [69]. It is important to curb or slow down the process of conversion of reactive astrocytes into scar-forming astrocytes via alternation of the microenvironment surrounding the cells. Expression of various genes in the entire genome was examined in naïve astrocytes transplanted in injured spinal cord. It was observed that genes of collagen type I (Coll-1) were expressed more in cells that were transplanted in injured spinal cord for the scar-forming duration, compared to those in naïve spinal cord [72]. The reactive astrocytes formed scars with coordinated expression of Coll-1; however, the reactive astrocytes remained in their form in the absence of expression of Coll-1 genes. These reactive astrocytes in the absence of Coll-1 expression reversed the spreading process and reduced the expression of GFAP. The same reactive astrocytes in contact with Coll-1 showed that they attached to the adjoining cells and upregulated the expression of GFAP and N-cadherin, which are properties of scar-forming astrocytes.

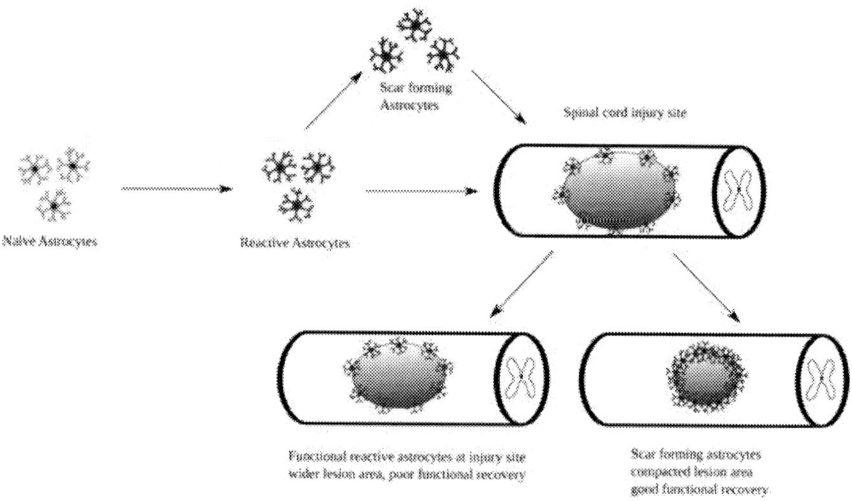

Figure 1. Reactive astrocyte's role in spinal cord injury repair.

Research studies involving impendence of the expression of Coll-1 with the addition of collagen-binding integrin, such as anti-integrin beta1 (anti-beta1) antibody, and promotion of N-cadherin neutralizing with antibodies have proven ways to prohibit the transition to scar-forming astrocytes from reactive astrocytes. It was also observed that the introduction of anti-beta1 antibody during the scar-forming phase post-SCI slowed the process and supported axonal regeneration at the site of injury in mice, thereby resulting in faster recuperation. This explains the significance of Coll-1 in the transformation of reactive astrocytes into scar-forming astrocytes and how this process could be regulated by use of environmental alteration methods that suppress scar formation and enhance axonal regeneration and functional recovery of damaged neurons [72].

Cell-to-Cell Communication of Astrocytes

Several types of astrocytes existing in the human brain can be recognized by the fusion of specific cell markers such as CD44, EAAT1, EAAT2, aquaporin (AQP), and GFAP [81]. Astrocytes perform many diversified functions, as mentioned above, such as modulating the activity of chemical synapses and supporting the delivery of substrates to neurons as needed. They can survive in a low-oxygen environment for longer periods than neurons due to their functioning by the process of anaerobic glycolysis. Cx30 and Cx43 astroglia allow the diffusion of glucose and lactate incorporated into metabolic networks and support distantly located neurons for their survival and regeneration. These molecules assist neurons by providing buffering molecules (glutamate, K+, nitric oxide, hydrogen peroxide, ammonia) for metabolic requirements, and they contribute to the formation of a BBB by setting up a primary defense at the site of injury [17]. To perform all these functions, it is essential for astrocytes to sense the signaling molecules and respond to them to communicate with adjacent astrocytes. Astrocytes demonstrate extended communication network levels by a direct cell-to-cell connection via gap junctions that comprise double-facing connexins developed by a hexameric ring of Cx30) and Cx43 [82]. Connexins are essential proteins that drive cell communication in astrocytes to accommodate and maintain physiological functioning of the CNS [82].

Migration of Astrocytes Essential for Repair of Neural Injury

Astrocyte migration is a critical process that contributes to the development, maintenance, and recuperation of neurons in the CNS. Under regular physiological conditions, astrocytes in the adult brain are inactive in terms of migration. Under pathological conditions such as trauma, ischemia, infection, inflammation, and neurodegeneration, however, they become activated and turn into migratory cells [83]. Several recent *in vivo* studies have shown that reactive astrocytes experience hypertrophy, followed by cell polarization and migration [73, 84]. Astrocytes migrate at the time of injury or pro-inflammatory conditions, and they form a glial scar to repair the site of injury and protect surrounding neurons from exposure to harmful chemicals resulting from disrupted tissue at that site [85].

In the adult mammalian CNS, astrocytes are distributed at specific sites, due to their connection with other cell types and the ECM. The basal lamina is covered by the astrocytes' endfeet, which protects the pial surface of the brain that is populated by blood vessels [86]. Because the basal lamina occupies a large surface area, an abundant number of astrocyte processes are necessary. Astrocytes also connect closely with neurons at the proximity of synapsis and at the nodes of Ranvier [87]. During their development, astrocytes form a widespread network of astrocytic spheres, which intersect with each other at the periphery and are linked through a series of gap junctions, thus facilitating the movement of ions and some molecules regulating cell-to-cell communication [88, 89]. Thus, newborn astrocytes (progenitors) are migratory during their development and differentiation, but become inactive after reaching a destined specific site under physiological conditions [7]. Astrocytes are aligned in a specific pattern, thereby prohibiting the association of their processes, and this is achieved through the contact-inhibition mechanism, which terminates the growth and migration of cells upon contact with other cells [90]. This mechanism is actively functional during postnatal development; however, it is dysfunctional during neural diseases and injuries [9]. At the beginning stage of neuronal injury, axons are unveiled to inhibitory molecules from the myelin sheath of oligodendrocytes. This interaction causes hinderance and slows down the axonal regeneration of damaged neurons [11]. Astrocytes that are present in the vicinity of the injury undergo multiple morphological and molecular alterations, converting their non-reactive nature to a reactive nature that proliferates and migrates towards the injury site and forms a glial scar [91]. Injured neural cells, blood cells, and inflammatory cells release several molecules, such as ATP, IL-6, IFN gamma, IL-1B, endothelin-1, and TNF [11, 12]. Depending on the distance of the astrocytes' location from the injury site, cells closer to the lesion become migratory as reactive astrocytes and experience cellular hypertrophy, thereby enhancing the expression of GFAP, vimentin, nestin, and iNOS [15–17].

After serious injury, astrocytes reach the injury site and proliferate, intensively overlapping their processes and forming glial scars that provide protection by secluding healthy neural tissue from injured tissue and harmful molecules that are secreted [19]. Astrocytes play a major role in containing the injury by absorbing extracellular signals such as glutamate, free iron, cytokines, ATP, and ADP, thus preventing its spread [20]. Because these are the same molecules that induce reactivity in astrocytes, astrogliosis also expel the detrimental effects on neuronal regeneration [20]. It has been observed that post-injury, astrocytes enhanced the secretion of chondritin sulfate proteoglycans (CSPGs) in the extracellular matrix, leaving an unfavorable environment for axonal repair when combined with released myelin-associated inhibitory molecules [22]. It is possible to categorize the reactive astrocytes into naïve-nonreactive astrocytes, scar-forming astrocytes that do not migrate, and expressing N-cadherin using various markers. Molecules such as MMP2, MMP13, and beta-catenin are expressed by reactive migratory astrocytes [92, 93]. After analyzing the detrimental effects of scar-forming astrocytes, the reversible process of transforming reactive astrocytes into naïve astrocytes can be used towards neural tissue by expanding the duration of reactive astrocytes. Hence, the migration of astrocytes is a significant modulator in terms of glial scar formation. Along with migration, astrocytes need to coordinate and communicate with each other through connexin channels, gap junctions, and hemichannels (HCs) that supply a path for release and absorption of ions and small molecules via extracellular compartments [94]. While GJs and HCs communicate with other cells about the damage, Cxs and HCs permit astrocytes to secrete signaling molecules that assist with astrocyte migration during the injury [94]. Several proteins such as a_vb_3 integrin, heparin sulfate syndecan-4 proteoglycan, purinergic P2X7 receptor, Cx43, and pannexin-1 (PX1) hemichannels are all upregulated during astrocyte migration [17].

Migration of Astrocytes and the Role of Connexins

Several recent *in vivo* studies have shown that reactive astrocytes experience hypertrophy, followed by cell polarization and migration [85, 95]. Astrocytes migrate upon injury or pro-inflammatory conditions, and form a glial scar to repair the site of injury and protect surrounding neurons from exposure to harmful chemicals [96]. Some *in vitro* studies have shown that in the presence of TNF and other cytokines, reactive astrocytes are the only cells to migrate in response to external stimuli [17]. Cx43 is an essential HC-forming protein that contributes to the migration of astrocytes because the inhibitory peptide Gap19 prohibits HC opening and cell migration induced by the neuronal protein Thy-1/CD90 [17, 94]. Pro-inflammatory signals that provoke astrocyte reactivity are vital to their migration as a response to extracellular cues along with the presence of Cx43. In TNF-treated astrocytes, Thy-1/CD90 activates its two receptors, a_vb_3 and syndecan-4, and their expressions are upregulated under pro-inflammatory conditions. Other essential proteins that are upregulated during TNF treatment are Cx43, Px1, P2x7r, GFAP, and iNOS

[17, 94]. In reactive astrocytes, the two receptors a_vb_3 integrin and syndecan-4 trigger intracellular signaling pathways including the release of $Ca2^+$ from the endoplasmic reticulum (ER); opening of Cx43; release of Px1, HCs, and ATPs; and activation of P2X7R, which elevates the intracellular concentrations of Ca2+ necessary for cell migration [17, 94].

Migration of Astrocytes under Physiological Conditions

The radial glia, which are progenitor cells of the astrocytes, are present in the SVZ of the fetal brains of mammals. They serve as a scaffold by extending their elongated ascending processes called radial fibers to the pial surface in order to facilitate the migration of progenitor cells and maintain them in a migratory and immature state [7]. These glial progenitors initially migrate to gray matter and differentiate into protoplasmic astrocytes, and then migrate into white matter to differentiate into fibrous astrocytes [38]. These cells migrate by using radial fibers and retract them and simultaneously elevate the cell soma from the VZ, the same movement as neuronal migration [97]. In the adult brain, some glial progenitors are non-migratory under regular conditions. In various pathological conditions such as ischemia, inflammation, neurodegeneration, and trauma, the non-migratory glial progenitors activate and move to the injury site for neural repair [98–100]. Although astrocytes are immobile during regular physiological conditions, they adapt a method of reversible cell process migration, controlling various functions of the CNS [101].

Migration of Astrocytes during Pathological Conditions

Astrogliosis is the process by which quiescent astrocytes regain the ability to migrate during pathological conditions such as injury or a diseased CNS [102]. The early stage of astrogliosis is highly significant in the repair of neural injury; however, the next stage of reactive astrocytes transforming into scar-forming astrocytes could lead to the release of various harmful chemicals that could be damaging to neurons around the injury site and the regeneration of axons [103, 104]. The scratch-wound assay is the model for a cell migration study that was performed to investigate the migration of astrocytes after traumatic injury [105]. In the culture plate, the injury was mimicked by scratching off the cells at the base, and then the degree of injury was evaluated based on the protein content left on the scratched culture plate in comparison with the unscratched plate. To track the intrinsic responses of the astrocytes, the medium was changed frequently to clear all debris from the scratch. To track both extrinsic and intrinsic responses of astrocytes during injury, media with the scratched cell debris was left on the culture plate to simulate the close conditioning of injury [106]. This experiment showed various properties of astrogliosis including hypertrophy (enlargement of cell size), hyperplasia (amplified cell production and number), and GFAP increase [107].

Cell adhesion is significant for cell motility, which is acquired by cell-to-cell or cell-to-ECM adhesion characteristics. Cell adhesion molecules (CAMs) are situated at the surface of cells, thereby facilitating them to attach with other cells or the ECM. CAMs are members of the main protein families, such as immunoglobulins, integrins, syndecans, cadherins, and selectins, and these vary functionally depending on the identification by other ligands. Thus, limitations with CAMs expression could impede cell adhesion and migration [108]. Many other adhesive molecules that are present in the ECM and necessary for migration are fibrous proteins, glycosaminoglycans, proteoglycans, and glycoproteins (fibronectin and integrins) [109].

Fibronectin is classified as one of the essential glycoproteins that assist with the organization of the matrix protein. It is released by cells as a protein dimer. When bound to integrins, the fibronectin is transformed into large insoluble fibrils via cell-mediated processes [80]. These accumulated fibronectins, which are critical for cell-to-cell or cell-to-ECM adhesion, are favorable for astroglial scar formation and injury repair by forming a substrate for astrocyte adhesion and migration [80, 110]. CAMs also include integrins and syndecans, which are cell receptors and are activated in the cell-adhesion process. They modify their activation depending on the surrounding mechanical forces and work as two-way mechanotransducers linking the cytoskeleton and ECM via Arg-Gly-Asp (RGD) tripeptides and syndecan-4 with heparin bonds [111, 112]. Fibronectin receptors such as a_5b_1 and a_vb_3 integrins are able to alter the composition of integrins, which in turn affect cell-to-ECM adhesion in various physiological and pathological conditions by initiating relevant signaling pathways activating Rho GTPases (RhoA and Rac1) [113]. Integrins and their signaling pathways instigate a reactive process in astrocytes, like proliferation and migration. The buildup of integrins is constantly altered in response to astrocyte migration. Targeted deletion of a certain integrin β_1 in astrocytes leads to migration [114, 115]. To initiate astrocyte migration at the quiescent stage, integrins portray the activity of transmembrane receptors and moderate Cdc42-regulated cell polarity [116].

Cytoskeleton elements such as actin filaments, intermediate filaments, and microtubules contribute to cell movement, which is modulated by GTPases like Rho, Rac, and Cdc42. Intermediate filaments (IFs) have a tendency to alter their composition based on specific events of the cell, such as development and repair [117]. Upon injury, astrocytes change their morphology and function, and produce IF proteins like GFAP, vimentin, and nestin in varied amounts. This shows the significant function of IF protein in astrocytic motility of both reactive and naïve astrocytes, as their downregulation could impede the elongation process and cell movement. Reduced IFs in astrocytes decrease the astrocytic migration rate, which further delays the glial scar formation promoting the injury-repair process [75]. Other transmembrane proteins like aquaporins facilitate the transfer of water through a selectively permeable membrane, which influences the cell migration in different cells [118]. AQP4 is expressed in the CNS (BBB and brain-cerebrospinal fluid barrier) and is a crucial water channel for astrocytes involved in cell migration [119]. The AQP4 isoform (M1 heterotetramer) moves freely in the plasma membrane and disperses into elongating lamellipodial regions to aid astrocytic migration [120]. The absence of these AQP4 proteins leads to slower migration, thus affecting the scar-formation process [120, 121].

Table 2. Molecules and genes involved in astrocyte migration towards neural repair

Molecule(s)	Function	Reference
Fibronectin (glycoprotein in ECM)	Helps with astroglial scar formation	[80, 111], [112]
Integrins (regulatory receptors involved in cell adhesion)	Instigate proliferation and migration in astrocytes; affect cell-to-cell and cell-to-ECM adhesion based on their alteration in composition	[114, 115]
Cdc42 and Other Transmembrane Receptors	Initiate migration of astrocytes	[116, 117]
Hyaluronan and CD44 Receptor	Are responsible for morphological changes in astrocytes; is highly expressed in reactive astrocytes	[73]
Rac1	Enhances astrocyte migration	[113]
Cell Adhesion Molecules (CAMs)	Adhere cells to cells or cells to surface	[80, 110]
Adenosine Triphosphate (ATP), Interleukin (IL)-6, Interferon (IFN) Gamma, IL-1B, Endothelin-1, Tumor Necrosis Factor (TNF)	Are secreted by blood cells and inflammatory cells during neural injury	[17, 122], [123]

Molecule(s)	Function	Reference
Connexin (Cx) Channels and Gap Junctions	Facilitate astrocytic communication and coordination	[17, 94]
Hemichannels (HCs)	Allow astrocytes to secrete signaling molecules to assist with migration	[21, 94]
Metalloproteinase (MMP)2, MMP13, beta-catenin	Are expressed in migratory reactive astrocytes	[17, 72, 94]
avb3 Integrin, Heparin Sulfate Syndecan-4 Proteoglycan, Purinergic P2X7 Receptor, Pannexin-1 (PX1)	Upregulate gene expression during migration of astrocytes	[14, 94]
Connexin (Cx) 43, Cx30	Are expressed in abundance in gray matter where astroglial endfeet are predominantly present (Cx30); also expressed in astrocytes (Cx43)	[17, 73, 94]
Aquaporin (AQP)4	Is expressed in astrocytes and ependymocytes of CNS and mostly at astrocyte endfeet	[118–120]
Sox 9 Transcriptional Factor	Is exclusively used to label nuclei of astrocytes present outside the neurogenic niches	[25–27]
Glutamate Transporters: EAAT-1 (GLAST), EAAT-2 (GLT-1)	Are specific to astroglia; EAAT-1 is expressed in cerebellum, label radial glia, fibrous protoplasmic astrocytes, cerebellar Bergmann glia, retinal Mullar glia, and SVZ of developing adult CNS; EAAT-2 shows neuronal expression during fetal development	[73]
Syndecans (regulating receptors)	Are activated to facilitate cell adhesion process	[80, 110]
Rho GTPases	Initiate signaling pathways that activate RhoA and Rac1; are necessary for cell-to-ECM adhesion	[113, 115]

Astrocytes play critical roles in acute brain injuries, influencing the uptake and release of glutamate and metabolic intermediates, limiting increased extracellular K+ concentrations, removing reactive oxygen species, and modulating the inflammatory response and activities of gliosis in acute brain injuries. Reactive astrocytes develop and migrate to spinal cord injury sites to assist in tissue repair and restoration of motor function. However, as they change into scar-forming astrocytes the activities of scar tissue formation can hinder functional recovery; thus, the microenvironment surrounding these cells should be controlled in order to slow this conversion process, for example through the transplantation of naïve astrocytes with upregulated expression of Coll-1 genes. Performance of cellular functions is due in part to their inherent capacity for cell-cell communications with adjacent astrocytes through gap junctions comprised of double-facing connexins.

The migratory role of astrocytes is essential for neural injury repair, because they must be present at the injury site to promote axonal regeneration. The migratory abilities of astrocytes in the adult brain are dormant under physiological conditions. However, during pathological conditions, astrocytes undergo hypertrophy, turning into reactive astrocytes and gaining cell polarization and migration towards the site of injury. Reactive astrocytes assist in neural repair, and scar-forming astrocytes protect healthy tissue surrounding the injury site from exposure to harmful chemicals from damaged tissue. The cause of changes in astrocytes and their activities in neural repair occurs at the molecular level, including MMP2, MMP13, and beta-catenin, expressed in migratory reactive astrocytes, the transmembrane receptor Cdc42 assisting the migration of astrocytes, syndecans regulating receptors to increase cell adhesion processes, and fibronectin in the ECM assisting with astroglial scar formation. The absence of AQP4 proteins leads to slower astrocyte migratory rates with subsequent slower formation of glial scar tissue. Astrocytes are specialized cells with an active role in brain and spinal cord homeostasis, participating in neuronal regulation for functional regeneration and repair of brain or spinal cord injuries. Future studies investigating the molecular and migratory roles of astrocyte function in CNS injuries may help elucidate the mechanism of controlling scar formation in order to optimize the time frame for neural regeneration to occur.

References

[1] Benjamin Kacerovsky J. and K. K. Murai, "Stargazing: Monitoring subcellular dynamics of brain astrocytes," *Neuroscience*, vol. 323, pp. 84–95, May 2016, doi: 10.1016/j.neuroscience.2015.07.007.

[2] Privat, A., M. Gimenez-Ribotta, and J.-C. Ridet, *Morphology of astrocytes*. New York: Oxford University Press, 1995.

[3] Ludwin, S. K., J. C. Kosek, and L. F. Eng, "The topographical distribution of S-100 and GFA proteins in the adult rat brain: An immunohistochemical study using horseradish peroxidase-labeled antibodies," *J. Comp. Neurol.*, vol. 165, pp. 197–207, 1976.

[4] Kang P., Lee H. K., Glasgow S. M., Finley M., Donti T., Gaber Z. B., Graham B. H., Foster A. E., Novitch B. G., Gronostajski, R. M., Deneen, B., "Sox9 and NFIA coordinate a transcriptional regulatory cascade during the initiation of gliogenesis," *Neuron*, vol. 74, pp. 79–94, 2012.

[5] Sloan S. A. and B. A. Barres, "Mechanisms of astrocyte development and their contributions to neurodevelopmental disorders," *Curr. Opin. Neurobiol.*, vol. 27, pp. 75–81, 2014, doi: 10.1016/j.conb.2014.03.005.

[6] Molofsky A. V., Krencik R., Ullian E. M., Tsai Hui-hsin, Dennen B., Richardson W. D., Barres B. A., Rowitch D. H., "Astrocytes and disease: A neurodevelopmental perspective," *Genes Dev.*, vol. 26, pp. 891–907, 2012.

[7] Goldman, J. E., M. Zerlin, S. Newman, L. Zhang, and J. Gensert, "Fate determination and migration of progenitors in the postnatal mammalian CNS," *Dev. Neurosci.*, vol. 19, no. 1, pp. 42–48, 1997, doi: 10.1159/000111184.

[8] Halassa, M. M., T. Fellin, H. Takano, J. H. Dong, and P. G. Haydon, "Synaptic islands defined by the territory of a single astrocyte," *J. Neurosci.*, vol. 27, no. 24, pp. 6473–6477, 2007, doi: 10.1523/JNEUROSCI.1419-07.2007.

[9] Sofroniew, M. V. "Molecular dissection of reactive astrogliosis and glial scar formation," *Trends Neurosci.*, vol. 32, no. 12, 2009, doi: 10.1016/j.tins.2009.08.002.

[10] Cao, Z., Y. Gao, K. Deng, G. Williams, P. Doherty, and F. S. Walsh, "Receptors for myelin inhibitors: Structures and therapeutic opportunities," *Mol. Cell Neurosci.*, vol. 43, no. 1, pp. 1–14, 2010, doi: 10.1016/j.mcn.2009.07.008.

[11] Giulian, D., J. Woodward, D. G. Young, J. F. Krebs, and L. B. Lachman, "Interleukin-1 injected into mammalian brain stimulates astrogliosis and neovascularization," *J. Neurosci.*, vol. 8, no. 7, pp. 2485–2490, 1988, doi: 10.1523/JNEUROSCI.

[12] Ahmed, S. M., B. A. Rzigalinski, K. A. Willoughby, H. A. Sitterding, and E. F. Ellis, "Stretch-induced injury alters mitochondrial membrane potential and cellular ATP in cultured astrocytes and neurons," *J. Neurochem.*, vol. 74, no. 5, 2000, doi: 10.1046/j.1471-4159.2000.741951000000000.

[13] John, G. R., S. C. Lee, and C. F. Brosnan, "Cytokines: powerful regulators of glial cell activation," *Neuroscientist*, vol. 9, no. 1, pp. 10–22, 2003, doi: 10.1177/1073858402239587.

[14] Gadea, A., S. Schinelli, and V. Gallo, "Endothelin-1 regulates astrocyte proliferation and reactive gliosis via a JNK/c-Jun signaling pathway," *J. Neurosci.*, vol. 28, no. 10, pp. 2394–2408, 2008, doi: 10.1523/JNEUROSCI.5652-07.2008.

[15] Miyake, T., T. Hattori, M. Fukuda, T. Kitamura, and S. Fujita, "Quantitative studies on proliferative changes of reactive astrocytes in mouse cerebral cortex," *Brain Res.*, vol. 451, no. 1–2, pp. 133–138, 1988, doi: 10.1016/0006-8993(88)90757-3.

[16] Clarke, S. R., A. K. Shetty, J. L. Bradley, and D. A. Turner, "Reactive astrocytes express the embryonic intermediate neurofilament nestin," *Neuroreport*, vol. 5, no. 15, pp. 1885–1888, 1994, doi: 10.1097/00001756-199410000-00011.

[17] Lagos-Cabre, R., A. Alvarez, M. Kong, F. Burgos-Bravo, A. Cardenas, and E. Rojas-Mancilla, "alphaVbeta3 Integrin regulates astrocyte reactivity," *J. Neuroinflammation*, vol. 14, no. 1, p. 194, 2017, doi: 10.1186/s12974-017-0968-5.

[18] Frisén, J. "Spinal Axons in central nervous system scar tissue are closely related to laminin-immunoreactive astrocytes," *Neuroscience*, vol. 65, no. 1, pp. 293–304, 1995, doi: 10.1016/0306-4522(94)00467-j.

[19] Homkajorn, B. "Connexin 43 Regulates Astrocytic Migration and Proliferation in Response to Injury," *Neurosci. Lett.*, vol. 486, no. 3, pp. 197–201, 2010, doi: 10.1016/j.neulet.2010.09.051.

[20] Bylicky, M. A., G. P. Mueller, and R. M. Day, "Mechanisms of endogenous neuroprotective effects of astrocytes in brain injury," *Oxid. Med. Cell Longev.*, p. 6501031, 2018, doi: 10.1155/2018/6501031.

[21] Pekny M. and M. Pekna, "Astrocyte reactivity and reactive astrogliosis: Costs and benefits," *Physiol. Rev.*, vol. 94, no. 4, pp. 1077–1098, 2014, doi: doi:

[22] Jones, L. L., R. U. Margolis, and M. H. Tuszynski, "The chondroitin sulfate proteoglycans neurocan, brevican, phosphacan, and versican are differentially regulated following spinal cord injury," *Exp. Neurol.*, vol. 182, no. 2, pp. 399–411, Aug. 2003, doi: 10.1016/s0014-4886(03)00087-6.

[23] Kriegstein A. and A. Alvarez-Buylla, "The glial nature of embryonic and adult neural stem cells," *Ann. Rev. Neurosci.*, vol. 32, pp. 149–184, 2009, doi: 10.1146/annurev.neuro.051508.135600.

[24] Montell, C. "The history of TRP channels, a commentary and reflection," *Pflugers Arch.*, vol. 461, pp. 499–506, 2011, doi: 10.1007/s00424-010-0920-3.

[25] He F., Ge W., Martinowich K., Becker-Catania S., Coskun V., Zhu W., Wu H., Castro D., Guillemot F., Fan G., de Vellis J., sun Y. E., "A positive autoregulatory loop of Jak-STAT signaling controls the onset of astrogliogenesis," *Nat. Neurosci.*, vol. 8, pp. 616–625, 2005, doi: 10.1038/ nn1440.

[26] Kanski, R., M. E. Strien, P. Tijn, and E. M. Hol, "A star is born new insights into the mechanism of astrogenesis," *Cell Mol. Life Sci.*, vol. 71, pp. 433–447, 2014, doi: doi:10.1007/ s00018-013-1435-9.

[27] Urayama S., Semi K., Sanosaka T., Hori Y., Namihira M., Kohyama J., Takizawa T., Nakashima K., "Chromatin accessibility at a STAT3 target site is altered prior to astrocyte differentiation," *Cell Struct. Funct.*, vol. 38, pp. 55–66, 2013, doi: 10.1247/csf.12034.

[28] Nakashima K., Wiese S., Yanagisawa M., Arakawa H., Kimura N., HIsatsune T., Yoshida K., Kishimoto T., Sendtner M., Taga T., "Developmental requirement of gp130 signaling in neuronal survival and astrocyte differentiation," *J. Neurosci.*, vol. 19, pp. 5429–5434, 1999.

[29] Bayraktar, O. A., L. C. Fuentealba, A. Alvarez-Buylla, and D. H. Rowitch, "Astrocyte development and heterogeneity," *Cold Spring Harb. Perspect. Biol.*, vol. 7, p. 020362, 2014, doi: 10.1101/cshperspect.a020362.

[30] Costa M. R., Kessaris N., Richardson W. D., Götz M., and Hedin-Pereira C., "The marginal zone/layer I as a novel niche for neurogenesis and gliogenesis in developing cerebral cortex," *J. Neurosci.*, vol. 27, pp. 11376–11388, 2007, doi: 10. 1523/JNEUROSCI.2418-07.

[31] Breunig J. J., Gate D., Levy R., Rodriguez Jr. J., Kim G. B., Danielpour M., Svendsen C. N., Town T., "Rapid genetic targeting of pial surface neural progenitors and immature neurons by neonatal electroporation," *Neural Dev.*, vol. 7, p. 26, 2012, doi: 10.1186/1749-8104-7-26.

[32] Ge, W. P., A. Miyawaki, F. H. Gage, Y. N. Jan, and L. Y. Jan, "Local generation of glia is a major astrocyte source in postnatal cortex," *Nature*, vol. 484, pp. 376–380, 2012, doi: 10.1038/nature10959.

[33] Schmechel D. E. and P. Rakic, "A Golgi study of radial glial cells in developing monkey telencephalon: Morphogenesis and transformation into astrocytes," *Anat. Embryol. Berl.*, vol. 156, pp. 115–152, 1979, doi: 10.1007/BF00300010.

[34] Voigt, T. "Development of glial cells in the cerebral wall of ferrets: Direct tracing of their transformation from radial glia into astrocytes," *J. Comp. Neurol.*, vol. 289, pp. 74-88, 1989, doi: 10.1002/cne.902890106.

[35] Nishiyama, A., L. Boshans, C. M. Goncalves, J. Wegrzyn, and K. D. Patel, "Lineage, fate, and fate potential of NG2-glia," *Brain Res. P.t B*, vol. 1638, pp. 116–128, 2016, doi: 10.1016/j.brainres.

[36] Lukaszevicz A. C., Sampaïo, N., Guégan, C., Benchoua A., Couriaud C., Chevalier E., Sola B., Lacombe P., Onténiente B., "High sensitivity of protoplasmic cortical astroglia to focal ischemia," *J. Cereb. Blood Flow Metab.*, vol. 22, pp. 289–298, 2002.

[37] Chen Y. and R. A. Swanson, "Astrocytes and Brain Injury," *J. Cereb. Blood Flow Metab.*, vol. 23, no. 2, pp. 137–149, Feb. 2003, doi: 10.1097/01.WCB.0000044631.80210.3C.

[38] Choi, D. W. "Glutamate neurotoxicity and diseases of the nervous system," *Neuron*, vol. 1, pp. 623–634, 1988.

[39] Anderson C. M. and R. A. Swanson, "Astrocyte glutamate transport: Review of properties, regulation, and physiological functions," *Glia*, vol. 32, pp. 1–14, 2000.

[40] Rosenberg P. A. and E. Aizenman, "Hundred-fold increase in neuronal vulnerability to glutamate toxicity in astrocyte-poor cultures of rat cerebral cortex," *Neurosci. Lett.*, vol. 103, pp. 162–168, 1989.

[41] Erecinska M. and I. A. Silver, "Metabolism and role of glutamate in mammalian brain," *Prog. Neurobiol.*, vol. 35, pp. 245–296, 1990.

[42] Szatkowski, M., B. Barbour, and D. Attwell, "Non-vesicular release of glutamate from glial cells by reversed electrogenic glutamate uptake," *Nature*, vol. 348, pp. 443–446, 1990.

[43] Longuemare M. C. and R. A. Swanson, "Excitatory amino acid release from astrocytes during energy failure by reversal of sodium dependent uptake," *J. Neurosci. Res.*, vol. 40, pp. 379–386, 1995.

[44] Bradford, H. F., H. K. Ward, and A. J. Thomas, "Glutamine—A major substrate for nerve endings," *J. Neurochem.*, vol. 30, pp. 1453–1459, 1978.

[45] Waniewski R. A. and D. L. Martin, "Exogenous glutamate is metabolized to glutamine and exported by rat primary astrocyte cultures," *J. Neurochem.*, vol. 47, pp. 304–313, 1986.

[46] Martin L. J., Brambrink A. M., Lehmann C., Portera-Cailliau C., Koehler R., Rothstein J., Traystman R. J., "Hypoxia-ischemia causes abnormalities in glutamate transporters and death of astroglia and neurons in newborn striatum," *Ann. Neurol.*, vol. 42, pp. 335–348, 1997.

[47] Rothstein J. D., Dykes-Hoberg M., Pardo C. A., Bristol L. A., Jin L., Kunci R. W., Kanai Y., Hediger M. A., Wang Y., Schielke J. P., Welty D. F., "Knockout of

glutamate transporters reveals a major role for astroglial transport in excitotoxicity and clearance of glutamate," *Neuro.*, vol. 16, pp. 675–686, 1996.

[48] Broer S. and N. Brookes, "Transfer of glutamine between astrocytes and neurons," *J. Neurochem.*, vol. 77, pp. 705–719, 2001.

[49] Paulsen R. E. and F. Fonnum, "Role of glial cells for the basal and Ca2+ dependent K+ evoked release of transmitter amino acids investigated by microdialysis," *J. Neurochem.*, vol. 52, pp. 1823–1829, 1989.

[50] Chan, P. H. "Role of oxidants in ischemic brain damage," *Stroke*, vol. 27, pp. 1124–1129, 1996.

[51] Dringen, R. "Metabolism and functions of glutathione in brain," *Prog. Neurobiol.*, vol. 62, pp. 649–671, 2000.

[52] Wilson, J. X. "Antioxidant defense of the brain: a role for astrocytes," *Can. J. Physiol. Pharmacol.*, vol. 75, pp. 1149–1163, 1997.

[53] Ben-Yoseph, O., P. A. Boxer, and B. D. Ross, "Assessment of the role of the glutathione and pentose phosphate pathways in the protection of primary cerebrocortical cultures from oxidative stress," *J. Neurochem.*, vol. 66, pp. 2329–2337, 1996.

[54] Walz, W. "Controversy surrounding the existence of discrete functional classes of astrocytes in adult gray matter," *Glia*, vol. 31, no. 2, pp. 95–103, Aug. 2000, doi: 10.1002/1098-1136(200008)31:2<95:aid-glia10>3.0.co;2-6.

[55] Karwoski, C. J., H. K. Lu, and E. A. Newman, "Spatial buffering of light evoked potassium increases by retinal Muller (glial) cells," *Science*, vol. 244, pp. 578–580, 1989.

[56] Giaume C. and K. D. McCarthy, "Control of gap-junctional communication in astrocytic networks," *Trends Neurosci.*, vol. 19, pp. 319–325, 1996.

[57] Nagy J. I. and W. E. Li, "A brain slice model for *in vitro* analyses of astrocytic gap junction and connexin43 regulation: Actions of ischemia, glutamate and elevated potassium," *Eur J Neurosci*, vol. 12, pp. 4567–4572, 2000.

[58] Martinez A. D. and J. C. Saez, "Regulation of astrocyte gap junctions by hypoxia-reoxygenation," *Brain Res. Brain Res. Rev.*, vol. 32, pp. 250–258, 2000.

[59] Cotrina M. L., Kang J., Lin Jane H-C, Bueno E., Hansen T. W., He L., Liu Y., Nedergaard M., "Astrocytic gap junctions remain open during ischemic conditions," *J. Neurosci.*, vol. 18, pp. 2520–2537, 1998.

[60] Klatzo, I. "Presidental address. Neuropathological aspects of brain edema," *J. Neuropathol. Exp. Neurol.*, vol. 26, pp. 1–14, 1967.

[61] Abbott, N. J. "Inflammatory mediators and modulation of blood-brain barrier permeability," *Cell Mol. Neurobiol.*, vol. 20, pp. 131–147, 2000.

[62] Dehouck, M. P., S. Meresse, P. Delorme, J. C. Fruchart, and R. Cecchelli, "An easier, reproducible, and mass-production method to study the blood-brain barrier *in vitro*," *J. Neurochem.*, vol. 54, pp. 1798–1801, 1990.

[63] Ridet, J. L., S. K. Malhotra, A. Privat, and F. H. Gage, "Reactive astrocytes: Cellular and molecular cues to biological function, *Trends Neurosci.*, vol. 20, pp. 570–577, 1997.

[64] Eng, L. F., R. S. Ghirnikar, and Y. L. Lee, "Glial fibrillary acidic protein: GFAP—Thirty-one years (1969–2000)," *Neurochem Res*, vol. 25, pp. 1439–1451, 2000.

[65] Campagne, M. V., H. Thibodeaux, N. Bruggen, B. Cairns, and D. G. Lowe, "Increased binding activity at an antioxidant-responsive element in the metallothionein-1 promoter and rapid induction of metallothionein-1 and -2 in response to cerebral ischemia and reperfusion," *J. Neurosci.*, vol. 20, pp. 5200–5207, 2000.

[66] Bush T. G., Puvanachandra N., Horner C. H., Polito A., Ostenfeld T., Svendsen C. N., Mucke L., Johnson M. H., Sofroniew M. V., "Leukocyte infiltration, neuronal degeneration, and neurite outgrowth after ablation of scar-forming, reactive astrocytes in adult transgenic mice," *Neuron*, vol. 23, pp. 297–308, 1999.

[67] Costa S., Planchenault T., Charriere-Bertrand C., Mouchel Y., Fages C., Juliano, S., Lefrançois T., Barlovatz-Meimon G., Tardy M., "Astroglial permissivity for neuritic outgrowth in neuron-astrocyte cocultures depends on regulation of laminin bioavailability," *Glia*, vol. 37, pp. 105–113, 2002.

[68] Kakinuma Y., Hama H., Sugiyama F., Yagami K., Goto K., Murakami K., Fukamizu A., "Impaired blood–brain barrier function in angiotensinogen-deficient mice," *Nat Med*, vol. 4, pp. 1078–1080, 1998.

[69] Okada S., Nakamura M., Katoh H., Miyao T., Shimazaki T., Ishii K., Yamane J., Yoshimura A., Iwamoto Y., Toyama Y., Okano H., "Conditional ablation of Stat3 or Socs3 discloses a dual role for reactive astrocytes after spinal cord injury," *Nat. Med.*, vol. 12, no. 7, pp. 829–834, Jul. 2006, doi: 10.1038/nm1425.

[70] Herrmann, J. E. "STAT3 is a critical regulator of astrogliosis and scar formation after spinal cord injury," *J. Neurosci.*, vol. 28, no. 28, pp. 7231–7243, 2008.

[71] Penkowa, M. "Astrocyte-targeted expression of interleukin-6 protects the central nervous system during neuroglial degeneration induced by 6-aminonicotinamide," *J. Neurosci. Res.*, vol. 73, no. 4, pp. 481–496, 2003.

[72] Hara M., Kobayakawa K., Ohkawa Y., Kumamaru H., Yokota K., Saito T., Kijima K., Yoshizaka S., Harimaya K., Nakashima Y., Okada S., "Interaction of reactive astrocytes with type I collagen induces astrocytic scar formation through the integrin-N-cadherin pathway after spinal cord injury," *Nat. Med.*, vol. 23, no. 7, pp. 818–828, Jul. 2017, doi: 10.1038/nm.4354.

[73] Bardehle, S., M. Kruger, F. Buggenthin, J. Schwausch, J. Ninkovic, and H. Clevers, "Live imaging of astrocyte responses to acute injury reveals selective juxtavascular proliferation," *Nat. Neurosci.*, vol. 16, no. 5, pp. 580–586, 2013, doi: 10.1038/nn. 3371.

[74] Miyake, T., T. Hattori, M. Fukuda, T. Kitamura, and S. Fujita, "Quantitative studies on proliferative changes of reactive astrocytes in mouse cerebral cortex," *Brain Res.*, vol. 451, no. 1–2, pp. 133–138, Jun. 1988, doi: 10.1016/0006-8993(88)90757-3.

[75] Lepekhin, E. A., C. Eliasson, C. H. Berthold, V. Berezin, E. Bock, and M. Pekny, "Intermediate filaments regulate astrocyte motility," *J. Neurochem.*, vol. 79, pp. 617–625, 2001.

[76] Silver J. and J. H. Miller, "Regeneration beyond the glial scar," *Nat. Rev. Neurosci.*, vol. 5, pp. 146–156, 2004.

[77] Cregg, J. M., DePaul M. A., Filous A. R., Lang B. T., Tran A., Silver J., "Functional regeneration beyond the glial scar," *Exp. Neurol.*, vol. 253, pp. 197–207, 2014.

[78] McKillop, W. M., M. Dragan, A. Schedl, and A. Brown, "Conditional Sox9 ablation reduces chondroitin sulfate proteoglycan levels and improves motor function following spinal cord injury," *Glia*, vol. 61, pp. 164–177, 2013.
[79] Hagino, S. "Slit and glypican-1 mRNAs are coexpressed in the reactive astrocytes of the injured adult brain," *Glia*, vol. 42, pp. 130–138, 2003.
[80] Hynes, R. O. "Integrins: bidirectional, allosteric signaling machines," *Cell*, vol. 110, pp. 673–687, 2002.
[81] Sosunov, A. A., X. Wu, N. M. Tsankova, E. Guilfoyle, G. M. McKhann, and J. E. Goldman, "Phenotypic heterogeneity and plasticity of isocortical and hippocampal astrocytes in the human brain," *J. Neurosci.*, vol. 34, no. 6, pp. 2285–2298, 2014, doi: 10.1523/JNEUROSCI.4037-13.2014.
[82] Anders, S., D. Minge, S. Griemsmann, M. K. Herde, C. Steinhauser, and C. Henneberger, "Spatial properties of astrocyte gap junction coupling in the rat hippocampus," *Philos. Trans. R. Soc. Lond. B Biol. Sci.*, vol. 369, 2014, doi: 10. 1098/rstb.2013.0600.
[83] Zhan, J. S., K. Gao, R. C. Chai, X. H. Jia, D. P. Luo, and G. Ge, "Astrocytes in migration," *Neurochem. Res.*, vol. 42, no. 1, pp. 272–282, 2017, doi: 10.1007/ s11064-016-2089-4.
[84] Sirko, S., G. Behrendt, P. A. Johansson, P. Tripathi, M. Costa, and S. Bek, "Reactive glia in the injured brain acquires stem cell properties in response to sonic hedgehog," *Corrected Cell Stem Cell*, vol. 12, no. 4, pp. 426–439, 2013, doi: 10. 1016/j.stem.2013.01.019.
[85] Chai R. C., Jiang J. H., Wong A. Y. K., Jiang F., Gao K., Vatcher G., Yu A. C. H., "AQP5 is differentially regulated in astrocytes during metabolic and traumatic injuries: AQP5 in astrocytic injuries," *Glia*, vol. 61, no. 10, pp. 1748–1765, Oct. 2013, doi: 10.1002/glia.22555.
[86] Peters, A., S. L. Palay, and H. deF Webster, *The fine structure of the nervous system: Neurons and their supporting cells*, 3rd ed. New York: Oxford University Press, 1991.
[87] Black J. A. and S. G. Waxman, "The perinodal astrocyte," *Glia*, vol. 1, no. 3, pp. 169–183, 1988, doi: 10.1002/glia.440010302.
[88] Butt A. M. and B. R. Ransom, "Visualization of oligodendrocytes and astrocytes in the intact rat optic nerve by intracellular injection of lucifer yellow and horseradish peroxidase," *Glia*, vol. 2, no. 6, pp. 470–475, 1989, doi: 10.1002/glia. 440020609.
[89] Comeli-Bell, A. H., S. M. Finkbeiner, M. S. Cooper, and S. J. Smith, "Glutamate induces calcium waves in cultured astrocytes: Long range glial signalling," *Science*, vol. 247, pp. 470–473, 1990.
[90] Lanosa X. A. and J. A. Colombo, "Cell contact-inhibition signaling as part of wound-healing processes in brain," *Neuron Glia Biol.*, vol. 4, no. 1, pp. 27–34, Feb. 2008, doi: 10.1017/S1740925X09000039.
[91] Burda J. E. and Sofroniew M. V., "Reactive Gliosis and the Multicellular Response to CNS Damage and Disease," *Neuron*, vol. 81, no. 2, pp. 229–248, Jan. 2014, doi: 10.1016/j.neuron.2013.12.034.

[92] Kanemaru K. "Calcium-dependent N-cadherin up-regulation mediates reactive astrogliosis and neuroprotection after brain injury," *Proc. Natl. Acad. Sci.*, vol. 110, no. 28, pp. 11612–17, 2013, doi: 10.1073/pnas.1300378110.

[93] Verslegers, M., K. Lemmens, I. Van Hove, and L. Moons, "Matrix metalloproteinase-2 and -9 as promising benefactors in development, plasticity, and repair of the nervous system," *Prog. Neurobiol.*, 2013, doi: 10.1016/j.pneurobio.2013.03.004.

[94] Retamal M. A., Froger N., Palacios-Prado N., Ezan P., Sáez P. J., Sáez J. C., Giaume C., "Cx43 hemichannels and gap junction channels in astrocytes are regulated oppositely by proinflammatory cytokines released from activated microglia," *J. Neurosci. Off. J. Soc. Neurosci.*, vol. 27, no. 50, pp. 13781–13792, Dec. 2007, doi: 10.1523/JNEUROSCI.2042-07.2007.

[95] Alvarez, A., R. Lagos-Cabre, M. Kong, A. Cardenas, F. Burgos-Bravo, and P. Schneider, "Integrin-mediated transactivation of P2X7R via hemichannel dependent ATP release stimulates astrocyte migration," *Biochim. Biophys. Acta*, vol. 1863, no. 9, pp. 2175–2188, 2016, doi: 10.1016/j.bbamcr.2016.05.018.

[96] Garré, J. M., G. Yang, F. F. Bukauskas, and M. V. Bennett, "FGF-1 Triggers pannexin-1 hemichannel opening in spinal astrocytes of rodents and promotes inflammatory responses in acute spinal cord slices," *J. Neurosci.*, vol. 36, no. 17, pp. 4785–4801, 2016, doi: 10.1523/JNEUR.

[97] Nadarajah, B., J. E. Brunstrom, J. Grutzendler, R. O. Wong, and A. L. Pearlman, "Two mode of radial migration in early development of the cerebral cortex," *Nat. Neurosci.*, vol. 4, pp. 143–150, 2001.

[98] Canoll P. and J. E. Goldman, "The interface between glial progenitors and gliomas," *Acta Neuropathol. Berl.*, vol. 116, pp. 465–477, 2008.

[99] Nait-Oumesmar B. et al., "Activation of the subventricular zone in multiple sclerosis: Evidence for early glial progenitors," *Proc. Natl. Acad. Sci. USA*, vol. 104, pp. 4694–4699, 2007.

[100] Parent, J. M., N. Bussche, and D. H. Lowenstein, "Prolonged seizures recruit caudal subventricular zone glial progenitors into the injured hippocampus," *Hippocampus*, vol. 16, pp. 321–328, 2006.

[101] Wang Y. F. and K. Hamilton, "Chronic vs. acute interactions between supraoptic oxytocin neurons and astrocytes during lactation: Role of glial ibrillary acidic protein plasticity," *Sci. World J.*, vol. 9, pp. 1308–1320, 2009.

[102] Sun D. and T. C. Jakobs, "Structural remodeling of astrocytes in the injured CNS," *Neuroscientist*, vol. 18, pp. 567–588, 2012.

[103] Rolls, A., R. Shechter, and M. Schwartz, "The bright side of the glial scar in CNS repair," *Nat. Rev. Neurosci.*, vol. 10, pp. 235–241, 2009.

[104] Davies, S. J., M. T. Fitch, S. P. Memberg, A. K. Hall, G. Raisman, and J. Silver, "Regeneration of adult axons in white matter tracts of the central nervous system," *Nature*, vol. 390, pp. 680–683, 1997.

[105] Yu, A. C., Y. L. Lee, and L. F. Eng, "Astrogliosis in culture: I. The model and the effect of antisense oligonucleotides on glial ibrillary acidic protein synthesis," *J. Neurosci. Res.*, vol. 34, pp. 295–303, 1993.

[106] Faber-Elman, A., A. Solomon, J. A. Abraham, M. Marikovsky, and M. Schwartz, "Involvement of wound-associated factors in rat brain astrocyte migratory response to axonal injury: *In vitro* simulation," *J. Clin. Invest.*, vol. 97, pp. 162–171, 1996.
[107] Gao K., Wang C. R., Jiang F., Wong A. Y. K., Su N., Jiang J. H., Chai R. C., Vatcher G., Teng J., Chen J., Jiang Y-W, Yu A. C. H., "Traumatic scratch injury in astrocytes triggers calcium influx to activate the JNK/c-Jun/AP-1 pathway and switch on GFAP expression," *Glia*, vol. 61, pp. 2063–2077, 2013.
[108] Gumbiner B. M. "Cell adhesion: The molecular basis of tissue architecture and morphogenesis," *Cell*, vol. 84, pp. 345–357, 1996.
[109] Boudreau N. and Bissell M. J., "Extracellular matrix signaling integration of form and function in normal and malignant cells," *Curr. Opin. Cell Biol.*, vol. 10, pp. 640–646, 1998.
[110] van Strien M. E., Brevé J. J. P., Fratantoni S., Schreurs M. W. J., Bol J. G. J. M., Jongenelen C. A. M., Drukarch B., van Dam A-M., "Astrocytederived tissue transglutaminase interacts with Fibronectin: A role in astrocyte adhesion and migration?" *PloS One*, vol. 6:e25037, 2011.
[111] Ginsberg M. H. "Integrin activation," *BMB Rep*, vol. 47, pp. 655–659, 2014.
[112] Nussinov R., Tsai C. J., and Liu J., "Principles of allosteric interactions in cell signaling," *J. Am. Chem. Soc.*, vol. 136, pp. 17692–17701, 2014.
[113] Cukierman E., Pankov R., Stevens D. R., and Yamada K. M., "Taking cell–matrix adhesions to the third dimension," *Science*, vol. 294, pp. 1708–1712, 2001.
[114] Wagner S., Tagaya M., Koziol J. A., Quaranta V., and Zoppo G. J., "Rapid disruption of an astrocyte interaction with the extracellular matrix mediated by integrin alpha 6 beta 4 during focal cerebral ischemia/reperfusion," *Stroke*, vol. 28, pp. 858–865, 1997.
[115] Robel S., Mori T., Zoubaa S., Schlegel J., Sirko S., Faissner A., Goebbels S., Dimou L., Götz M., "Conditional deletion of beta1-integrin in astroglia causes partial reactive gliosis," *Glia*, vol. 57, pp. 1630–1647, 2009.
[116] Etienne-Manneville S. and Hall A., "Integrin-mediated activation of Cdc42 controls cell polarity in migrating astrocytes through PKCzeta," *Cell*, vol. 106, pp. 489–498, 2001.
[117] Bershadsky A. D., Vaisberg E. A., and Vasiliev J. M., "Pseudopodial activity at the active edge of migrating ibroblast is decreased after drug-induced microtubule depolymerization," *Cell Motil. Cytoskelet.*, vol. 19, pp. 152–158, 1991.
[118] Papadopoulos M. C., Saadoun S., and Verkman A. S., "Aquaporins and cell migration," *Plugers Arch.*, vol. 456, pp. 693–700, 2008.
[119] Verkman A. S., Binder D. K., Bloch O., Auguste K., and Papadopoulos M. C., "Three distinct roles of aquaporin-4 in brain function revealed by knockout mice," *Biochim. Biophys. Acta*, vol. 1758, pp. 1085–1093, 2006.
[120] Smith A. J., Jin B. J., Ratelade J., and Verkman A. S., "Aggregation state determines the localization and function of M1- and M23-aquaporin-4 in astrocytes," *J. Cell Biol.*, vol. 204, pp. 559–573, 2014.
[121] Papadopoulos M. C. and A. S. Verkman, "Potential utility of aquaporin modulators for therapy of brain disorders," *Prog. Brain Res.*, vol. 170, pp. 589–601, 2008.

[122] Miyake T., Hattori T., Fukuda M., Kitamura T., and Fujita S., "Quantitative studies on proliferative changes of reactive astrocytes in mouse cerebral cortex," *Brain Res.*, 1988, doi: 10.1016/0006-8993(88)90757-3.

[123] Clarke, S. R., Shetty A. K., Bradley J. L., and Turner D. A. "Reactive astrocytes express the embryonic intermediate neurofilament nestin," *Neuroreport*, vol. 5, pp. 1885–1888, Oct. 1994, doi: 10.1097/00001756-199410000-00011.

Chapter 5

Molecular Role of Schwann Cell Migration in Repair and Regeneration of Nervous Tissue

Haneesha Vishwa Sai, Ryan Brice and Li Yao*
Department of Biological Sciences, Wichita State University,
Wichita, Kansas, USA

Abstract

Schwann cells (SCs) myelinate neurons in the peripheral nervous system (PNS), thereby facilitating saltatory conduction via the myelination of axons, as well as digesting damaged axons and subsequently forming a tube-like structure to guide neural regeneration. During neural injury, Schwann cells migrate, proliferate, and assist the impaired neurons at injury site by engulfing damaged myelin and axon endings, and forming an endoneural tube connecting the neural cell body to the ends. They also secrete several neural growth factors promoting axon elongation. Motility and migration of Schwann cells are critical for remyelination of neurons after neural injury. SCs are reprogrammed by their dedifferentiation and activation, further initiating neural repair functionality, which results in down regulation of myelin genes and upregulation of trophic factors, thereby leading to the removal of damaged myelin. In this review, we will discuss the development, functionality, myelination, pathologies, and molecular regulation of SC motility, further elucidating the significant role that migration plays in the repair of damaged nervous tissue.

Keywords: Schwann cells, motility, migration, neural regeneration

* Corresponding Author's Email: li.yao@wichita.edu.

In: Horizons in Neuroscience Research. Volume 48
Editors: Andres Costa and Eugenio Villalba
ISBN: 979-8-88697-230-6
© 2022 Nova Science Publishers, Inc.

Schwann Cell Development and Origin

Schwann cells (SCs) are the primary glial cells of the peripheral nervous system (PNS), comprised of myelinating and non-myelinating cells [1, 2]. They assist in the migratory direction of neurons; regulate axonal diameter, phosphorylation, and neurofilament spacing; eliminate cellular debris; and can continually divide throughout their lifespan [3]. Myelinating Schwann cells form a non-continuous myelin sheath in myelinated axons, resulting in the formation of gaps between the SCs, known as nodes of Ranvier [4], thus facilitating saltatory conduction at increased velocities as an economical means of transferring action potentials. This function is analogous to oligodendrocytes in the central nervous system (CNS) [5]. Non-myelinating Schwann cells are involved in the maintenance of axons and are vital for neuronal persistence, with some assembling around smaller axons and forming Remak bundles [2, 6]. In the PNS, myelinating Schwann cells are out-numbered by their non-myelinating counterparts in a ratio of 3–4:1 [7].

The majority of SCs are derived early in embryonic development from neural crest cells (NCCs) [1, 8] that migrate during embryonic development and can differentiate into other cell types including pigment cells, smooth muscle, glial cells, and cartilage [9]. Induction of the neural crest is derived from ectoderm, a process that requires signaling of bone morphogenetic protein (BMP), Wnt signaling pathways, and fibroblast growth factor (FGF) [10]. Neural crest-derived boundary cap cells are another source of SCs. These progenitor cells are located at the dorsal root entry and embryonic motor areas [11].

Neural crest cells mature through several stages, first developing into precursor cells, followed by transformation into immature SCs until birth [12]; post birth, the immature cells will differentiate into non-myelinating or myelinating SCs. These immature cells first go through the myelination pathway at birth and then go through the non-myelin pathway later in development [9, 13]. Neural crest cells will travel along two developmentally discrete pathways: the ventral pathway, whereby they move ventrally through the anterior sclerotome from which SCs will be derived, and the dorsolateral pathway, which lies between the epidermis and dermis [10, 14]. Each developmental stage in the SC line is regulated by different signaling responses, tissue associations, and the presence of certain transcription factors [15]. NCCs become SC progenitor cells, in turn becoming immature SCs and then maturing into non-myelin-forming or myelin-forming SCs [16].

Table 1. Schwann cell developmental lineage markers

Lineage Marker	Functional Information	Schwann Cell Development Stage(s)	References
Growth associated protein 43 (GAP43)	Plasticity, neurite formation	Progenitor	[6, 13]
Krox-20, early growth response protein 2 (EGR2)	Zinc-finger protein transcription factor, also known as early growth response protein 2 (EGR2)	Immature, myelinating	[15, 24]
Myelin-associated glycoprotein (MAG)	Transmembrane glycoprotein critical for myelin formation and maintenance	Myelinating	[28, 29]
Myelin basic protein (MBP), P1	Important for myelin formation and maintenance, as well as role in membrane lipid interaction	Myelinating	[6, 27]
Myelin protein zero (P0)	Major structural membrane component of myelin sheath	Myelinating	[1, 26]
Neuregulin 1 type 3 (NRG1-III)	Promotes myelination in low concentrations, inhibits in higher concentrations, inhibits neurogenesis at neural crest cell stage	Progenitor, immature, myelinating, non-myelinating	[10, 30]
Oct6, POU domain class 3 transcription factor 1	Protein transcription factor, also known as POU domain, class 3, transcription factor 1	Immature	[17, 19]
P75, low-affinity nerve growth factor receptor	Stimulates neuronal cells to differentiate and survive in general	Immature, non-myelinating	[15, 19]
Peripheral myelin protein 22 kD (PMP22)	Formation of myelin and subsequent maintenance, also known as growth arrest-specific protein 3 (GAS-3)	Myelinating	[25, 31]
S100 protein	Normally present in neural crest-derived cells, cell growth and differentiation, regulation of transcription factors	Immature, myelinating, non-myelinating	[1, 22]
SRY-related HMG-box 10 (Sox10)	Cell fate determinant, transcriptional activator	Progenitor, immature, myelinating, non-myelinating	[17, 23]

Several markers facilitate characterization of the SC development stages. The calcium-binding growth-associated protein 43 (GAP43) is present at the SC progenitor stage [6]. The presence of transcription factor Sox10 plays a critical role in SC differentiation from NCCs into SC progenitor cells [1]. Mice with mutations of Sox10 have shown that while neuronal cells will still form in dorsal root ganglia, SCs will not be generated [17, 18]. Transcription factors Sox10, the zinc-finger protein Krox20, and Oct6 are found at the immature SC stage, along with S100 low molecular weight proteins and a low-affinity neurotrophin receptor P75 [15, 19]. Neuregulins (NRGs) are a family of four proteins derived from the epidermal growth factor family [20]. NRG1 isoform type III assists in the differentiation from NCCs to SC progenitor cells [21]: axons smaller than one micrometer will secrete NRG1-III at low levels to direct ensheathment, whereas axons greater than one micrometer will secrete NRG1-III at comparatively higher levels, which will assist in the direction of myelination. Once the SC has reached a stage of being either myelinating or non-myelinating, it has the ability to revert back to an immature SC, if needed [1]. Non-myelinating SCs will express S100 [22], Sox10 [23], and P75 [15] markers. Myelinating SCs will express S100 [1], Sox10 [17], and Krox20 [24] as well as myelination-specific markers, including peripheral myelin protein 22 kD (PMP22) [25], myelin protein zero (P0) [26], myelin basic protein (MBP) [27], and myelin-associated glycoprotein (MAG) [28].

Schwann Cell Myelination

Myelin provides the essential function of protecting nervous tissue in the peripheral nervous system, connecting organs and limbs with the brain and spinal cord of the central nervous system, as well as facilitating the saltatory conduction of action potentials [29]. The initial development of myelin is in early gnathostome precursor glial cells that myelinate axons that are later distinguished into oligodendrocytes in the CNS and Schwann cells in the PNS [29]. SCs and oligodendrocytes essentially perform a similar myelination function; however, they differ in the activation of transcriptional cascades, extrinsic signals responsible for myelination, and some cytoskeletal changes that guide the wrapping of glial membranes throughout the axon [29].

Myelinating SCs are radially and longitudinally polarized cells that arrange themselves into specific membrane domains with a unique set of proteins and a collection of cytoplasmic compartments for communication. Axon and myelinating SCs are organized into nodal, paranodal, juxtaparanodal and internodal compartments through longitudinal polarity [32]. Radial polarity distinguishes inner (adaxonal) and outer (abaxonal) membrane surfaces. The periaxonal space (approximately 15 nm) between adaxonal and abaxonal membranes is flush with adhesion molecules, such as pals1, which regulates the extension of the myelin sheath in the PNS [33], and receptors [34]. Adhesion molecules present along the internode consist of myelin-associated glycoprotein (MAG) and nectin-like proteins such as Necl-2 (CADM1) [35] and Necl-4 (CADM4) [36]. The abaxomal membrane interacts with laminin in the basal lamina where integrins α6β1, α6β4, and 4dystroglycan are expressed and upregulated with myelination [37, 38]. Between the abaxonal membrane and outer wrap of the compact myelin sheath lie periodic appositions rich in dystroglycan complex comprised of dystrophin-related protein 2 (Drp2) and periaxin, which are abundant scaffolding proteins in myelinating SCs [39, 40]. A network displayed by cytoplasmic channels and anatomoses called Cajal bands contain a huge array of cytoskeletal proteins such as microtubules, intermediate filaments, actin, and spectrin complexes [41, 42].

The specific myelination process in the PNS begins with a 1:1 association of SCs with axons to be myelinated, triggered by a molecular signal from the axon, which results in SC linking with the axon [43]. The SCs wrap around one end of the axon, with one end of the SC membrane slipping under the other as it continues to encircle the axon, progressing as multiple concentric membrane lamellae form around ten layers, which will compact and form the myelin sheath [23]. Myelin supplies a high-resistance and low-capacitance sheath, crucial for the impulse propagation by saltatory conduction, and alone consists of more than 40 lamellae [44]. Myelin is rich in lipid content, which is about 70% of the membrane, and also contains an abundance of glycosphingolipids, saturated long-chain fatty acids cholesterol, which plays an important role in the assembly of the myelin sheath [45].

Initially, myelin forms loose wraps of a non-compact membrane, and with the initiation of myelin transcription, the myelin proteins are upregulated [29]. The main components of compact myelin are myelin basic protein, peripheral myelin protein 22 kD, and myelin protein zero (P0) [6]. P0 is the most plentiful protein in PNS myelin, comprised of tetramers that interact in trans and cis, holding the shape of the extracellular space between intraperiod lines of compact myelin. MS-based quantification shows that P0 comprises 21% of myelin proteins, followed by periaxin at 16%, MBP at 8%, and fatty acid synthase at 1% [46]. The electrostatic interaction of MBP with a phospholipic bilayer mediates the tight apposition of cytoplasmic leaflets via interaction with the P0 cytoplasmic tail [29].

Table 2. Molecules related to myelination

Molecule	Function	Reference
Dystrophin-related protein 2 (Drp2)	Abundant scaffolding protein in myelinating SCs; stabilizes and limits myelin radial growth	[40]
E-cadherin (CDH1)	Calcium-dependent cell-adhesion protein	[53]
Fatty acid synthase	Catalyzes synthesis of palmitate from acetyl-CoA and malonyl-CoA in presence of NADPH into long-chain saturated fatty acids	[54]
Galactocerebroside	Marker for myelin formation found in compact myelin	[48]
Integrins α6β1 and α6β4	Mediates laminin activity during myelination; α6β1 may favor deposition of immature basal lamina in pre-myelinating SCs, while α6β4 stabilizes mature basal lamina in myelinating SCs	[38]
Krox-20, early growth response protein 2 (EGR2)	Transcription factor, zinc-finger protein, involved in differentiation of Schwann cells	[24]
Myelin-associated glycoprotein (MAG)	Adhesion molecule that mediates interactions between myelinating cells and neurons by binding to neuronal sialic acid-containing gangliosides and to glycoproteins RTN4R and RTN4RL2; not required for initial myelination but seems to play a role in the maintenance of normal axon myelination	[55]
Myelin basic protein (MBP), P1	Major component of myelin sheath, compact myelin, plays role in both its formation and stabilization	[56]
Myelin protein zero (P0)	Holding the shape of the extracellular space between intraperiod lines of compact myelin,	[57]
Nectin-like cell adhesion molecule 4 (Necl-4)	Main protein expressed by SCs, serving as binding partner with Necl-1 on axons; disruption of this binding inhibits myelination	[36]
Neuregulin 1 type 3 (NRG1-III)	Promotes Schwann cell growth and survival, migration along extending axon, and myelination; alters expression of multiple genes including myelin lamellae constituents as well as signaling SCs to express transcription factors Oct6 and Krox-20	[21]
Nuclear factor kappa-light-chain-enhancer of activated B cells (NF-κB)	Transcription factor, essential differentiation signal, highly upregulated in pre-myelinating Schwann cells	[58]
Oct6, POU domain class 3 transcription factor 1	Transcription factor, POU domain protein, involved in differentiation of Schwann cells, regulates a set of downstream genes that includes Krox-20	[59]
Periaxin	Scaffolding protein, functions as part of a dystroglycan complex in Schwann cells, required for maintenance of peripheral myelin sheath	[39]
Peripheral myelin protein 22 kD (PMP22)	Component of compact myelin, facilitates protein-protein interactions with P0	[60]
Protein associated with lin7 1 (Pals1)	Cell polarity protein involved in regulation of PNS myelin sheath extension	[33]

Molecule	Function	Reference
Rapamycin complex 1 (mTORC1)	Promotes Schwann cell cycling and myelinogenesis	[51]
Spectrin	Cytoskeletal protein on intracellular side of plasma membrane in SCs; modulates PNS myelination, its loss reduces Necl-4, prevents myelination and remyelination activities	[41]
SRY-related HMG-box 10 (Sox10)	Transcription factor, Sry box protein, key regulator in differentiation of peripheral glial cells	[18]
Sulphatide	Found in compact myelin; assists in glial-axon interactions and neural plasticity, stimulates myelination	[61]
Vimentin	Negative regulator of PNS myelination, with loss resulting in hypermyelination, related to neuron-autonomous increase in NRG1-III	[52]

The glycolipids galactocerebroside and sulfatide are found in abundance in compact myelin, which makes up most of the myelin lamellae, with the remainder consisting of non-compact myelin containing MAG, Cx32, Cx29, claudins 1 and 5, and E-cadherin [47]. Galactocerebroside is involved in signaling myelin formation and likely has other functions [48], whereas sulfatide assists in multiple glial-axon interactions and neural plasticity, including the initiation of basement membrane formation. Sulfatide also stimulates myelination to occur via a multiple step process, beginning with the molecular binding of sulfatide to laminin or tenascin-R in the extracellular matrix [49]. This leads to the binding of integrins and F3 signaling molecules in the glial membrane. The laminin $\alpha6\beta1$-integrin will complex with focal adhesion kinase and fyn kinase, which in turn will trigger myelination signaling [50].

The axonal signal NRG1-III alters the expression of multiple genes including myelin lamellae constituents, as well as signaling SCs to express transcription factors Brn-5, Oct6, and Krox-20 [6]. Rapamycin complex 1 (mTORC1) promotes SC myelinogenesis and cycling [51]. The first PNS myelin proteome compendium resulted in 462 proteins found, not including those also present in known classes of nuclear, hair, blood, and mitochondrial proteins [46]. The interconnection between myelin sheath thickness and axon diameter provides an idea of the limiting factors of myelination. Promyelinating signaling compounds in the NRG1/erbB signaling pathway are downregulated, and negative regulators are upregulated. Through the neuron-autonomous effect of vimentin, NRG1 activity will operate towards negative regulation of the myelination process [52].

In-depth knowledge of these numerous proteins and their multiple functions in PNS myelin is lacking, thus further studies in this area have potential towards better understanding aspects of myelin-related disease and targets for novel therapeutics, the process of myelination itself, and analysis of glia-axonal interactions.

Pathological Process of Schwann Cells in Neural Injury

Axons can become damaged through mechanical injury, diseases which can cause axon demyelination, autoimmune disorders, and genetic mutations [62, 63]. This section will survey these conditions and the molecules involved as well as processes and methods for repair and remyelination. The molecules involved in these conditions are summarized in Table 3.

When a nerve sustains damage, the injury site will undergo Wallerian degeneration as a form of the innate immune response, recruiting SCs to assist in phagocytizing the damaged myelin and axonal ends, creating an environment for regeneration to occur [64]. This degenerative process takes place two to four days post injury, though SCs have been detected in the lesion within a matter of hours, such that the damaged axons may be signaling the quick recruitment of SCs to the site via an unelucidated mechanism [65]. Secretion of upregulated cytokine innate immune response factors by SCs, including LIF, MCP-1, Il-1α/1β, and TNFα, will recruit and facilitate communications with macrophages in the injured site to clear myelin and axonal debris [66].

Schwann cells will dedifferentiate into a distinct repair phenotype with an elongated bipolar morphology, migrate into the nerve gap, and proliferate, forming an endoneurial tube-bridge known as the band of Büngner, connecting the damaged end with the cell body [1]. The tubular structure formation and SC phenotype plasticity are critical, because they provide an appropriate environmental substrate for the damaged axon to regenerate. The dedifferentiation phenotype change occurs via the upregulation of immature SC characterization molecules, including GFAP, NCAM, p75NTR, and L1 [65], whereas genes associated with myelination are downregulated including P0, MBP, MAG, and Krox20 [67]. The up-regulating and secretion of nerve growth factors by SC can promote axon elongation and survival, including artemin, pleiotrophin, BDNF, GDNF, VEGE, NGF, and NT3 [68]. A study involving the axotomy of adult rat sciatic nerves found that SC also secrete F-spondin, an extracellular matrix protein, post injury [69]. Upregulation of both F-spondin protein and mRNA was found distal to the lesion site, serving to promote neurite outgrowth. The complex microenvironment of the lesion likely lacks proper guidance cues for the regrowing axons to properly migrate, and as such, SCs provide another critical role in carrying these axons along the tube-bridge, with the migratory behavior activated via upregulation of Sox2, N-cadherin, and EphB2 [67]. Here, EphB2 on SCs activates the movement of N-cadherin to SC junctions, via Sox2, creating an attractive behavior and allowing formation of migratory cords that will cross the tubular peripheral nerve bridge and connect the damaged nerve endings.

Injury to the nerve can trigger the conversion of myelin and non-myelin SCs to specialize in repair of the myelin; SCs also provide the necessary cellular signaling to promote neuronal survival, reinnervation targeting, and axonal regeneration [70]. Reprogramming begins via dedifferentiation and activation of alternative differentiations into repairing functionality via downregulation of myelin genes and upregulation of trophic factors, myelin autophagy and recruitment of macrophages, formation of regeneration tracks in the form of Büngner's bands, spindle-shaped assemblies of SCs in the act of proliferation, and elevation of cytokines as part of the innate immune response [67]. Transcriptional control of this mechanism involves the c-Jun transcription factor, which is quickly upregulated after nerve injury [2]. While this factor is unnecessary for normal SC development, its absence results in an inability to form a functional repair form of the SC. This is crucial because SCs provide biomechanical support at the level of single nerve fibers through the joint action of PMP22 and the basal lamina [2].

Post nerve injury, axons downstream of the damaged site will degenerate, otherwise known as Wallerian degeneration (WD) [71]. Levels of fibroblast growth factor 9 (FGF9) have been shown to decrease in SCs in the presence of WD, with FGF9 also inhibiting the dedifferentiation of SCs into their repair phenotype and accelerating the aggregation of macrophages in the injured area [72]. The repair process will work to repair the damaged axons and direct them towards the correct targets via migration through two environments: the area of new tissue called the bridge region, which forms to repair the damaged site, and the distal stump, which will require a remodeling step in order for axonal regrowth to occur [73].

Table 3. Molecules involved in Schwann cell pathologies and repair

Molecule	Function	Reference
c-Jun	Transcription factor involved in reprogramming of myelin and non-myelin (Remak) Schwann cells to repair cells after injury	[2]
Fibroblast growth factor 9 (FGF9)	Growth factor also known as a glia-activating factor; stimulates growth of glial cells; inhibits dedifferentiation of SCs into their repair phenotype at decreased levels	[72]
F-spondin	Extracellular matrix protein promoting neurite outgrowth of sensory neurons; likely plays a role in promoting axonal regeneration after peripheral nerve injury; is also present in peripheral nerve during embryonic development	[69]
Immunoglobulin G (IgG)	Most common antibody in human serum; in GBS patients, binds to four different PNS gangliosides (GD1a, GM1, GQ1b, and GT1a), leading to demyelination	[78]
Mitofusin 2 (MFN2)	Mediator of mitochondrial outer membrane fusion; results in larger than normal mitochondrial groups in mutations in CMT patients, impeding their movement along axons, leading to nonfunctional PNS synapses	[81]
N-acetyl-5-methoxy tryptamine (Melatonin)	Potential solution for DN via inhibition of high glucose-induced reactive oxygen species (ROS) and restoration of mitochondrial membrane potential in the PNS	[84]
Neuregulin 1 type 3 (NRG1-III)	SC growth promoter of cell survival and myelination growth, potential means of PNS remyelination with a soluble form	[23]
Peripheral myelin protein 22 kD (PMP22)	Constituent protein of compact myelin; provides biomechanical support at level of single nerve fibers, is encoded by PMP2 gene, causes HNPP if only one copy present, results in CMT 1A if three copies present	[6]
Polydimethylsiloxane (PDMS)	Biocompatible silicone-based neural scaffold material with features such as optical transparency, chemical inertness, oxygen permeability, viscoelasticity	[75]
Polylactic-co-glycolic acid (PLGA)	Copolymer neural scaffold material that is 100% biodegradable	[85]
SRY-related HMG-box 10 (Sox10)	Encoded by the Sox10 gene; genetic defects lead to non-development of SCs and satellite cells, resulting in severe motor and sensory neuron degeneration	[18]

Other demyelinating disorders include Charcot-Marie-Tooth disease (CMT), leprosy caused by *Mycobacterium leprae* infection, and neurofibromatosis type 1 and 2 tumor formation [1]. CMT is a hereditary disease caused by mutations leading to defective myelinogenesis, characterized by progressive touch sensation and motor loss across the body [80]. Mutations on chromosome 17, which usually affect the gene PMP22 and in some cases MFN2, which will lead to mitochondrial formation in larger than normal groups, will impede their movement and lead to nonfunctional synapses in the PNS [81]. If only one copy of the PMP gene is present, then hereditary neuropathy with liability to pressure palsies (HNPP) develops; if three copies of the PMP22 gene are present, then this leads to development of CMT type 1A [6]. Remyelination may be possible via the supplementation of soluble NRG1-III [23].

Defects in Sox10 can lead to the development of neuronal cells in the dorsal root ganglia; however, SCs and satellite cells will not be generated, thereby resulting in severe motor and sensory neuron degeneration [18]. Heterozygous Sox10 mutations lead to Waardenburg syndrome due to defects in the neural crest, which are also present in dysfunctions in pigmentation and the megacolon [82].

Diabetic patients often exhibit neuropathic complications; diabetic neuropathy (DN) is caused by apoptosis of SCs due to long-term exposure to oxidative stress and high glucose concentrations [83]. Treatment with melatonin may be an effective solution for DN, which has shown to inhibit high glucose-induced reactive oxygen species (ROS) generation and helped to restore the membrane potential of mitochondria in the PNS, thereby preventing SC apoptosis [84] via alterations to the Bcl-2, NF-κB, mTOR, and Wnt signaling pathways.

An interesting area of research in PNS repair is through the creation of specifically engineered scaffolds that allow for the implantation of SCs into damaged areas to facilitate axonal repair. These scaffolds provide shelter from the actions of inflammatory cytokines and oxidative stress, allowing for SCs to carry out repair and continue to secrete nerve growth factors. One material researched in scaffold fabrication is polydimethylsiloxane (PDMS), a silicone-based material with qualities that include biocompatibility, optical transparency, chemical inertness, oxygen permeability, viscoelasticity, and ease of construction [75]. Polylactic-co-glycolic acid (PLGA), a copolymer material that has been shown to safely guide nerve repair, is 100% biodegradable [85]. In addition, studies have utilized electrical stimulation in conjunction with electrically conductive scaffolds seeded with SC stem cells which have proven beneficial for axonal regeneration and neurite migration [86].

Role of Schwann Cell Migration in Neural Repair

The highly plastic Schwann cells, derived from neural crest progenitors, are the primary glial cells of the PNS and essential in the development and regeneration of PNS axons. Myelinating SCs wrap around axons of motor and sensory neurons to form the myelin sheath, a layer of insulation comprised of fatty substances and proteins that facilitate efficient, rapid transmission of electrical impulses in a step-wise process regulated by transcription factors and extracellular signaling [87]. Under polarized light, myelin exhibits a birefringence that is both protein and lipid dependent, correlating with X-ray diffraction studies of myelin with resultant electron-density plots of protein and lipid repeating units comprised of three peaks corresponding to lipid and protein polar groups, and two troughs corresponding to lipid hydrocarbon chains [88].The diameter of the axon is related directly to the amount of compacted myelin lamellae and the velocity of action potential propagation via saltatory conduction [89]. Larger sensory fibers, for example, can have upwards of 100 spirals of compact myelin lamellae.

If damage occurs to the myelin, the conductive velocity of the impulses decreases. Repairs over short distances seem to be more effective than those over long distances, which correlate with increased amounts of errors and specificity not being maintained [90]. In the PNS, SCs will migrate towards and contact an axon, forming a singular sheath of myelin; if they are stopped from associating with and guiding axons in the regeneration process, then axons are not able to reconnect by themselves, and repair will not take place. As such, the process of myelination is critical for repair of peripheral nerve damage [91]. When damage is sustained, SCs assist in the phagocytosis of the damaged axons. Once the debris has been removed from the area, SCs dedifferentiate, morphing into a repair phenotype, proliferating and forming an endoneural tube-like structure known as the band of Büngner [87]. Differentiation of SCs to a myelinating type is inducible *in vitro* via the addition of dibutyryl cAMP (db-cAMP), expressing transcription factors Krox-20 and Oct-6, and myelin sheath proteins MBP, P0, PMP22, and periaxin [92]. This process thus provides a protective and conducive habitat for the regeneration of the damaged axons.

In addition to the application of myelin, regenerative SCs secrete various neurotrophic and synaptogenic factors that facilitate the formation and repair of chemical synapses, including fibroblast growth factor, nerve growth factor, brain-derived neurotrophic factor, and transforming growth factor-β1 [91, 93]. In a study of synapses of the neuromuscular junction, Xenopus nerve-muscle cocultures treated with SC-conditioned medium for four days exhibited acetylcholine receptor clusters in nerve-muscle contacts visualized via Alexa Fluor 594 α-BTX staining that doubled in size compared with controls [93]. Activation of Raf kinase signaling has been found to inhibit SC differentiation

[92]. Here, an *in vitro* culture of primary SCs infected via retrovirus to encode the inducible Raf fusion protein (NSΔRafER) was treated with tamoxifen for 48 hours to activate Raf signaling. The resultant cells had a refractile, elongated morphology like Raf-transformed cells, yet no induction of differentiation markers. In comparison, treatment of these cells with db-cAMP resulted in a strong induction of periaxin, MBP, P0, and PMP22. SCs were also differentiated with the application of db-cAMP for three days, followed by treatment with tamoxifen for 48 hours, resulting in the switching off of markers for SC differentiation determined via western blotting, thus showing that the signaling ability of Raf can both inhibit and reverse SC differentiation. An *in vivo* Sprague-Dawley (SD) rat model study investigated the SC migratory effects on sciatic nerve crush injury combined with treatments of cytochalasin D, an actin polymerization inhibitor [94]. After the sciatic nerve crush, rats were injected with 6 μl of cytochalasin D at a concentration of either 400 nM or 1000 nM, with subsequent tissue sampling and immunohistochemistry staining at three and five days. The data showed that the SC migratory distance was significantly less at the 1000 nM concentration, while at the 400 nM concentration, the migration was equal to the controls. Similarly, the measured length of regenerated nerve fibers was shorted in the 1000 nM treatment group. Electrophysiological parameters were assessed at four weeks post injury with compound muscle action potential (CMAP) recording. A significantly lower cAMP amplitude was observed for the 1000 nM treatment group, with the 400 nM treatment near control levels. Inhibition of the actin cytoskeleton in this study provides data indicating that delaying SC migration hinders the rate of peripheral nerve regeneration.

Molecular Regulation of Schwann Cell Motility in Neural Repair

In order for Schwann cells to effectively regenerate neural damage, movement towards the injury site is critical [65]. To myelinate axons along their entire longitudinal axis, matching numbers of SCs to axons must migrate long distances from nerve roots to the site of ensheathment [95]. The capability and quality of SC motility is therefore an essential aspect for axonal repair, for without their physical presence remyelination will not occur, and the damage remains as is. Furthermore, following spinal cord injury, endogenous SCs are able to penetrate, via an unknown molecular mechanism of migration, into the spinal cord tissues, appearing to provide damaged axons a substrate for remyelination [96]. As such, a significant number of studies have been carried out in order to determine, at the molecular level, which molecules are the determinants of motility and migration. Herein, twelve such molecules will be discussed that have experimentally demonstrated a modulation effect on these properties.

Betacellulin (BTC) is a protein that is part of the family of epidermal growth factors, functioning as a ligand for the epidermal growth factor receptor [97]. An *in vitro* study determined, via enzyme-linked immunosorbent assay (ELISA), that BTC is secreted by SCs and acts as a regenerative neurotrophic factor; transfecting against BTC resulted in a decreased rate of SC migration, determined by the transwell migration assay [98]. After a forceps-induced sciatic nerve crush injury in an SD rat model study, the exogenous application of BTC itself was found to increase SC migration. Additionally, neurites grew longer in SCs compared with non-BTC-expressing SCs.

Ephrin receptors mediate many developmental processes, especially in the nervous system. B class ephrin receptors (EphB) are transmembrane proteins [99]. An SD rat model study investigating the effects of EphB signaling on SC behavior after left sciatic nerve hemi-transection and injection of control or inhibitor proteins with a mini-osmotic pump found changes in motility by modulation of the actin cytoskeleton via the transcription factor Sox2 [100]. The Sox2-dependent EphB2 variant demonstrated migratory sorting of SCs, which is mediated through the redistribution of N-cadherin to cell-to-cell junctions, believed to hold potential for promoting neural regeneration through the maintenance of SC migration in groups. Lack of the EphB2 variant decreased this organized migration, leading to misdirected axonal growth *in vivo*.

Sox2, also known as SRY (sex-determining region Y)-box 2, belongs to the Sox family of transcription factors and plays an essential role in the maintenance of neural stem cells [101]. Through the use of rat RSC96 SCs in culture, a line of spontaneously transformed immortal cells, Sox2 itself was found to control the expression of fibronectin fibrillogenesis [102]. The fibronectin binding site was located 200 nucleotides upstream from the transcription starting site in the rat fn1, with the use of the MatInspector software. Chromatin immunoprecipitation assays located an enrichment of Sox2 at this location. This fn1 promoter binding site was found to be conserved in several species, including humans. Through the upregulation of genes responsible for the formation of focal adhesions and migration, the

Sox2-dependent fibronectin matrix mediates the axonal-oriented growth of neurons. Comparatively, the knockout loss of fibronectin in SCs impaired their ability to migrate directionally *in vitro*.

The family of fibroblast growth factor (FGF) polypeptides plays a key role in promoting tissue repair [103]. In a study of two-month-old C57BL/6 mice, post right sciatic nerve transection injury, FGF5 was found to be upregulated in SCs [104]. FGF receptors 1/2 were highly expressed in SCs both before and after injury. As part of the same study, day three SD rat SCs were harvested and cultured, and treated with 10 ng/ml of FGF5, with treatment wells lysed for analysis after 0, 5, 10, 20, 30, and 60 minutes post FGF5 application. With no resultant activation of ERK1/2 after any of these time points, another time point of 120 minutes was tested, finally showing rapid SC migration, demonstrating that FGF5 inhibits ERK1/2 MAP kinase activity while promoting an increased migratory and adhesion in SCs through upregulation of N-cadherin.

Hyaluronic acid (HA) receptors cluster of differentiation 44 (CD44) and CD168, also known as hyaluronan-mediated motility receptor (RHAMM) have been established as both playing a role in cell motility in various cell types [105]. A study using SC-like cells derived from adipose-derived mesenchymal stem cells (dAD-MSCs) confirmed that RHAMM is highly expressed via flow cytometry [106]. Fat tissue surrounding the stomach and intestines was harvested from male SD rats and cultured in glial differentiation medium to attain a SC-like phenotype. Furthermore, antibody-blocking of RHAMM in a scratch wound assay followed by 24 h monitoring of cell motility from the edge to the center of the scratch via a Leica AS MDW live cell imaging system completely immobilized the SC-like cells, whereas blocking of only CD44 caused a decrease in motility. These data suggest that both RHAMM and CD44 may share some similar means of controlling motility.

One unique *in vitro* migration SD rat model study looked at identifying elements produced by astrocytes of the CNS that may inhibit SC migration, as they considered the possibilities of transplanting SCs into the CNS for neural regenerative purposes [107]. SCs were harvested from days 1–3 SD rat sciatic nerves and mixed with astrocytes or aggrecan knockdown astrocytes, with a migration assay performed on inverted coverslips. After treatment conditions of 24 h and 48 h, the cells were stained and fixed with 4% paraformaldehyde, and their travel distance was measured. Here, data showed that aggrecans produced by astrocytes inhibited migration via disruption of SC integrin function. SC migration was improved through aggrecan knockdown.

Developing haptotactic strategies for SC migration can assist in understanding the driving forces for facilitating the movement into injured nerve site. An SD rat model study utilized a series of tethered laminin-derived peptides aligned in a gradient on microscope glass coverslips, as a substrate for assessing SC migration [108]. Peptides of interest for this study were synthesized with Fmoc solid-phase chemistry, with gradients of peptides created using vacuum-away confined channel deposition. SCs were obtained from adult female SD rat sciatic nerves, whereas rat fibroblasts were purchased and cultured until passage 3. A cell front migration assay was performed, taking an image every 15 m for 24 h using a time-lapse phase-contrast microscope, with image analysis performed by ImageJ. The YIGSR (Cys-Tyr-Ile-Gly-Ser-Arg) sequence demonstrated a higher SC velocity and a concentration-dependent directional movement, whereas the fibroblasts migrated in random directions. Utilizing materials coated with such peptide sequences may hold promise as a means of facilitating SC migration into an injury site.

The leukemia inhibitory factor (LIF) is a pleiotropic cytokine that stimulates neuronal development and survival [109]. An SD rat study showed that the LIF protein is highly expressed in SCs post-sciatic nerve injury [110]. Adult male SD rats weighing 180–220 g were inflicted with sciatic nerve crush injuries. Segments of these nerves were then collected, as well as segments from uninjured rats at days 1, 4, 7, and 14 after injury. A transwell migration assay was performed, incubating the SCs for 24 h to allow for migration from the upper well to the lower well, and imaged with a Leica Microsystems imager. Decreasing the LIF increased the proliferation and migration rate of SCs, while increasing the LIF decreased both. In a separate assay, a group of adult SD rats were subjected to the same sciatic nerve crush injury. The direct *in vivo* application of 5 μl LILF-siRNA on this peripheral nerve injury, followed by SC samples taken at days 1, 4, and 7 after injury, stained and analyzed with ImageJ, resulted in increased SC proliferation and migration velocity to this area, with data showing higher levels of myelin and the amount of lipid debris removed from the site.

Through the development of high-throughput analytical techniques, long noncoding RNAs (lncRNAs) have been recognized for taking part in diverse biological processes and diseases [111]. Using microarray analysis, long non-coding RNA (lncRNA) BC088259 was investigated to determine its potential role in nerve regeneration [112]. In this adult male SD rat post sciatic nerve crush injury model study, lncRNA BC088259 was found to be upregulated as a result of microarray analysis of RNA samples taken from SCs treated with

BC088259-specific siRNAs, with subsequent KEGG pathway analysis performed on significantly different expressed genes (FC > 2). Silencing this lncRNA inhibited SC migration, whereas overexpression of BC088259 increased the rate of migration. Additionally, the direct *in vivo* injection of lncRNA BC088259 into a transected rat sciatic nerve injury with a 5 mm gap filled with a silicon conduit, and Cy5-BC088259 siRNA or Cy5-siRNA control, and harvested for immunostaining four days post injury also demonstrated a higher SC migratory rate with the Cy5-BC088259 treatment, suggesting the modulating capability of this lncRNA on SC migration and axon repair.

An adult male SD rat study showed that matrix metalloproteinase 7 (MMP-7), an SC-secreted proteolytic enzyme, is upregulated in sciatic nerve tissue post injury [113]. These rats were subjected to a forceps-based sciatic nerve crush injury, with nerve tissue samples taken from groups at days 1, 4, 7, and 14 post injury. RNA from the samples was extracted with Trizol, and transcriptome analysis was performed on an Illumina Hiseq 2000 system. Downstream bioinformatic analysis was performed with Online Ingenuity pathway analysis software, providing the data on MMP-7 upregulation. In a separate study by the same group, the presence of MMP-7 showed a higher migration and myelination rate in SCs harvested from neonatal SD rats in a nerve crush model [114]. The cells were analyzed for motility ability in a transwell migration assay, with groups stained with 0.1% crystal violet and imaged with a Leica Microsystems DMR inverted microscope at 12 h and 24 h of culturing. In contrast, SCs transfected against MMP-7 showed a decrease in migration rate but no effect in their proliferation.

Tau is a critical protein for the stability and assembly of the microtubule, as well as the functional maintenance of the nervous system. Tau is abundant in astrocytes, oligodendrocytes, and neurons [115]. An SD rat model study investigated the presence of tau and its encoding gene MAPT in SCs [116]. Primary SCs were cultured, with RT-PCR performed to determine if MAPT, the mRNA for tau, was present. Data confirmed the presence of tau in SCs and showed a significantly higher Ct value for MAPT in comparison with the GAPDH control; via gene silencing of MAPT, SCs demonstrated an increased level of proliferation and differentiation, while decreasing migration. MAPT-knockout mice similarly showed higher proliferation of SCs and reduced migration, with nerve tissue samples taken four days post injury for immunofluorescence labeling with the anti-S100β antibody. The relative intensity of S100β fluorescence was significantly less in MAPT-knockout mice in comparison with the wild type. In a similar *in vivo* adult SD rat nerve crush injury model study, direct application of MAPT siRNA resulted in decreased SC migration post injury, with nerve stump samples taken four days post injury and analyzed via the same immunofluorescence labeling method with anti-S100β.

Last, the effects of transforming growth factor β1 (TGF-β1) on SC migration has not yet been fully understood. In an adult rat SC RSC96 *in vitro* wound-healing assay, application of TGF-β1 resulted in an increase in SC migration and invasion into the damaged tissue [117]. Here, RSC96 cells were purchased from ATCC, seeded in 12-well plates, and cultured until confluent, with subsequent scraping of a 500 μm diameter line with a 20 μl pipette tip in each well. This higher rate of migration was found to be blockable via inhibition of matrix metalloproteinase 2/9 (MMP-2/9), either by transfection with an siRNA sequence specific for MMP-2/9 or via pretreatment with MMPi, an inhibitor of MMP-2/9. Another study applied various concentrations of TGF- β1 to SCs *in vitro*, with samples analyzed at time points of 0, 10, 15, 30, and 60 m post treatment. Analysis was performed with western blotting using anti-MMP-2/9 antibodies. Data demonstrated that TGF-β1 increased the levels of MMP-2/9 mRNA and proteins in a time- and concentration-dependent manner, with a maximum level of MMP-2/9 reached at 10 ng/ml of TGF- β1. In particular, MMP-2 expression was reduced post injury but was still present during neural repair, suggesting a role in facilitating axon elongation. MMP-9 promotes SC migration, myelination, and differentiation [118]. As a result, the data suggests that TGF-β1 plays a role in the stimulation of SCs via MMP-2/9, towards effecting the repair of neural injury.

Schwann cells originate in the neural crest, migrating extensively and associating with developing axons along their entire length prior to myelination. Aside from nerve development, the motility and migratory activity of SCs is also an important aspect of remyelination after nerve injury. SCs play a crucial role in the internal repair of peripheral axons by virtue of their ability to dedifferentiate and proliferate as a repair phenotype, migrate extensively, express appropriate growth factors, and conduct activities of remyelination to effectively repair damaged axons. Thus, the motile character of SCs and their ability to migrate across vast distances is a paramount facet of neural regeneration. Working towards an understanding of the molecules and mechanisms involved in the processes of SC motility, myelin pathogenesis, and diseases of the PNS has important implications for improving treatments for nerve and tissue regeneration. Future studies analyzing the SC repair phenotype can lead to the development of novel pharmacological tools that could improve the signaling properties of transcription factors such as c-Jun. Additional work should be directed to PNS neuropathies connected to SCs and PMP22, especially regarding their biomechanical properties, to advance the treatment strategies for PNS injuries. Further proteomic analysis of PNS myelin can deepen the understanding of the myelination process and myelin-related pathogenesis. Electrically stimulated SC scaffolds have potential as a role in facilitating axonal regeneration. Motility and migration of SCs are critical to affect neural repair. Focusing future studies on molecules, such as BTC, FGF5, and MMP-7, which have shown increasing effects on migration rates, may prove useful in optimizing treatments for neural regeneration.

Table 4. Molecules affecting Schwann cell motility and migration

Molecule	Model	Result	Reference
Betacellulin (BTC)	Sprague-Dawley (SD) rat	Secreted by SCs; transfection against BTC impeded SC migration while application of exogenous BTC increased it, neurites grew longer in length versus non-BTC SCs	[98]
Ephrin receptor B (EphB)	SD rat	EphB signaling elicits changes in SC behavior via modulation of transcription factor Sox2; Sox2-dependent, EphB2-mediated SC sorting induced via redistribution of N-cadherin to cell-to-cell junctions, likely to promote regeneration through maintaining migration of SCs in groups	[100]
Fibroblast growth factor 5 (FGF5)	SD rat and C57BL/6 mouse	Highly upregulated in SCs of mouse distal sciatic nerve; in rats, inhibits ERK1/2 activation and increases SC migration and adhesion	[104]
Hyaluronan-mediated motility receptor (RHAMM)	SC-like cells derived from adipose-derived mesenchymal stem cells (dAD-MSCs)	Upregulated upon differentiation of progenitor cells to dAD-MSCs; antibody blocking of CD168 effectively immobilized dAD-MSCs	[106]
Integrin	SD rat	Aggrecans produced by astrocytes inhibit SC motility, via disrupting SC integrin function; can be reversed by activating integrins with manganese	[107]

Table 4. (Continued)

Molecule	Model	Result	Reference
Laminin-derived peptides	SD rat	Concentration gradients demonstrated increased haptotactic response, with SCs traveling with higher velocity	[108]
Leukemia inhibitory factor (LIF)	SD rat	Upregulated post nerve injury and expressed by SCs; application of LIF-siRNA to peripheral nerve injury accelerated SC migration and proliferation, contributing to increased levels of lipid debris removal and myelin formation	[110]
Long non-coding RNA (LncRNA) BC088259	SD rat	Silencing LncRNA BC088259 inhibited SC migration, whereas overexpression increased it, suggesting its ability to modulate SC migration as well as axon regeneration	[112]
Matrix metalloproteinase 7 (MMP-7)	SD rat	Promotes SC migration and formation of myelin post treatment but no effect on SC proliferation	[114]
Sox2	Rat RSC96 Schwann cells	Controls expression of fibronectin fibrillogenesis in RSC96 SCs, mediating their axonal-oriented growth via upregulation of migration genes and formation of focal adhesions	[102]
Tau protein	SD rat	Is expressed in SC and contributes to SC phenotype modulation; silencing MAPT gene encoding Tau increases SC proliferation and decreases migration and differentiation	[116]
Transforming growth factor β1 (TGF-β1)	Rat RSC96 Schwann cells	Stimulates SC migration, whereas this enhanced migration blocked via inhibition of MMP2/9	[117]

References

[1] Bhatheja, K. and J. Field, Schwann cells: Origins and role in axonal maintenance and regeneration. *The International Journal of Biochemistry & Cell Biology,* 2006. 38(12): p. 1995-1999.

[2] Rosso, G., P. Young, and V. Shahin, Implications of Schwann Cells Biomechanics and Mechanosensitivity for Peripheral Nervous System Physiology and Pathophysiology. *Frontiers in Molecular Neuroscience,* 2017. 10: p. 345.

[3] Hsieh, S. T., Kidd, G. J., Crawford, T. O., Xu, Z., Lin, W. M., Trapp, B. D., Cleveland, D. W., Griffin, J. W., Regional modulation of neurofilament organization by myelination in normal axons. *The Journal of Neuroscience,* 1994. 14(11): p. 6392.

[4] Poliak, S. and E. Peles, The local differentiation of myelinated axons at nodes of Ranvier. *Nature Reviews Neuroscience,* 2003. 4(12): p. 968-980.

[5] Kuhn, S., Gritti, L, Crooks, D., Dombrowski, Y., Oligodendrocytes in Development, Myelin Generation and Beyond. *Cells,* 2019. 8(11): p. 1424.

[6] Armati, P., *The Biology of Schwann Cells: Development, Differentiation and Immunomodulation.* 2007, Cambridge: Cambridge University Press.

[7] Jacobs, J. M. and S. Love, Qualitative and Quantitative Morphology of Human Sural Nerve at Different Ages. *Brain,* 1985. 108(4): p. 897-924.

[8] Le Douarin, N. M., Cell line segregation during peripheral nervous system ontogeny. *Science,* 1986. 231(4745): p. 1515.

[9] Jessen, K. R. and R. Mirsky, The origin and development of glial cells in peripheral nerves. *Nature Reviews Neuroscience,* 2005. 6(9): p. 671-682.

[10] Monk, K. R., M. L. Feltri, and C. Taveggia, New insights on Schwann cell development. *Glia,* 2015. 63(8): p. 1376-1393.

[11] Maro, G. S., Vermeren, M., Voiculescu O., Melton, L., Cohen, J., Charnay, P., Topilko, P., Neural crest boundary cap cells constitute a source of neuronal and glial cells of the PNS. *Nature Neuroscience*, 2004. 7(9): p. 930-938.

[12] Bronner, M. E. and M. Simões-Costa, The Neural Crest Migrating into the Twenty-First Century. *Current topics in developmental biology,* 2016. 116: p. 115-134.

[13] Jessen, K. R., Brennan, A., Morgan, L., Mirsky, R., Kent, A., Hashimoto, Y., Gavrilovic J., The schwann cell precursor and its fate: A study of cell death and differentiation during gliogenesis in rat embryonic nerves. *Neuron,* 1994. 12(3): p. 509-527.

[14] Le Douarin, N. M. and M. A. M. Teillet, Experimental analysis of the migration and differentiation of neuroblasts of the autonomic nervous system and of neurectodermal mesenchymal derivatives, using a biological cell marking technique. *Developmental Biology,* 1974. 41(1): p. 162-184.

[15] Woodhoo, A. and L. Sommer, Development of the Schwann cell lineage: From the neural crest to the myelinated nerve. *Glia,* 2008. 56(14): p. 1481-1490.

[16] Stolt, C. C. and M. Wegner, Schwann cells and their transcriptional network: Evolution of key regulators of peripheral myelination. *Brain Research,* 2016. 1641: p. 101-110.

[17] Yao, L. and P. Priyadarshani, Application of Schwann Cells in Neural Tissue Engineering, in *Glial Cell Engineering in Neural Regeneration,* L. Yao, Editor. 2018, Springer International Publishing: Cham. p. 37-57.

[18] Britsch, S., Goerich, D. E., Riethmacher, D., Peirano, R. I., Rossner, M., Nave, K. A., Birchmeier, C., Wegner, M., The transcription factor Sox10 is a key regulator of peripheral glial development. *Genes & development,* 2001. 15(1): p. 66-78.

[19] Jessen, K. R. and R. Mirsky, Schwann cells and their precursors emerge as major regulators of nerve development. *Trends in Neurosciences,* 1999. 22(9): p. 402-410.

[20] Geissler, A., S. Ryzhov, and D. B. Sawyer, Neuregulins: protective and reparative growth factors in multiple forms of cardiovascular disease. *Clinical science* (London, England : 1979), 2020. 134(19): p. 2623-2643.

[21] Birchmeier, C. and K. A. Nave, Neuregulin-1, a key axonal signal that drives Schwann cell growth and differentiation. *Glia,* 2008. 56(14): p. 1491-7.

[22] Marenholz, I., C. W. Heizmann, and G. Fritz, S100 proteins in mouse and man: from evolution to function and pathology (including an update of the nomenclature). *Biochemical and Biophysical Research Communications,* 2004. 322(4): p. 1111-1122.

[23] Syed, N. and H. A. Kim, Soluble Neuregulin and Schwann Cell Myelination: a Therapeutic Potential for Improving Remyelination of Adult Axons. *Mol Cell Pharmacol,* 2010. 2(4): p. 161-167.

[24] Topilko, P., Schneider-Maunoury, S., Levi, G., Baron-Van Evercooren, A., Chennoufi, A. B., Seitanidou, T., Babinet, C., and Charnay, P., Krox-20 controls myelination in the peripheral nervous system. *Nature,* 1994. 371(6500): p. 796-799.

[25] Sango, K. and J. Yamauchi, *Schwann Cell Development and Pathology*. 2014 ed. 2014, Tokyo: Springer Verlag.

[26] Lemke, G., E. Lamar, and J. Patterson, Isolation and analysis of the gene encoding peripheral myelin protein zero. *Neuron,* 1988. 1(1): p. 73-83.

[27] Lutz, D., Kataria, H., Kleene, R., Loers, G., Chaudhary, H., Guseva D., Wu, B., Jakovcevski, I., Schachner M., Myelin Basic Protein Cleaves Cell Adhesion Molecule L1 and Improves Regeneration After Injury. *Molecular Neurobiology,* 2016. 53(5): p. 3360-3376.

[28] Chaudhry, N., Bachelin, C., Zujovic, V., Hilaire, M., Baldwin, K. T., Follis, R. M., Giger, R., Carter, B. D., Baron-Van Evercooren, A., Filbin, M., Myelin-Associated Glycoprotein Inhibits Schwann Cell Migration and Induces Their Death. *The Journal of neuroscience: the official journal of the Society for Neuroscience,* 2017. 37(24): p. 5885-5899.

[29] Salzer, J. L., *Schwann Cell Myelination.* Cold Spring Harbor Perspectives in Biology, 2015. 7(8).

[30] Huang, L. L., Liu, Z-Y., Huang, J-H., Luo, Z-J., Expression pattern of neuregulin-1 type III during the development of the peripheral nervous system. *Neural Regen Res,* 2015. 10(1): p. 65-70.

[31] Mittendorf, K. F., Marinko, J. T., Hampton, C. M., Ke, Z., Hadziselimovic, A., Schlebach, J. P., Law, C. L., Li, J., Wright, E. R., Sanders, C. R., Peripheral myelin protein 22 alters membrane architecture. *Science advances,* 2017. 3(7): p. e1700220-e1700220.

[32] Salzer, J. L., Polarized Domains of Myelinated Axons. *Neuron,* 2003. 40(2): p. 297-318.

[33] Ozçelik, M., Cotter, L., Jacob, C., Pereira, J. A., Relvas, J. B., Suter, U., Tricaud, N., Pals1 is a major regulator of the epithelial-like polarization and the extension of the myelin sheath in peripheral nerves. *The Journal of neuroscience: the official journal of the Society for Neuroscience,* 2010. 30(11): p. 4120-4131.

[34] Pereira, J. A., F. Lebrun-Julien, and U. Suter, Molecular mechanisms regulating myelination in the peripheral nervous system. *Trends in Neurosciences,* 2012. 35(2): p. 123-134.

[35] Maurel, P., Einheber, S., Galinska, J., Thaker, P., Lam, I., Rubin, M. B., Scherer, S. S., Murakami, Y., Gutmann, D. H. and Salzer, J. L., Nectin-like proteins mediate axon Schwann cell interactions along the internode and are essential for myelination. *The Journal of cell biology,* 2007. 178(5): p. 861-874.

[36] Spiegel, I., Adamsky, K., Eshed, Y., Milo, R., Sabanay, H., Sarig-Nadir, O., Horresh, I., Scherer, S. S., Rasband, M. N., Peles, E., A central role for Necl4 (SynCAM4) in Schwann cell-axon interaction and myelination. *Nature neuroscience,* 2007. 10(7): p. 861-869.

[37] Einheber, S., M. A. Bhat, and J. L. Salzer, Disrupted axo-glial junctions result in accumulation of abnormal mitochondria at nodes of ranvier. *Neuron glia biology,* 2006. 2(3): p. 165-174.

[38] Previtali, S. C., Nodari, A., Taveggia, C., Pardini, C., Dina, G., Villa, A., Wrabetz, L., Quattrini, A., and Feltri, M. L., Expression of laminin receptors in schwann cell differentiation: evidence for distinct roles. *The Journal of neuroscience : the official journal of the Society for Neuroscience,* 2003. 23(13): p. 5520-5530.

[39] Boerkoel, C. F., Takashima, H., Stankiewicz, P., Garcia, C. A., Leber, S. M., Rhee-Morris, L., and Lupski, J. R., Periaxin Mutations Cause Recessive Dejerine-Sottas Neuropathy. *American Journal of Human Genetics,* 2001. 68(2): 325-333.

[40] Sherman, D. L., Wu, L. M. N., Grove, M., Gillespie, C. S., and Brophy, P. J., Drp2 and Periaxin Form Cajal Bands with Dystroglycan But Have Distinct Roles in Schwann Cell Growth. *The Journal of Neuroscience,* 2012. 32(27): p. 9419.

[41] Susuki, K., Raphael, A. R., Ogawa, Y., Stankewich, M. C., Peles, E., Talbot, W. S. and Rasband, M. N., Schwann cell spectrins modulate peripheral nerve myelination. *Proceedings of the National Academy of Sciences of the United States of America,* 2011. 108(19): p. 8009-8014.

[42] Kidd, G. J., N. Ohno, and B. D. Trapp, Chapter 5 - Biology of Schwann cells, in *Handbook of Clinical Neurology,* G. Said and C. Krarup, Editors. 2013, Elsevier. p. 55-79.

[43] Salzer, J. L. and B. Zalc, Myelination. *Current Biology,* 2016. 26(20): p. R971-R975.

[44] Peters, A., S. L. Palay, and H. Webster, The fine structure of the nervous system, Third edition, in: *Neurons and their supporting cells.* Oxford University Press (1991), 494 pages. £80.00., 0-19-506571-9. *Cell Biology International Reports,* 1992. 16: p. 2-3.

[45] Saher, G. and M. Simons, *Cholesterol and Myelin Biogenesis, in Cholesterol Binding and Cholesterol Transport Proteins: Structure and Function in Health and Disease*, J. R. Harris, Editor. 2010, Springer Netherlands: Dordrecht. p. 489-508.

[46] Patzig, J., Jahn, O., Tenzer, S., Wichert, S. P., de Monasterio-Schrader, P., Rosfa, S., Kuharev, J., Yan, K., Bormuth, I., Bremer, J., Aguzzi, A., Orfaniotou, F., Hesse, D., Schwab, M. H., Möbius, W., Nave, K-A. and Werner, H. B., Quantitative and integrative proteome analysis of peripheral nerve myelin identifies novel myelin

proteins and candidate neuropathy loci. *The Journal of neuroscience: the official journal of the Society for Neuroscience,* 2011. 31(45): p. 16369-16386.

[47] Scherer, S. S. and E. J. Arroyo, Recent progress on the molecular organization of myelinated axons. *Journal of the Peripheral Nervous System,* 2002. 7(1): p. 1-12.

[48] Jessen, K. R., Morgan, L., Brammer, M. and Mirsky, R., Galactocerebroside is expressed by non-myelin-forming Schwann cells in situ. *The Journal of cell biology,* 1985. 101(3): p. 1135-1143.

[49] Roberts, D. D., Rao, C. N., Magnani, J. L., Spitalnik, S. L., Liotta, L. A. and Ginsburg, V., Laminin binds specifically to sulfated glycolipids. *Proceedings of the National Academy of Sciences of the United States of America,* 1985. 82(5): p. 1306-1310.

[50] Eckhardt, M., The Role and Metabolism of Sulfatide in the Nervous System. *Molecular Neurobiology,* 2008. 37(2): p. 93-103.

[51] Beirowski, B. and K. M. Wong, mTORC1 promotes Schwann cell cycling and myelinogenesis. *Cell cycle* (Georgetown, Tex.), 2017. 16(18): p. 1637-1638.

[52] Triolo, D., Dina, G., Taveggia, C., Vaccari, I., Porrello, E., Rivellini, C., Domi, T., La Marca, R., Cerri, F., Bolino, A., Quattrini, A. and Previtali, S. C., Vimentin regulates peripheral nerve myelination. *Development,* 2012. 139(7): p. 1359-1367.

[53] Singhai, R., Patil, V. W., Jaiswal, S. R., Patil, S. D., Tayade, M. B. and Patil, A. V., E-Cadherin as a diagnostic biomarker in breast cancer. *North American journal of medical sciences,* 2011. 3(5): p. 227-233.

[54] Nisthul A., A., Retnakumari, A. P., A, Shabna, Anto, R. J. and Sadasivan, C., In silico screening for identification of fatty acid synthase inhibitors and evaluation of their antiproliferative activity using human cancer cell lines. *Journal of Receptors and Signal Transduction,* 2018. 38(4): p. 335-341.

[55] Lossos, A., Elazar, N., Lerer, I., Schueler-Furman, O., Fellig, Y., Glick, B., Zimmerman, B-E., Azulay, H., Dotan, S., Goldberg, S., Gomori, J. M., Ponger, P., Newman, J. P., Marreed, H., Steck, A. J., Schaeren-Wiemers, N., Mor, N., Harel, M., Geiger, T., Eshed-Eisenbach, Y., Meiner, V. and Peles, E., Myelin-associated glycoprotein gene mutation causes Pelizaeus-Merzbacher disease-like disorder. *Brain: a journal of neurology,* 2015. 138(Pt 9): p. 2521-2536.

[56] Nye, S. H., Pelfrey, C. M., Burkwit, J. J., Voskuhl, R. R., Lenardo, M. J. and Mueller, J. P., Purification of immunologically active recombinant 21.5 kDa isoform of human myelin basic protein. *Molecular Immunology,*V 32, 1995(14): p. 1131-1141.

[57] Lagueny, A., Latour, P., Vital, A., Rajabally, Y., Le Masson, G., Ferrer, X., Bernard, I., Julien, J., Vital, C. and Vandenberghe, A., Peripheral myelin modification in CMT1B correlates with MPZ gene mutations. *Neuromuscul Disord,* 1999. 9(6-7): p. 361-7.

[58] Nickols, J. C., Valentine, W., KAnwal, S. and Carter, B. D., Activation of the transcription factor NF-κB in Schwann cells is required for peripheral myelin formation. *Nature Neuroscience,* 2003. 6(2): p. 161-167.

[59] Jaegle, M., Ghazvini, M., Mandemakers, W., Piirsoo, M., Driegen, S., Levavasseur, F., Raghoenath, S., Grosveld, F. and Meijer, D., The POU proteins Brn-2 and Oct-

6 share important functions in Schwann cell development. *Genes & Development,* 2003.

[60] D'Urso, D., P. Ehrhardt, and H. W. Muller, Peripheral myelin protein 22 and protein zero: a novel association in peripheral nervous system myelin. *J Neurosci,* 1999. 19(9): p. 3396-403.

[61] Xiao, S., C. V. Finkielstein, and D. G. Capelluto, The enigmatic role of sulfatides: new insights into cellular functions and mechanisms of protein recognition. *Adv Exp Med Biol,* 2013. 991: p. 27-40.

[62] Kira, J. I., R. Yamasaki, and H. Ogata, Anti-neurofascin autoantibody and demyelination. *Neurochemistry International,* 2019. 130: p. 104360.

[63] Park, H. T., Kim, Y. H., Lee, K. E. and Kim, J. K., Behind the pathology of macrophage-associated demyelination in inflammatory neuropathies: demyelinating Schwann cells. *Cellular and molecular life sciences: CMLS,* 2020. 77(13): p. 2497-2506.

[64] Rotshenker, S., Wallerian degeneration: the innate-immune response to traumatic nerve injury. *Journal of neuroinflammation,* 2011. 8: p. 109-109.

[65] Jessen, K. R., R. Mirsky, and A. C. Lloyd, Schwann Cells: Development and Role in Nerve Repair. *Cold Spring Harbor perspectives in biology,* 2015. 7(7): p. a020487-a020487.

[66] Min, Q., D. B. Parkinson, and X. P. Dun, Migrating Schwann cells direct axon regeneration within the peripheral nerve bridge. *Glia,* 2021. 69(2): p. 235-254.

[67] Jessen, K. R. and R. Mirsky, The repair Schwann cell and its function in regenerating nerves. *The Journal of Physiology,* 2016. 594(13): p. 3521-3531.

[68] Brushart, T. M., Aspalter, M., Griffin, J. W., Redett, R., Hameed, H., Zhou, C., Wright, M., Vyas, A. and Höke, A., Schwann cell phenotype is regulated by axon modality and central-peripheral location, and persists in vitro. *Experimental neurology,* 2013. 247: p. 272-281.

[69] Burstyn-Cohen, T., Frumkin, A., Xu, Y. T., Scherer, S. S. and Klar, A., Accumulation of F-Spondin in Injured Peripheral Nerve Promotes the Outgrowth of Sensory Axons. *The Journal of Neuroscience,* 1998. 18(21): p. 8875.

[70] Ma, K. H., H. A. Hung, and J. Svaren, Epigenomic Regulation of Schwann Cell Reprogramming in Peripheral Nerve Injury. *The Journal of neuroscience : the official journal of the Society for Neuroscience,* 2016. 36(35): p. 9135-9147.

[71] Koliatsos, V. E. and A. S. Alexandris, Wallerian degeneration as a therapeutic target in traumatic brain injury. *Current opinion in neurology,* 2019. 32(6): p. 786-795.

[72] Lv, W., Deng, B., Duan, W., Li, Y., Song, X., Ji, Y., Li, Z., Liu, Y., Wang, X. and Li, C., FGF9 Alters The Wallerian Degeneration Process by Inhibiting Schwann Cell Transformation and Accelerating Macrophage Infiltration. *Brain Research Bulletin,* 2019.

[73] Stierli, S., V. Imperatore, and A. C. Lloyd, Schwann cell plasticity-roles in tissue homeostasis, regeneration, and disease. *Glia,* 2019. 0(0).

[74] Nocera, G. and C. Jacob, Mechanisms of Schwann cell plasticity involved in peripheral nerve repair after injury. *Cellular and molecular life sciences: CMLS,* 2020. 77(20): p. 3977-3989.

[75] Lotfi, L., Khakbiz, M., Moghaddam, M. M. and Bonakdar, S., A biomaterials approach to Schwann cell development in neural tissue engineering. *Journal of Biomedical Materials Research Part A,* 2019. 0(0).

[76] Jasti, A. K., Selmi, C., Sarmiento-Monroy, J. C., Vega, D. A., Anaya, J-M. and Gershwin, M. E., Guillain-Barré syndrome: causes, immunopathogenic mechanisms and treatment. *Expert Review of Clinical Immunology,* 2016. 12(11): p. 1175-1189.

[77] Dimachkie, M. M. and R. J. Barohn, Guillain-Barré syndrome and variants. *Neurologic clinics,* 2013. 31(2): p. 491-510.

[78] Yuki, N. and H. P. Hartung, Guillain–Barré Syndrome. *New England Journal of Medicine,* 2012. 366(24): p. 2294-2304.

[79] Scheidl, E., Diez Canseco, D., Hadji-Naumov, A. and Bereznai, B., Guillain-Barré syndrome during SARS-CoV-2 pandemic: A case report and review of recent literature. *Journal of the peripheral nervous system: JPNS,* 2020. 25(2): p. 204-207.

[80] Barreto, L. C. L. S., Santos Oliveira, F., Santos Nunes, P., Pinheiro de França Costa, I. M., Andrade Garcez, C., Mattos Goes, G., Aquino Neves, E. L., de Souza Siqueira Quintans, J., and Antunes de Souza Araújo, A., Epidemiologic Study of Charcot-Marie-Tooth Disease: A Systematic Review. *Neuroepidemiology,* 2016. 46(3): p. 157-165.

[81] Baloh, R. H., Schmidt, R. E., Pestronk, A. and Milbrandt, J., Altered Axonal Mitochondrial Transport in the Pathogenesis of Charcot-Marie-Tooth Disease from Mitofusin 2 Mutations. *The Journal of Neuroscience,* 2007. 27(2): p. 422.

[82] Southard-Smith, E. M., Angrist, M., Ellison, J. S., Agarwala, R., Baxevanis, A. D., Chakravarti, A. and Pavan, W. J., The Sox10Dom Mouse: Modeling the Genetic Variation of Waardenburg-Shah (WS4) Syndrome. *Genome Research,* 1999. 9(3): p. 215-225.

[83] Feldman, E. L., Callaghan, B. C., Pop-Busui, R., Zochodne, D. W., Wright, D. E., Bennett, D. L., Bril, V., Russell, J. W. and Viswanathan V., Diabetic neuropathy. *Nature reviews. Disease primers,* 2019. 5(1): p. 42-42.

[84] Tiong, L. Y., Ng, K. Y., Koh, R. Y., Ponnudurai, G. and Chye, S. M., Melatonin Prevents Oxidative Stress-Induced Mitochondrial Dysfunction and Apoptosis in High Glucose-Treated Schwann Cells via Upregulation of Bcl2, NF-κB, mTOR, Wnt Signalling Pathways. *Antioxidants,* 2019. 8(7).

[85] Hadlock, T., Sundback, C., Hunter, D., Cheney, M. and Vacanti, J. P., A Polymer Foam Conduit Seeded with Schwann Cells Promotes Guided Peripheral Nerve Regeneration. *Tissue Engineering,* 2000. 6(2): p. 119-127.

[86] Moskow, J., Ferrigno, B., Mistry, N., Jaiswal, D., Bulsara, K., Rudraiah, S. and Kumbar, S. G., Review: Bioengineering approach for the repair and regeneration of peripheral nerve. *Bioactive Materials,* 2019. 4(1): p. 107-113.

[87] Glenn, T. D. and W. S. Talbot, Signals regulating myelination in peripheral nerves and the Schwann cell response to injury. *Current opinion in neurobiology,* 2013. 23(6): p. 1041-1048.

[88] Morell, P. and R. H. Quarles, The Myelin Sheath. *Basic Neurochemistry: Molecular, Cellular and Medical Aspects*. 6th edition, 1999.

[89] Armati, P. J. and E. K. Mathey, An update on Schwann cell biology — Immunomodulation, neural regulation and other surprises. *Journal of the Neurological Sciences,* 2013. 333(1): p. 68-72.

[90] Carlson, N. R., *Physiology of behavior.* Ninth edition ed. 2007, Boston, MA: Pearson/A&B Allyn and Bacon.

[91] Wang, C., Lu, C-f., Peng, J., Hu, C-d. and Wang, Y., Roles of neural stem cells in the repair of peripheral nerve injury. *Neural regeneration research,* 2017. 12(12): p. 2106-2112.

[92] Harrisingh, M. C., Perez-Nadales, E., Parkinson, D. B., Malcolm, D. S., Mudge, A. W. and Lloyd, A. C., The Ras/Raf/ERK signalling pathway drives Schwann cell dedifferentiation. *The EMBO journal,* 2004. 23(15): p. 3061-3071.

[93] Feng, Z. and C. P. Ko, Schwann cells promote synaptogenesis at the neuromuscular junction via transforming growth factor-beta1. *The Journal of neuroscience: the official journal of the Society for Neuroscience,* 2008. 28(39): p. 9599-9609.

[94] Wang, Y., Shan, Q., Pan, J. and Yi, S., Actin Cytoskeleton Affects Schwann Cell Migration and Peripheral Nerve Regeneration. *Frontiers in physiology,* 2018. 9: p. 23-23.

[95] Heermann, S. and M. H. Schwab, Molecular control of Schwann cell migration along peripheral axons. *Cell Adhesion & Migration,* 2013. 7(1): p. 18-22.

[96] Oudega, M. and X. M. Xu, Schwann Cell Transplantation for Repair of the Adult Spinal Cord. *Journal of Neurotrauma,* 2006. 23(3-4): p. 453-467.

[97] Oh, Y. S., Shin, S., Lee, Y-J., Kim, E. H. and Jun, H-S., Betacellulin-Induced Beta Cell Proliferation and Regeneration Is Mediated by Activation of ErbB-1 and ErbB-2 Receptors. *PLOS ONE,* 2011. 6(8): p. e23894.

[98] Wang, Y., Zhang, F., Zhang, Y., Shan, Q, Liu, W., Zhang, F., Zhang, F. and Yi, S., Betacellulin regulates peripheral nerve regeneration by affecting Schwann cell migration and axon elongation. *Molecular medicine* (Cambridge, Mass.), 2021. 27(1): p. 27-27.

[99] Arcas, A., D. G. Wilkinson, and M. Á. Nieto, The Evolutionary History of Ephs and Ephrins: Toward Multicellular Organisms. *Molecular biology and evolution,* 2020. 37(2): p. 379-394.

[100] Parrinello, S., Napoli, I., Ribeiro, S., Digby, P. W., Fedorova, M., Parkinson, D. B., Doddrell, R. D. S., Nakayama, M., Adams, R. H. and Lloyd, A. C., EphB Signaling Directs Peripheral Nerve Regeneration through Sox2-Dependent Schwann Cell Sorting. *Cell,* 2010. 143(1).

[101] Zhang, S. and W. Cui, Sox2, a key factor in the regulation of pluripotency and neural differentiation. *World journal of stem cells,* 2014. 6(3): p. 305-311.

[102] Torres-Mejía, E., Trümbach, D., Kleeberger, C., Dornseifer, U., Orschmann, T., Backer, T., Brenke, J. K., Hadian, K., Wurst, W., López-Schier, H. and Desbordes, S. C., Sox2 controls Schwann cell self-organization through fibronectin fibrillogenesis. *Scientific Reports,* 2020. 10.

[103] Ornitz, D. M. and N. Itoh, The Fibroblast Growth Factor signaling pathway. *WIREs Developmental Biology,* 2015. 4(3): p. 215-266.

[104] Chen, B., Hu, R., Min, Q., Li, Y., Parkinson, D. B. and Dun, X-p., FGF5 Regulates Schwann Cell Migration and Adhesion. *Frontiers in cellular neuroscience,* 2020. 14: p. 237-237.

[105] Hiraga, T., S. Ito, and H. Nakamura, Cancer Stem–like Cell Marker CD44 Promotes Bone Metastases by Enhancing Tumorigenicity, Cell Motility, and Hyaluronan Production. *Cancer Research,* 2013. 73(13): p. 4112.

[106] Ouasti, S., Faroni, A., Kingham, P. J., Ghibaudi, M., Reid, A. J. and Tirelli, N., Hyaluronic Acid (HA) Receptors and the Motility of Schwann Cell(-Like) Phenotypes. *Cells,* 2020. 9(6).

[107] Afshari, F. T., Kwok, J. C., White, L. and Fawcett, J. W., Schwann cell migration is integrin-dependent and inhibited by astrocyte-produced aggrecan. *Glia,* 2010. 58(7): p. 857-869.

[108] Motta, C. M. M., Endres, K. J., Wesdemiotis, C., Willits, R. K. and Becker, M. L., Enhancing Schwann Cell Migration Using Concentration Gradients of Laminin Derived-peptides. *Biomaterials,* 2019. 218: p. 119335.

[109] Cheema, S. S., Richards, L., Murphy, M. and Bartlett, P. F., Leukemia inhibitory factor prevents the death of axotomised sensory neurons in the dorsal root ganglia of the neonatal rat. *Journal of Neuroscience Research,* 1994. 37(2): p. 213-218.

[110] Chen, Q., Liu, Q., Zhang, Y., Li, S. and Yi, S., Leukemia inhibitory factor regulates Schwann cell proliferation and migration and affects peripheral nerve regeneration. *Cell death & disease,* 2021. 12(5): p. 417-417.

[111] Yang, L., J. E. Froberg, and J. T. Lee, Long noncoding RNAs: fresh perspectives into the RNA world. *Trends in Biochemical Sciences,* 2014. 39(1): p. 35-43.

[112] Yao, C., et al., LncRNA BC088259 promotes Schwann cell migration through Vimentin following peripheral nerve injury. *Glia,* 2020. 68(3): p. 670-679.

[113] Qin, J., Zha, G-B., Yu, J., Zhang, H-H. and Yi, S., Differential temporal expression of matrix metalloproteinases following sciatic nerve crush. *Neural Regeneration Research,* 2016. 11(7): p. 1165-1171.

[114] Wang, H., Zhang, P., Yu, J., Zhang, F., Dai, W. and Yi, S., Matrix metalloproteinase 7 promoted Schwann cell migration and myelination after rat sciatic nerve injury. *Molecular Brain,* 2019. 12.

[115] Elie, A., Prezel, E., Guérin, C., Denarier, E., Ramirez-Rios, Serre, L., Andrieux, A., Fourest-Lieuvin, A., Blanchoin, L. and Arnal, I., Tau co-organizes dynamic microtubule and actin networks. *Scientific reports,* 2015. 5: p. 9964-9964.

[116] Yi, S., Liu, Q., Wang, X., Qian, T., Wang, H., Zha, G., Yu, J., Wang, P., Gu, X., Chu, D. and Li, S., Tau modulates Schwann cell proliferation, migration and differentiation following peripheral nerve injury. *Journal of Cell Science,* 2019. 132(jcs222059).

[117] Muscella, A., Vetrugno, C., Cossa, L. G. and Marsigliante, S., TGF-β1 activates RSC96 Schwann cells migration and invasion through MMP-2 and MMP-9 activities. *Journal of Neurochemistry,* 2020. 153(4): p. 525-538.

[118] Kobayashi, H., Chattopadhyay, S., Kato, K., Dolkas, J., K. S-I., Myers, R. R. and Shubayev, V. I., MMPs initiate Schwann cell-mediated MBP degradation and mechanical nociception after nerve damage. *Molecular and Cellular Neuroscience,* 2008. 39(4): p. 619-627.

Chapter 6

Longitudinal Progression of Non-Interventional Traumatic Brain Injury: Resting-State Functional Reorganization and Neuropsychological Assessments

Muhammad Riddha Abdul Rahman[1,2,3], Aini Ismafairus Abd. Hamid[1,3,4], Hazim Omar[1,3,4], Wan Nor Azlen Wan Mohamad[1,3,4], Mohamed Faiz Mohamed Mustafar[1,3,4], Mohd Faizal Mohd Zulkifly[1,3,4], Azizah Othman[5] and Jafri Malin Abdullah[1,3,4]

[1]Department of Neurosciences, School of Medical Sciences, Universiti Sains Malaysia, Kubang Kerian, Malaysia
[2]School of Medical Imaging, Faculty of Health Sciences, Universiti Sultan Zainal Abidin, Kuala Nerus, Malaysia
[3]Brain and Behaviour Cluster, School of Medical Sciences, Universiti Sains Malaysia, Kubang Kerian, Malaysia
[4]Department of Neurosciences, Hospital Universiti Sains Malaysia, Kubang Kerian, Malaysia
[5]Department of Paediatrics, School of Medical Sciences, Universiti Sains Malaysia, Kubang Kerian, Malaysia

Abstract

In this chapter, we discuss a case series involving three traumatic brain injury (TBI) participants who underwent resting-state functional MRI scanning and neuropsychological assessments at two-time points, at one-

In: Horizons in Neuroscience Research. Volume 48
Editors: Andres Costa and Eugenio Villalba
ISBN: 979-8-88697-230-6
© 2022 Nova Science Publishers, Inc.

month and twelve-month post-TBI. Longitudinal studies of TBI can reveal important information regarding the reorganization of the functional aspect of the brain. Untreated head injuries can take a long time to heal, affecting their physical and cognitive activities. This chapter focuses on neuropsychological performance and reorganization in functional connectivity. We discuss work with participants who are in the sub-acute and chronic phases of TBI without intervention. Despite no rehabilitation being given, neuropsychological scores appeared to have the potential to improve over time, although lower scores in a few domains were recorded. Functional connectivity (FC) reveals alteration in the Default Mode Network (DMN) connectivity with other regions. Additionally, there is an alteration in FC within temporal regions involved in working memory and visual processing, as well as between visual areas and superior temporal areas involved in sound processing. Findings from a case series showed that neuropsychological performance and FC alterations at the onset of TBI can still improve without intervention but at a slower rate. Several studies show that cognitive training approaches promote better recovery than the no-intervention group. Rehabilitation or treatment is needed to help people recover quickly and get back to their normal lives.

Introduction

Debilitating effects of traumatic brain injury (TBI) can last for a long time and have a negative impact on the quality of life of its survivors, regardless of age [1–3]. TBI, which was becoming more common around the world, posed a significant burden on public healthcare and the socioeconomic aspect. The goal is to reintegrate TBI survivors into society, so understanding the mechanism of recovery after TBI is critical. Longitudinal assessment of TBI can shed a light on how this disease affects the functional aspect of the brain over time. In this chapter, we presented three case studies of non-severe TBI survivors from motor-vehicle accidents. The participants were scanned at one-month and twelve-month post-injury intervals to document the progression of TBI using functional MRI. Following that, we examined and discussed the brain activation, functional connectivity, and effective connectivity of the default mode network associated with TBI, as well as the reorganization of functional connectivity.

Quality of Life in TBI Patients

TBI can be caused by a variety of head injuries, including motor vehicle accidents, blast injuries, and falls. The likelihood of the TBI survivors being successfully rehabilitated often depends on the severity of the injury and care provided in the acute and chronic phases, which can last years. Longitudinal TBI research can help researchers better understand how the condition progress over time. The nature of TBI is heterogeneous, and the recovery projection can vary between each individual. Nevertheless, a general recovery trend can be established to guide the healthcare provider on the expected prognosis, allowing TBI survivors to be rehabilitated to a better quality of life. A few TBI studies follow up the TBI survivors that received no intervention [2, 4–6], while others investigate the efficacy and positive effect on the recovery of experimental interventional procedures [7–11]. Findings from previous studies demonstrate different recovery rates and performance for different intervention approaches.

Recovery with Intervention

Intervention following TBI often involves rehabilitation using cognitive, memory, or attention training. Studies have shown that with training, TBI survivors perform better post-training compared to before. For example, attentional performance was reportedly improved after intense cognitive training [10], while trail-making scores were positively correlated with increased global and local efficiency post-training [7]. Another study showed that with rehabilitation, TBI patients displayed improved behavioral and communication performance [11]. Structural recovery was also accompanied by better balance control, improved with 8-week training sessions [9]. However, it can be argued that the resolution of structural and functional connectivity may have influenced the improved scores regardless of the training. Therefore, it is imperative to compare with studies that did not incorporate any intervention.

Recovery without Intervention

The following studies are observational studies that track the changes in functional connectivity in TBI survivors as time progress. Among these studies, TBI cases involving the veterans of war are often not followed by any intervention [12], especially those in the mild spectrum as impairments went undiagnosed [13, 14]. Non-intervened survivors of TBI still report some cognitive impairments even after years [15–17], with the effects more pronounced if TBI was acquired at a young age, due to the developing brain [18]. However, improvements without intervention were also reported [19, 20], albeit with the neural compensatory mechanism in the form of increased activation [21]. Those with persistent symptoms also demonstrated aberrant functional connectivity that lasts for years [22].

The Advantages of Brain Imaging

Technology advancements in healthcare have paved the path for a deeper understanding of the brain. Neuroimaging research, in particular, has ceased the need to dissect the brain to determine the cause of illness, as brain imaging can offer precise data of physiological and psychological abnormalities in vitro, non-invasively, and promptly.

Neuroimaging modalities range from ionizing radiation-based imaging such as computed tomography (CT) and positron emission tomography (PET), electrophysiological imaging such as electroencephalography (EEG) and magnetoencephalography (MEG), and non-ionizing radiation-based imaging such as functional magnetic resonance imaging (fMRI). Each of these modalities has its advantages, either excellent spatial or temporal resolution, fast acquisition, relatively cheaper, easier to carry out experiments, simpler setup, and so forth. It can be argued that no single neuroimaging modality has the best advantages all around, therefore multi-modalities imaging has been adopted to overcome the limitation of one modality and integrate findings [23]. In this case, a wide range of modalities can be used simultaneously to meet the specific diagnostic need [24]. However, trade-offs of these modalities must be carefully weighed so that the benefit always outweighs the risk when selecting a suitable neuroimaging modality.

One of the most widely used neuroimaging modalities is the fMRI, which is the modality used in this case study. fMRI detects brain activity by using the magnetic properties of oxygenated and deoxygenated blood as it circulates in the brain. When neural activity increases, this results in a subtle increase in the local magnetic resonance signal, which is known as the blood oxygenation level-dependent (BOLD) effect [25]. The fMRI is excellent in terms of spatial resolution; however, its temporal resolution is relatively poor compared to electrophysiological neuroimaging such as electroencephalography (EEG), with a response time of up to one second compared to milliseconds in EEG.

To elicit the functional aspect of the brain, the resting-state fMRI is one of the most widely used neuroimaging paradigms. Participants are only required to relax inside the scanner when using this procedure. The lack of tasks that require responses thus allowed a wide range of patients, including those who were unconscious or unable to respond, to be recruited and diagnosed.

Reorganization of Functional Network Over Time

When the brain is injured, its structure could be altered. Structural aberrations can range from subtle traumatic axonal injuries to more widespread diffuse axonal injuries. Subtle injuries, most often seen in the mild TBI spectrum, can be undetected under a CT scan. Therefore, using sufficiently sensitive modalities such as MRI is imperative to avoid misdiagnosis, as even mild TBI can have deleterious effects on brain function.

At the onset of the injury, functional connectivity suffered losses since the transfer pathway was disconnected. To resolve this, the brain would compensate by finding multiple pathways so that brain processes can reach the intended region [4]. This would culminate in hyperconnectivity, that would persist for months [19]. While this may seem ideal to preserve brain functionality, it increases metabolic costs and is taxing to the overall network [26]. Over time, the brain tries to balance the need to identify the optimal route for information processing i.e., transfer efficiency with network metabolic costs [27]. As a result, most of the hyperconnectivity would resolve in the chronic phase of TBI, some with no significant differences recorded between the TBI and healthy population [22], although some may still present for years resulting in persistent symptoms exhibited by the TBI survivors [20, 22].

Case Descriptions

Functional magnetic resonance imaging (fMRI), a neuroimaging method that offers detailed functional data of the resting brain, was used to scan the TBI cases. The resting-state paradigm was used to assess the Default Mode Network (DMN) of our participants. Other than fMRI scans, a series of neuropsychological assessments were administered to assess the cognitive domains that are frequently affected after a TBI. We used the Wechsler Abbreviated Scale of Intelligence 1st edition (WASI; block design and matrix reasoning) to estimate general cognitive ability [28], Rey Auditory Verbal Learning Test (RAVLT; immediate and delayed recall) to assess the verbal memory function [29, 30], Rey Complex Figure Test and Recognition Trial (RCFT; immediate and delayed recall) to assess the visual memory and perception [31], Comprehensive Trail-Making Test (CTMT) to assess the psychomotor speed and cognitive flexibility [32, 33], and Wisconsin Card Sorting Test (WCST) to measure the executive functioning [34]. The results are based on standard scores that have been adjusted for age and education level.

Case 1

A 20-year-old gentleman was admitted to the emergency department after suffering a head injury in a motor vehicle accident. Initial assessment categorized him as moderate TBI with a GCS score of 11. Computerized tomography (CT) scanning revealed a contusion in the bilateral temporal and left frontal area. At one-month post-injury, the participant performed worse compared to HC in matrix reasoning and CTMT, where scores in both tests correspond to the impairment in the cognitive domain. At twelve months post-injury, the participant performed better in matrix reasoning, RCFT immediate and delayed recall, WCST, and CTMT, whereas Block Design and RAVLT immediate recall performed worse.

Case 2

A 53-year-old gentleman suffered a moderate TBI due to a motor vehicle accident, with a GCS score of 10. CT scanning revealed bilateral frontal and occipital contusion, as well as a left temporal contusion. At one-month post-injury, the participant performed comparatively similar to the healthy population in all domains of neuropsychological tests. At twelve months post-injury, the participant performed better compared to the first visit, as depicted in the scores on all neuropsychological tests except for both RAVLT tests.

Case 3

A 29-year-old gentleman was admitted to the emergency department following a head injury sustained during a motor vehicle accident. Initial assessments revealed that he had a mild TBI with a GCS score of 15. Contusions were discovered on CT scans in the left frontal and right temporal areas. At one-month post-injury, the participant performed poorly compared to the HC in all domains. However, his neuropsychological performance improved significantly in his second visit compared to the first. This participant performed better in all neuropsychological tests, except in RCFT delayed recall.

Overall Neuropsychological Progression

In this preliminary case, the independent samples Kruskal-Wallis test was used to assess the neuropsychological progression. Overall neuropsychological assessment revealed that the participants performed worse on all tests when compared to healthy controls. However, there are significant differences between healthy controls and TBI participants at their one-month post-TBI timepoint, in the overall IQ score and matrix reasoning component. Time progression reveals no significant differences between the TBI participants, although improvements in raw scores were recorded at the individual level. Table 1 outline the mean scores of all groups.

For the matrix reasoning component, the significant difference in the first visit scores between the TBI participants and HC was not found during the twelve months visit, indicating that the patients' scores improved. Table 2 outlined the comparison between all groups, showing the significant difference between HC and first visit TBI. Figure 1 shows the boxplot of the score comparison between all groups.

Table 1. Neuropsychological characteristics of the participants

Neuropsychological test	Mean HC (SD)	Mean TBI-1 (SD)	Mean TBI-2 (SD)	Statistic	p
Block Design	51.42 (8.28)	45.00 (2.00)	44.33 (7.37)	4.10	0.129
Matrix Reasoning	50.75 (11.95)	28.00 (11.36)	34.00 (16.46)	7.79	0.020*
RAVLT – immediate	45.71 (10.90)	43.67 (7.77)	45.33 (2.31)	0.25	0.883
RAVLT – delayed	9.71 (3.13)	8.67 (2.89)	8.33 (1.53)	1.03	0.597
RCFT – immediate recall	50.10 (13.74)	38.33 (18.15)	49.00 (11.79)	1.98	0.372
RCFT – delayed recall	45.04 (15.28)	37.33 (5.03)	44.67 (15.31)	1.08	0.583
WCST	85.38 (20.83)	74.33 (11.24)	92.00 (11.14)	1.27	0.530
CTMT	36.54 (8.32)	27.67 (10.26)	32.00 (9.85)	2.39	0.303

HC, healthy cotrols; TBI-1, 1-month visit; TBI-2, 12 months visit.
*Significant at $p < 0.05$.

Table 2. Matrix reasoning scores were analyzed using multiple comparisons

Groups	Statistic	Std. Error	p
TBI-1 – TBI-2	-3.333	7.179	0.642
TBI-1 – HC	12.708	5.384	0.018*
TBI-2 – HC	9.375	5.384	0.082

HC, healthy controls; TBI-1, 1-month visit; TBI-2, 12 months visit.
*Significant at $p < 0.05$.

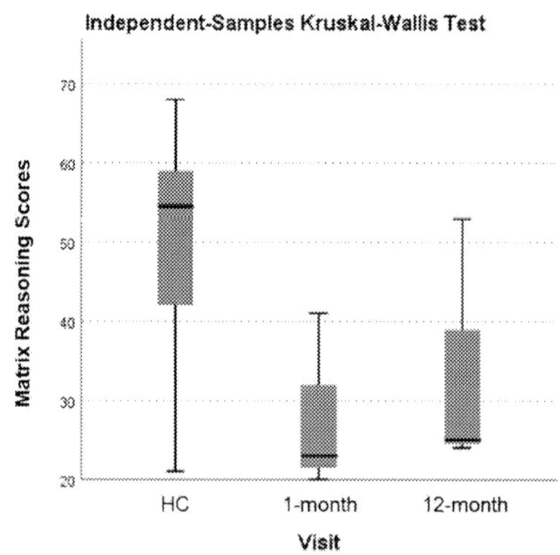

Figure 1. Matrix reasoning boxplot showed a significant difference in scores between HC and TBI participants at the 1-month visit, which was improved at the twelve months visit.

Functional Connectivity Results

We analyzed the resting-state network connectivities between HC and one-month TBI groups, with emphasis on the DMN at the seed level. For analytical purposes, we thresholded the peak activation for seed-based analysis at $p_{unc} < 0.001$, while controlling for multiple comparisons at the cluster level $p_{FDR} < 0.05$. For the ROI-based analysis, we thresholded the connectivity at $p_{FDR} < 0.05$.

Seed-based connectivity analysis revealed that compared to the HC, subacute TBI participants had increased connectivity involving the nodes of the DMN, specifically between: 1) MPFC and Precentral gyri (PreCG, right $p_{FDR} = 0.000$, left $p_{FDR} = 0.012$), right inferior lateral occipital (iLOC, $p_{FDR} = 0.001$), putamen ($p_{FDR} = 0.009$), and right superior temporal gyrus (STG, $p_{FDR} = 0.016$), 2) right LP and right occipital pole (OP, $p_{FDR} = 0.001$), right precentral gyrus (PreCG, $p_{FDR} = 0.011$), and left frontal pole (FP, $p_{FDR} = 0.044$), and 3) posterior cingulate cortex and left superior lateral occipital cortex (sLOC, $p_{FDR} = 0.010$) (Figure 2). At the same time, decreased connectivity was observed between MPFC and the right sLOC ($p_{FDR} = 0.009$) (Figure 3). Table 3 outlined the results.

Table 3. Seed-based analysis showing the regions with significant activation in TBI > HC at one-month post-injury

Seed	to	Cluster size	pFDR*
Increased FC			
MPFC	R PreCG	289	0.000
	R iLOC	169	0.001
	R Putamen	121	0.009
	L PreCG	110	0.012
	R STG	96	0.016
RLP	R OP	196	0.001
	R PreCG	121	0.011
	L FP	82	0.044
PCC	L sLOC	123	0.010
Decreased FC			
MPFC	R sLOC	125	0.009

MPFC, medial prefrontal cortex; PreCG, precentral gyrus; iLOC, inferior lateral occipital cortex; STG, superior temporal gyrus; LP, latral parietal; OP, occipital pole; FP, frontal pole; PCC, posterior cingulate cortex; sLOC, superior lateral occipital cortex; R, right; L, left.

*Significant at $p < 0.05$.

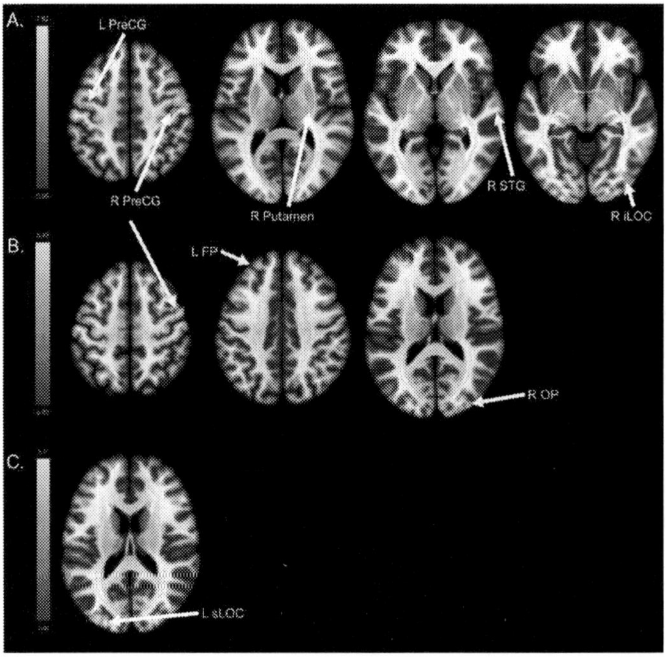

Figure 2. Areas with significant activations due to hyperconnectivity from A) MPFC, B) LP, and C) PCC in the TBI group at one-month post-injury. Results are thresholded at voxel level $p_{unc} < 0.001$ and cluster size $p_{FDR} < 0.05$. the color bar represents the T-score.

Table 4. ROI-based analysis shows the node pairs with increased connectivity in TBI > HC at one-month post-injury

Node	To	T-score	pFDR*
Visual occipital (VN)	R insula	3.99	0.037
R SFG (DAN)	R thalamus	4.84	0.008
R pSTG (LN)	L fusiform	4.66	0.012

VN, visual network; SFG, superior frontal gyrus; DAN, dorsal attention network; pSTG, posterior superior temporal gyrus; LN, language network; R, right; L, left.
*significant at $p < 0.05$.

In addition, we performed an ROI-based analysis using the resting state networks set a priori in the CONN toolbox. We found increased FC involving the visual network (between visual occipital and right insula, $p_{FDR} = 0.037$), dorsal attention network (between and right thalamus, $p_{FDR} = 0.008$), and language network (between posterior STG and left temporal occipital fusiform, $p_{FDR} = 0.012$). The results are outlined in Table 4.

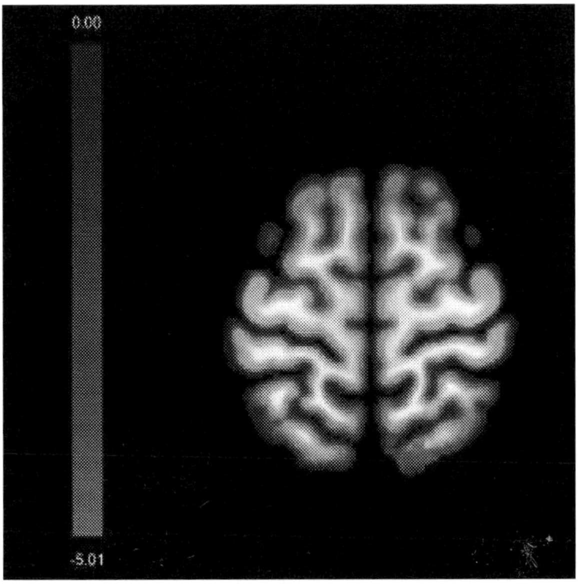

Figure 3. Areas with significant activations due to hypoconnectivity from MPFC in the TBI group at one-month post-injury. Results are thresholded at voxel level $p_{unc} < 0.001$ and cluster size $p_{FDR} < 0.05$. the color bar represents the T-score.

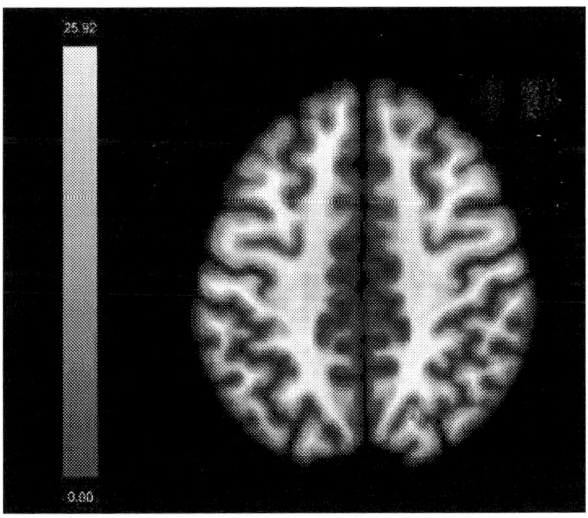

Figure 4. Areas with significant activations due to hyperconnectivity from MPFC in the TBI group at twelve months post-injury. Results are thresholded at voxel level $p_{unc} < 0.001$ and cluster size $p_{FDR} < 0.05$. the color bar represents the T-score.

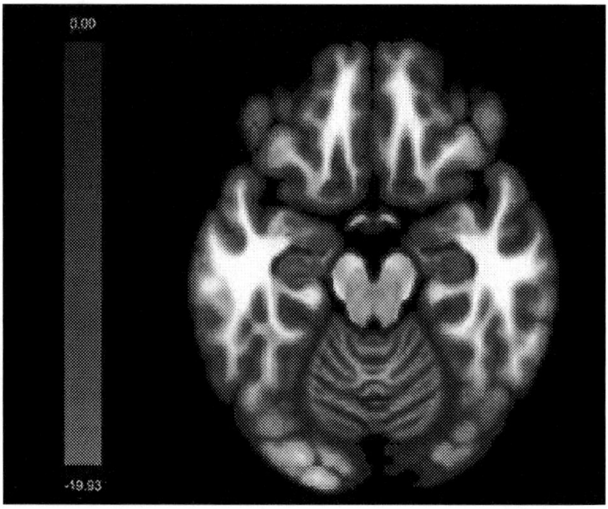

Figure 5. Areas with significant activations due to hypoconnectivity from PCC in the TBI group at twelve months post-injury. Results are thresholded at voxel level $p_{unc} <$ 0.001 and cluster size $p_{FDR} < 0.05$. the color bar represents the T-score.

Subsequently, we performed both seed-based and ROI-based analyses on the comparison of one month and twelve months post-injury. Seed voxel analysis of the DMN nodes revealed increased FC within the TBI group after twelve months between MPFC and left superior lateral occipital area (pFDR = 0.000) (refer to Figure 4) and between PCC and precuneus (pFDR 0.018) and decreased FC between PCC and frontal orbital area (pFDR 0.040) (refer to Figure 5).

Table 5 outlines the statistical results. There are no significant differences in seed-based connectivity between TBI and HC.

Table 5. Seed-based analysis showing the regions with significant activation in TBI > HC at twelve months post-injury

Seed	to	Cluster size	pFDR
Increase FC			
MPFC	L sLOC	57	0.000
PCC	Precuneus	24	0.018
Decrease FC			
PCC	L Frontal orbital	20	0.040

Table 6. ROI-based analysis shows the node pairs with decreased connectivity in TBI > HC at twelve months post-injury

Node	To	T-score	pFDR
Visual occipital	R aSTG	-12.00	0.045
MTG	L anterior ITG	-24.33	0.003

RSNs ROI-based analysis between one month and twelve months post-TBI revealed that the FC between the visual occipital and the right anterior superior temporal gyrus (aSTG) was decreased over time ($p_{FDR} = 0.045$), as well as between the middle temporal gyrus (MTG) and left inferior temporal gyrus (ITG) ($p_{FDR} = 0.003$). Table 6 outlines the statistical results.

Discussion

In this chapter, we longitudinally analyzed the functional connectivity of TBI survivors and compared them to the connectivity profile of the healthy control (HC). In addition, we evaluated the performance of cognitive, memory, and attention tasks and subsequently correlate them with functional connectivity observed one month and twelve months post-TBI.

Analysis of the neuropsychological scores revealed that TBI participants displayed score progress in several domains of neuropsychological assessments, while others had lower scores. When compared to the HC, subacute TBI showed multiple hyperconnectivity between the nodes of the DMN and other parts of the brain. Three DMN nodes were implicated, with connection to the precentral gyri, lateral occipital gyri, putamen, and the frontal pole. In fact, we observed hyperconnectivity between two nodes of the DMN with the precentral gyri. The hyperconnectivity in the DMN and precentral gyrus was expected at the acute stage of the injury [35]. Indeed, increased connectivity between the DMN and precentral gyrus is negatively associated with IQ [36], which may contribute to the poor performance in the matrix reasoning component, a subset of WASI tests designed to measure IQ. However, increased connectivity between the DMN and precentral gyri is also associated with improved attention [37].

The putamen is a component of the basal ganglia network, which is typically anti-correlated with the DMN in healthy populations [38, 39]. Increased connectivity and activation of the putamen during activation of the DMN component may have a negative impact on the scores for the CTMT test among the TBI participants, which measures cognitive flexibility [40]. At rest, the connectivity between the DMN and lateral occipital areas is not normally observed, since the LOC is part of the DAN. The LOC is more likely to form connectivity with the FPN at rest, whereas the connectivity involving DMN and LOC is usually observed during focused perception [41]. Reflecting on hyperconnectivity observed between the DMN and precentral gyri, improved attention may play a role in the increased connectivity between DMN and LOC.

During the twelve months visit, most of the scores improved compared to the one-month visit. It is common for neuropsychological test scores to return to normal over time [42]. Resolved connectivity over time may play a role in improving the scores. It is interesting to note that there are no significant differences in FC between the HC and TBI groups after twelve months, suggesting that the hyperconnectivity eventually subsided during the chronic phase of the injury. However, when compared to the subacute phase, there is a significant alteration in connectivity involving two major DMN nodes: the MPFC and PCC. In addition, TBI participants reported increased scores in the visual memory domain that was accompanied by an increase in FC between MTG and ITG. The MTG is implicated in working memory for the visual maintenance of information [43]. The visual area of the occipital lobe was also increased in FC with the STG, the area that was implicated in the processing of sound and acoustic [43]. Moreover, FC between nodes of the DMN and the occipital area was also increased. The occipital area is known as the main visual center of the brain [44], therefore further corroborating our findings on the affected visual memory domain and visual processing observed between the DMN and MTG.

Conclusion

TBI is a heterogeneous disease that has a wide spectrum of effects and recovery projections. However, patterns begin to emerge at a single-TBI participant level that relatively fit into the evidence found in the literature. Even without intervention, the brain compensated for the loss of structural connections by rerouting the functional connectivity through network hubs, trading off the network cost with improved performance. Literature covering longitudinal cases of TBI up to twelve months is quite scarce, thus we suggest that the findings could be extrapolated to get a better insight into how TBI affects the general population. However, as with any case study, extrapolation should be done with caution and supported by a future study with a bigger sample size.

As we have shown in this chapter, there is evidence of neural plasticity in TBI patients in the form of functional connectivity improvement. Furthermore, our findings from the neuropsychological assessments and neuroimaging data are consistent with the theory of compensatory mechanisms exhibited by the brain in the event of injury. From what we have observed and evidence from the literature, without intervention, either through medication or cognitive training, the survivors of TBI would recover much slower than those with intervention. As a result, the quality of life will be affected as a longer time were needed for recovery. Therefore, a suitable intervention can be suggested to be applied to the TBI survivors, such as a cognitive training regimen tailored to the deficiencies experienced by the patient. This can aid their recovery and return to a quality and productive life.

References

[1] Mckee, A. C. and Daneshvar, D. H. (2015) The neuropathology of traumatic brain injury. *Handb. Clin. Neurol.* 127, 45–66.

[2] Tuerk, C., Dégeilh, F., Catroppa, C., Dooley, J. J., Kean, M., Anderson, V., & Beauchamp, M. H. (2020) Altered resting-state functional connectivity within the developing social brain after pediatric traumatic brain injury. *Hum. Brain Mapp.* 41, 561–576.

[3] Stephens, J. A., Jaclyn A. Stephens, Cynthia F. Salorio, Anita D. Barber, Sarah R. Risen, Stewart H. Mostofsky, Stacy J. Suskauer (2017) Preliminary findings of altered functional connectivity of the default mode network linked to functional outcomes one year after pediatric traumatic brain injury. *Dev. Neurorehabil.* doi: 10.1080/17518423.2017.1338777.

[4] Dall'Acqua, P., Johannes, S., Mica, L., Simmen, H.-P., Glaab, R., Fandino, J., Schwendinger, M., Meier, C., Ulbrich, E. J., Müller, A., Baetschmann, H., Jäncke, L., & Hänggi, J. (2017) Functional and Structural Network Recovery after Mild Traumatic Brain Injury: A 1-Year Longitudinal Study. *Front. Hum. Neurosci.* doi: 10.3389/fnhum.2017.00280.

[5] Messé, A., Caplain, S., Pélégrini-Issac, M., Blancho, S., Lévy, R., Aghakhani, N., Montreuil, M., Benali, H., & Lehéricy, S. (2013) Specific and Evolving Resting-State Network Alterations in Post-Concussion Syndrome Following Mild Traumatic Brain Injury. *PLoS One* 8, 1–10.

[6] Abbas, K., Shenk T. E., Poole V. N., Breedlove E. L., Leverenz L. J., Nauman E. A., Talavage T. M., Robinson M. E. (2015) Alteration of Default Mode Network in High School Football Athletes Due to Repetitive Subconcussive Mild Traumatic

Brain Injury: A Resting-State Functional Magnetic Resonance Imaging Study. *Brain Connect.* 5, 91–101.

[7] Han, K., Chapman, S. B., & Krawczyk, D. C. (2020) Cognitive Training Reorganizes Network Modularity in Traumatic Brain Injury. *Neurorehabil. Neural Repair* 34, 26–38.

[8] Han, K., Chapman, S. B., & Krawczyk, D. C. (2018) Neuroplasticity of cognitive control networks following cognitive training for chronic traumatic brain injury. *NeuroImage Clin.* doi: 10.1016/J.NICL.2018.01.030.

[9] Drijkoningen, D., Caeyenberghs, K., Leunissen, I., Vander Linden, C., Leemans, A., Sunaert, S., Duysens, J., & Swinnen, S. P. (2015) Training-induced improvements in postural control are accompanied by alterations in cerebellar white matter in brain injured patients. *NeuroImage Clin.* 7, 240–251.

[10] Kim, Y. H., Yoo, W. K., Ko, M. H., Park, C., Sung Tae Kim, & Na, D. L. (2009) Plasticity of the Attentional Network After Brain Injury and Cognitive Rehabilitation. *Neurorehabil. Neural Repair* 23, 468–477.

[11] Sacco, K., Gabbatore, I., Geda, E., Duca, S., Cauda, F., Bara, B. G., & Bosco, F. M. (2016) Rehabilitation of Communicative Abilities in Patients with a History of TBI: Behavioral Improvements and Cerebral Changes in Resting-State Activity. *Front. Behav. Neurosci.* 10, 48.

[12] Franke, L. M., Walker, W. C., Hoke, K. W., & Wares, J. R. (2016) Distinction in EEG slow oscillations between chronic mild traumatic brain injury and PTSD. *Int. J. Psychophysiol.* 106, 21–29.

[13] Huang, M. X., Nichols, S., Robb-Swan, A., Angeles-Quinto, A., Harrington, D. L., Drake, A., Huang, C. W., Song, T., Diwakar, M., Risbrough, V. B., Matthews, S., Clifford, R., Cheng, C. K., Huang, J. W., Sinha, A., Yurgil, K. A., Ji, Z., Lerman, I., Lee, R. R., & Baker, D. G. (2020) Marked Increases in Resting-State MEG Gamma-Band Activity in Combat-Related Mild Traumatic Brain Injury. *Cereb. Cortex* 30, 283–295.

[14] Arciniega, H., Shires, J., Furlong, S., Kilgore-Gomez, A., Cerreta, A., Murray, N. G., & Berryhill, M. E. (2021) Impaired visual working memory and reduced connectivity in undergraduates with a history of mild traumatic brain injury. *Sci. Rep.* 11.

[15] De Simoni, S., Grover, P. J., Jenkins, P. O., Honeyfield, L., Quest, R. A., Ross, E., Scott, G., Wilson, M. H., Majewska, P., Waldman, A. D., Patel, M. C., & Sharp, D. J. (2016) Disconnection between the default mode network and medial temporal lobes in post-traumatic amnesia. *Brain* 139, 3137–3150.

[16] Alhourani, A., Wozny, T. A., Krishnaswamy, D., Pathak, S., Walls, S. A., Ghuman, A. S., Krieger, D. N., Okonkwo, D. O., Richardson, R. M., & Niranjan, A. (2016) Magnetoencephalography-based identification of functional connectivity network disruption following mild traumatic brain injury. *J. Neurophysiol.* 116, 1840–1847.

[17] Vakhtin, A. A., Calhoun, V. D., Jung, R. E., Prestopnik, J. L., Taylor, P. A., & Ford, C. C. (2013) Changes in intrinsic functional brain networks following blast-induced mild traumatic brain injury. *Brain Inj.* 27, 1304–1310.

[18] Galicia-Alvarado, M., Alducin-Castillo, J., Ramírez-Flores, M. J., Sánchez Quezada, A. L., Yáñez-Suárez, O., & Flores-Ávalos, B. (2019) Cognitive and

spectral coherence of EEG alterations in resting state in children with chronic TBI. *Salud Ment.* 42, 91–100.

[19] Meier, T. B., Bellgowan, P. S. F., & Mayer, A. R. (2017) Longitudinal assessment of local and global functional connectivity following sports-related concussion. *Brain Imaging Behav.* 11, 129–140.

[20] Madhavan, R., Joel, S. E., Mullick, R., Cogsil, T., Niogi, S. N., Tsiouris, A. J., Mukherjee, P., Masdeu, J. C., Marinelli, L., & Shetty, T. (2019). Longitudinal resting state functional connectivity predicts clinical outcome in mild traumatic brain injury. *Journal of Neurotrauma*, 36(5), 650–660. https://doi.org/10.1089/neu.2018.573936.

[21] Rajesh, A., Cooke, G. E., Monti, J. M., Jahn, A., Daugherty, A. M., Cohen, N. J., & Kramer, A. F. (2017) Differences in Brain Architecture in Remote Mild Traumatic Brain Injury. *J. Neurotrauma* 34, 3280–3287.

[22] Van Der Horn, H. J., Myrthe E. Scheenen, Myrthe E. de Koning, Edith J. Liemburg, Jacoba M. Spikman, Joukje van der Naalt. (2017) The Default Mode Network as a Biomarker of Persistent Complaints after Mild Traumatic Brain Injury: A Longitudinal Functional Magnetic Resonance Imaging Study. *J. Neurotrauma* 34, 3262–3269.

[23] Tsuchimoto, S., Shibusawa, S., Mizuguchi, N., Kato, K., Ebata, H., Liu, M., Hanakawa, T., & Ushiba, J. (2017) Resting-State Fluctuations of EEG Sensorimotor Rhythm Reflect BOLD Activities in the Pericentral Areas: A Simultaneous EEG-fMRI Study. *Front. Hum. Neurosci.* 11, 356.

[24] Narayana, P. A., Yu, X., Hasan, K. M., Wilde, E. A., Levin, H. S., Hunter, J. V., Miller, E. R., Patel, V. K. S., Robertson, C. S., & McCarthy, J. J. (2015) Multi-modal MRI of mild traumatic brain injury. *NeuroImage Clin.* doi: 10.1016/j.nicl.2014.07.010.

[25] Medaglia, J. D. (2017) Functional neuroimaging in traumatic brain injury: From nodes to networks. *Front. Neurol.* doi: 10.3389/fneur.2017.00407.

[26] Hillary, F. G., Roman, C. A., Venkatesan, U., Rajtmajer, S. M., Bajo, R., & Castellanos, N. D. (2015) Hyperconnectivity is a fundamental response to neurological disruption. *Neuropsychology* 29.

[27] Roy, A., Bernier, R. A., Wang, J., Benson, M., French, J. J., Good, D. C., & Hillary, F. G. (2017) The evolution of cost-efficiency in neural networks during recovery from traumatic brain injury. *PLoS One.* doi: 10.1371/journal.pone.0170541.

[28] McCrimmon, A. W. and Smith, A. D. (2013) Review of the Wechsler Abbreviated Scale of Intelligence, Second Edition (WASI-II). *J. Psychoeduc. Assess.* 31, 337–341.

[29] Bean, J. (2011) Rey Auditory Verbal Learning Test, Rey AVLT. In *Encyclopedia of Clinical Neuropsychology* (Kreutzer, J. S. et al., eds), pp. 2174–2175, Springer New York.

[30] Khosravi Fard, E., Jennifer L Keelor, Alireza Akbarzadeh Bagheban, Robert W Keith. (2016) Comparison of the Rey Auditory Verbal Learning Test (RAVLT) and Digit Test among Typically Achieving and Gifted Students. *Iran. J. child Neurol.* 10, 26–37.

[31] Sargénius, H. L., Bylsma, F. W., Lydersen, S., & Hestad, K. (2017) Visual-Constructional Ability in Individuals with Severe Obesity: Rey Complex Figure Test Accuracy and the Q-Score. *Front. Psychol.* 8, 1629.

[32] Gray, R. (2006) Comprehensive Trail Making Test. *J. Psychoeduc. Assess.* 24, 88–91.

[33] Beratis, I. N., Andronas, N., Fragkiadaki, S., Kontaxopoulou, D., Pavlou, D., Papantoniou, P., Stamelou, M., Stefanis, L., Yannis, G., & Papageorgiou, S. G. (2018) Exploring the association of the Comprehensive Trail Making Test with driving indexes in patients with Parkinson's disease. *Transp. Res. Part F Traffic Psychol. Behav.* 59, 535–544.

[34] Kolakowsky-Hayner, S. A. (2011) Wisconsin Card Sorting Test. In *Encyclopedia of Clinical Neuropsychology* (Kreutzer, J. S. et al., eds), pp. 2719–2720, Springer New York.

[35] Bharath, R. D., Munivenkatappa, A., Gohel, S., Panda, R., Saini, J., Rajeswaran, J., Shukla, D., Bhagavatula, I. D., & Biswal, B. B. (2015) Recovery of resting brain connectivity ensuing mild traumatic brain injury. *Front. Hum. Neurosci.* 9, 513.

[36] DeSerisy, M., Ramphal, B., Pagliaccio, D., Raffanello, E., Tau, G., Marsh, R., Posner, J., & Margolis, A. E. (2021) Frontoparietal and default mode network connectivity varies with age and intelligence. *Dev. Cogn. Neurosci.* 48, 100928.

[37] Shumskaya, E., van Gerven, M. A. J., Norris, D. G., Vos, P. E., & Kessels, R. P. C. (2017) Abnormal connectivity in the sensorimotor network predicts attention deficits in traumatic brain injury. *Exp. Brain Res.* 235, 799–807.

[38] Rektor, I., Tomčík, J., Mikl, M., Mareček, R., Brázdil, M., & Rektorová, I. (2013) Association between the basal ganglia and large-scale brain networks in epilepsy. *Brain Topogr.* 26, 355–362.

[39] Li, J., Curley, W. H., Guerin, B., Dougherty, D. D., Dalca, A. V., Fischl, B., Horn, A., & Edlow, B. L. (2021) Mapping the subcortical connectivity of the human default mode network. *Neuroimage* 245.

[40] Vatansever, D., Manktelow, A. E., Sahakian, B. J., Menon, D. K., & Stamatakis, E. A. (2016) Cognitive Flexibility: A Default Network and Basal Ganglia Connectivity Perspective. *Brain Connect.* 6, 201–207.

[41] Karten, A., Pantazatos, S. P., Khalil, D., Zhang, X., & Hirsch, J. (2013) Dynamic Coupling Between the Lateral Occipital-Cortex, Default-Mode, and Frontoparietal Networks During Bistable Perception. *Brain Connect.* 3, 286–293.

[42] Kaltiainen, H., Liljeström, M., Helle, L., Salo, A., Hietanen, M., Renvall, H., & Forss, N. (2019) Mild traumatic brain injury affects cognitive processing and modifies oscillatory brain activity during attentional tasks. *J. Neurotrauma* 36, 2222–2232.

[43] Patel, A., Grace Marie Nicole R. Biso, James B. Fowler. (2021) Neuroanatomy, Temporal Lobe. *StatPearls* at https://www.ncbi.nlm.nih.gov/books/NBK519512.

[44] Moini, J. and Piran, P. (2020) *Cerebral cortex.*

Chapter 7

A Review on the Effect of Deep Breathing Exercises on Stress Reduction

G. Sridevi[*], PhD
Department of Physiology, SRM Dental College and Hospital,
Chennai, Tamil Nadu, India

Abstract

Breathing is a subconscious phenomenon that needs to be accurately regulated. Improper breathing patterns can lead to improper exchange of oxygen and carbon dioxide transport at the alveolar level. There are two types of breathing patterns: Diaphragmatic (abdominal) breathing and Thoracic (chest) breathing. Chest breathing is characterized by an upward and outward movement of the chest wall. Abdominal Breathing is purely a diaphragmatic breathing; the diaphragm moves down and flattens, sucking the air into the lungs during inspiration and the diaphragm moves down pushing the abdominal wall out during expiration. Deep Breathing exercises are techniques that can help a person to relax, and to make a person feel comfortable. Deep breathing exercise is one of the effective and best ways to reduce the stress level in the body. Breathing exercises in the form laughter, paced breathing, abdominal breathing, yoga breathing is found to be beneficial. Deep breathing exercises are a part of relaxation strategy. It calms down the mind and balances your hormones- lowering down cortisol levels, increasing endorphin rush in the body. It helps to give a better sleep-in case of insomnia. Stress may invoke many cardiovascular problems, anxiety depression, immunosuppression and many pathological changes in the body. Deep breathing is considered as one of the best ways to lower

[*] Corresponding Author's Email: sridevig.sdc@saveetha.com.

In: Horizons in Neuroscience Research. Volume 48
Editors: Andres Costa and Eugenio Villalba
ISBN: 979-8-88697-230-6
© 2022 Nova Science Publishers, Inc.

stress in the body. They encourage full oxygen exchange at lung and tissue level and also it is a beneficial import and export of incoming oxygen for outgoing carbon dioxide. This effect can slow the heartbeat and lower or stabilize blood pressure.

Keywords: deep breathing exercises, types, stress reduction

Introduction

Breathing is a very essential process that the body undergoes for the survival of an organism. During the process of breathing, the air containing the essential nutrient oxygen is inhaled and the waste product carbon di oxide is exhaled out of the lungs. Breathing is a subconscious phenomenon that need to be accurately regulated. Improper breathing patterns can lead to improper exchange of oxygen and carbon do oxide transport at the alveolar level. This improper oxygenation can lead to anxiety related disturbances, panic attacks, physical and emotional disorders [1].

Ventilation is a process of air movement in and out of the lungs and is considered as a precise modality that takes into account significant markers of gas exchange like PaO_2, $PaCO_2$, and pH. Maintenance of accurate control on the proper ventilation is regulated by central respiratory pacemaker cells present in the dorsal respiratory group of neurons (DRGN) from the medulla oblongata of the brain stem. Motor efferents from the DRGN supply the inspiratory muscles of respiration and regulate the inspiratory ramp signal. This signal stops inspiration and expiration occurs passively. Thus, the respiratory rhythmic pattern is controlled by the DRGN, but these neurons are indirectly controlled by the pontine centre called the Pneumotaxic centre. Thus, adjustments in ventilation like the rate of breathing, length and duration of breath, and intensity of neural impulses from the pacemaker are controlled and properly executed [2].

Disturbances in Breathing Patterns

The variations in respiratory rate and altered patterns of breathing are associated with variety of disease patterns and diseased states. It also alters the feed-back patterns controlled by the central respiratory centres and significantly alters the PaO_2, $PaCO_2$, or pH. The alterations might lead to acute hypoxaemia with PaO_2 lower than 55 to 60 mm Hg, increased $PaCO_2$, and lowered pH. This stimulates the chemoreceptors and causes significant and rapid changes in minute ventilation. But if the improper ventilation continues, it can lead to elevated $PaCO_2$, CO_2 narcosis that can cause depression of the respiratory centers of the medulla. It also causes metabolic acidosis with a drop in pH and kussmaul breathing resulting from ketoacidosis in diabetes mellitus [2].

There are two types of breathing patterns: Diaphragmatic (abdominal) breathing and Thoracic (chest) breathing. Chest breathing is characterised by an upward and outward movement of the chest wall. This type of breathing occurs during vigorous exercise, or emergency situations. Thoracic breathing can disturb the pattern of breathing, improper oxygenation, decreased carbon di oxide elimination, increased muscle tension, dizziness and tachycardia. Abdominal Breathing is purely a diaphragmatic breathing the diaphragm moves down and flattens sucking the air into the lungs during inspiration and the diaphragm moves down pushing the abdominal wall out during expiration. Abdominal (diaphragmatic) breathing is the most effectual way of breathing air into the lungs. This breathing can reduce the heartbeat and can also stabilize the blood pressure [3].

Simple breathing exercises: A simple relaxation exercise consists of two important aspects: Step 1: Inhale a slow and deep breath through the nose in such a way the abdomen should expand and chest should raise. Step 2: Exhale slowly through the mouth. Keep the lips pursed and jaw relaxed while expiration. Repeat these two steps for several minutes [4].

Benefits of Deep Breathing Exercises

Deep breathing exercises significantly relieves pain and triggers the release of endorphins, increases the energy caused by good oxygenation of blood, lowers the blood pressure, heart rate and improves circulation, improves digestion, maintenance of correct posture, decreases the stress levels.

Stress and Anxiety

Stress is a state of physical and mental exhaustion that produces profound effects on the body. The stress hormone cortisol causes significant changes like tachycardia, hypertension and ischemic heart diseases, weakened immune system, hyperglycemia, heart burns, insomnia, fertility problems, missed periods, tensed muscles. Deep controlled breathing can calm the mind and maintain it in good-relaxed state and shape. It can also reduce the BP and reduce anxiety. It also promotes a feeling of calmness, relaxes the mind and thereby relieves stress.

The different types of breathing exercised are mindful breathing, square breathing, mantra breathing, pranayama breathing and nostril breathing. Mindful breathing is a type where a person is always aware of the breath and it is a slow pattern of breathing that makes a person relaxed. Meditation procedures that incorporate mindfulness have been useful to reduce stress, anxiety, depression and other negative emotions. Square breathing is a technique that creates a focus on visualization of one side of a square. Mantra breathing is a technique that focusses on breath using mantras. This technique relaxes the person and helps in meditation. Pranayama breathing uses the practice of yoga as a power to cleanse the body. It uses the technique to inhale with mouth closed and exhale through the nose. This method allows good clean oxygen for the heart and brain. Nostril breathing is a technique to breathe in with one nostril closed and take in air slowly and then switch off closing the second nostril and continue breathing through the first nostril. This method reduces anxiety, irritation and agitation [5]. Yoga breathing is another technique that relaxes the mind and can be used anytime to help with a relaxation response, including when stretching during yoga. This technique works to tune in to the way breath is taken. Inhale and exhale naturally through the nose for a few minutes, noticing the slight rise and fall of the hands [5].

Stress Management and Breathing Exercises

Deep Breathing exercises are techniques that can help a person to relax, and to make a person feel comfortable. Deep breathing exercise is one of the effective and best ways to reduce the stress level in the body. This is because when you take a deep breath, it carries impulses to the brain and reduces the anxiety and calms down and relax. Breath focus is an important feature of many techniques that evoke the relaxation response. Deep breathing is the keystone of several relaxation protocols that is usually combined with other relaxing therapies like aromatherapy and music, etc.

Types of Deep Breathing Exercises for Stress Reduction

Stress is a physiological condition that disrupts the homeostasis of the body affecting all the organ systems of the body like central nervous system, cardiovascular system and musculoskeletal system. The cause of stress and stress related diseases may be multiple but stress reduction protocols would help to overcome the stress. One such protocol is deep breathing exercises for stress reduction.

Laughter

Laughter is an efficient and stronger medicine that can influence and induce a healthy physical condition and psychological changes in the body. Laughter is a technique that boosts mood, diminishes pain, strengthens immune system and protects from damaging effects of stress. This technique lightens burdens that created the stress, gives good connectivity, makes us focused and alert, reduces anger and promotes sense of forgiveness. It triggers the release of endorphins and promotes a good sense of well-being and can even relieve pain temporarily [6].

Paced Breathing

Paced Breathing is a method that helps to activate mechanisms that cause stress reduction in the body. It promotes a harmonious state to prevail between the respiration system and cardiovascular system. This technique involves inhalation for 2-4 seconds and exhalation for 4-6 seconds. The method focuses the attention on a specific object or image and even sound to avoid distractions and maintain concentration. If there is difficulty in concentration, the mind is redirected to focus back on counting and breathing [7].

Abdominal Breathing

This Technique is an automatic type of breathing. This technique creates a good feeling of calm composure, renews the energy processes and brings a better focus. The procedure involves sitting with one hand on the chest and other hand on the belly, a deep breath is taken in through the nose is such a way the diaphragm alone inflates with enough air so as to create a stretch in the lungs. Exhalation is done slowly through pursed lips. The process is repeated for next 3 times. This follows for 6-10 deep, slow breaths per minute for 2-3 minutes [7].

Yoga Breathing

Yoga breathing is a relaxation technique that can be used to help to create calmness to mind and relaxation and is done during stretching while performing yoga. The person is made to sit comfortably resting the hands below the navel and inhale and exhale normally through the nose for a few minutes and observing the slight rise and fall of your hands while breathing. Consider the way the air feels as it enters and exits your nostrils. Counting is done silently as 1 2 3 and then backwards ass 3 2 1 during inspiration and expiration. The expiration is made such that exhalation is twice as long as each inhalation and exhalation must be slow and smooth [7].

4-4-8 Breathing

The 4-4-8 Breathing technique is a good and efficient procedure for stress relaxation and creates calmness to the mind during periods of stress and helps to avoid distractions and gives a soothing effect on brain. The procedure involves a sitting position and breathe in through the nostrils for a count of 4, taking good air into the lungs, hold the breath for a count of 4 and release the breath through mouth for a count of 8 with a whooshing sound. Again immediately without a break, breath is taken in again for a count of 4. The process is repeated for the entire technique for 3-4 times in a row. During the whole process, focusing on counting when breathing in, holding the breath, and breathing out is carried out [7].

Psychological stress is considered as an important and major risk factor progression of diseases like cardiovascular disease, cancer, arthritis, and major depression. So a study led by Valentina Perciavalle 2016, used samples of 38 university students Experimental Group (N = 19) and the Control Group (N = 19) to assess the effect of relaxing technique called deep breathing as a stress Intervention Functional protocol to reduce the perceived stress and improve the mood. Subjects (aged between 18 and 28 years) volunteered the study. Ten treatment sessions of Anti-stress Protocol, each lasting 90 mins for the experimental groups and Control Group sat ten times for 90 min, once per week, without following any treatment. The psychological assessment of the subjects by measurement of Psychological Stress (MSP) and Profile of Mood State (POMS) and autonomic functional status of mind was detected by measuring the heart rate and biological stress assessment was done by determining salivary cortisol. The results of the study revealed that deep breathing techniques has proved to be effective in improving the mood and stress by improving MPS and POMS and improvement in objective parameters, such as heart rate and salivary cortisol levels [8].

Another study investigated the effect of diaphragmatic breathing on cognition, affect, and cortisol responses to stress. Forty participants were assigned randomly as a control group and breathing intervention group. The breathing intervention group underwent breathing training for 8 weeks in 20 sessions using a real-time feedback device. The average respiratory rate of 4 breaths/min was assigned. The control group did not receive this treatment. All participants completed pre- and post-tests with good concentration and attention. Also, the stress indicators pre and post-test salivary cortisol concentrations were determined in both groups. The results of the study showed that breathing intervention group showed a significant decrease in negative affect caused by stress compared to baseline. Breathing intervention showed significant and increased sustained attention after breathing training when compared to baseline. Breathing intervention also significantly lowered the cortisol levels after training and control group did not show any significant change in cortisol levels [9].

A research study by Singh et al., 2017 [10] investigated the effect of slow and deep voluntary breathing exercise blood pressure both systolic as well as diastolic. Regular practice of breathing exercise (Pranayama) on increases parasympathetic tone, decreases sympathetic activity and simultaneously improves cardiovascular and respiratory functions. It also decreases the effects of stress and strain on the body and improves the physical and mental health. This study was done to find out the effect of simple slow and deep voluntary breathing on body and mind which was evaluated by recording blood pressure (BP) with the help of sphygmomanometer and stethoscope. The study involved healthy volunteers from Nepal Medical College and Teaching Hospital in the age group 18-25 years. The breathing technique used Sukhasan where the person was made to sit in a steady posture with head, neck and trunk erect in a straight line and the person takes slow deep inspiration followed by slow deep expiration for 5 minutes at approximately 4 times per minute. BP was recorded using a sphygmomanometer and stethoscope were used to measure blood pressure. The results showed a significant reduction in systolic as well as diastolic blood pressure 5 minutes post slow deep voluntary breathing exercise. The decrease of diastolic blood pressure and mean blood pressure were significant [10].

Deep Breathing Exercises - A Part of Relaxation Strategy

Mindfulness exercises based on deep breathing are a part of relaxation exercises. These techniques that use mindfulness skills have originated from Buddhist meditation practices. It has been reviewed and used by many psychologists and physicians in recent decades. These techniques helps a person to regulate his emotions and calm his mind. The technique involves sitting quietly with your feet on the floor or take a lying position and relax the body. The person is asked to begin slow, diaphragmatic breathing. The mind is must focus on the breath as air flows in and out of your nostrils. This technique is continued for a period as long as the person is able to do. During this time the mind might wander a memory or a worry or it may ger distracted with an itch or pain. Gently the person is asked to remind those distractions later and focus the mind on breathing. This technique can be followed for 10 minutes.

The breathing pattern followed during relaxation protocols is a "Slow Diaphragmatic Breathing". In a sitting position or lying a person can fold his hands on the belly and a normal breath is taken slowly and calmly in such a way the belly is filled up with a normal breath. Breathing must be slowly paced but not heavily. Also that while breathing lifting the shoulders during inhalation should be avoided. This is followed by an expiration for a count of 5 and after exhalation hold for 2-3 seconds before inhaling again. The speed of the breath is considered as more important compared to the depth of breathing [11].

How Do Deep Breathing Exercises Reduce Stress

The term stress is a "fight or flight" response that prepares a person to confront or avoid danger. Stress may invoke many cardiovascular problems, anxiety depression, immune-suppression and many pathological changes in the body.

Deep breathing is considered as one of the best ways to lower stress in the body. The reason being breathing deeply sends a message to the brain to calm down and relax. The brain in turn sends this message to your body. Deep abdominal breathing exercises encourages a full oxygen exchange at lung level and tissue levels and it is a beneficial import and export of incoming oxygen for outgoing carbon dioxide. This effect can slow the heartbeat and lower or stabilize blood pressure. Also, That Breath focus is a common feature of several techniques that evoke the relaxation response. So getting a breath focus, helps to keep the mind away from distractions and diversions [12]. A study by Hayama et al. 2012 [13] showed a reduction of 'tension anxiety' and fatigue through the use of deep breathing [13]. Another esystematic reviewed the development of stress in dental students and the intervention of deep breathing exercises significantly improved the mental state of the students [14].

Proper deep breathing allows air to enter all areas of the lungs. This breathing improves chest expansion and strengthens the chest wall muscles. This type of breathing increases the alveolar ventilation and improves oxygenated of the blood at the alveolar level. These breathing exercises also helps to decrease your rate of breathing, pain, and risk for lung infections. It is also recommended that breathing exercises can be practiced 5-10 times, three times each day. The more the practice of deep breathing exercise, the more natural it would be and improves the mind and body's internal rhythm.

Deep Breathing Exercises - A Part of Chest Physiotherapy

The Active Cycle of Breathing Techniques are used by a physiotherapist that helps to clear sputum from your chest. ACBT is a set of breathing exercises loosen and moves the sputum from your airways. These exercises are best taught by a physiotherapist and used with postural drainage to clear the sputum from the airways. The ACBT exercises also helps for breathing control, deep breathing and huffing which are performed in a cycle until the chest becomes clear. Breathing control can also help you when you are short of breath or feeling fearful, anxious or in a panic [6].

Deep breathing exercises act as Natural painkillers that help the body to release endorphins, and act as natural pain killer created by the body itself. It also improves blood flow and helps to remove the toxins from the body promoting better blood flow. It also improves immunity and ensures smoother functioning of your vital organs, including the immune system. A cleaner, toxin-free and healthier blood supply help ward off infection-causing germs from the base and strengthens your immunity. Deep breathing also functions to relieve toxins from the body. It also causes good absorption of vitamins as well as essential nutrients in the body and recovers the body to a normal state. It calms down the mind and also balances your hormones - lowering down cortisol levels, increasing endorphin rush in the body. It helps to give a better sleep in cases of insomnia. It increases the energy level due to increased blood flow and better oxygenation. It also improves the posture of the trunk. It Stimulates lymphatic system to have a good flow. Shallow breathing can lead to a sluggish lymphatic system which will not detoxify properly. Deep breathing will help you get the lymph flowing properly so that your body can work more efficiently. Dee breathing improves digestion and make the visceral system function effectively. The increased blood flow due to deep breathing also encourages intestinal action which further improves your overall digestion. In addition, deep breathing results in a calmer nervous system, which in turn also enhances optimal digestion [7].

Conclusion

Thus researchers reported that the use of deep breathing techniques has led to an effective improvement in the management of stress in our daily life. It could also exert positive impacts on the stress conditions that every person had to face during the entire course of his life. In the present scenario with the increased risk of COVID-19 infection, it is important to be proactive in maintaining a healthy and clear chest by completing regular breathing exercises.

References

[1] Paulus MP. The breathing conundrum-interoceptive sensitivity and anxiety. *Depress. Anxiety*. 2013;30(4):315-320. doi:10.1002/da.22076.

[2] Braun SR. Respiratory Rate and Pattern. In: Walker HK, Hall WD, Hurst JW, editors. *Clinical Methods: The History, Physical, and Laboratory Examinations*. 3rd edition. Boston: Butterworths; 1990. Chapter 43. Available from: https://www.ncbi.nlm.nih.gov/books/NBK365/.

[3] https://www.google.com/search?q=two+types+of+breathing&oq=TWO+TYPES+OF+BREATHING&aqs=chrome.0.0i457j0l2j0i395l2j0i22i30i395l5.5188j1j7&sourceid=chrome&ie=UTF-8.

[4] Cleaveland Clinic. *Diaphragmatic breathing*; 2018.

[5] https://homecareassistance.com/e-books/ultimate-guide-self-care/mindful-breathing-can-achieve-tremendous-health-benefits.

[6] https://www.helpguide.org/articles/mental-health/laughter-is-the-best-medicine.htm.

[7] https://uhs.berkeley.edu/sites/default/files/breathing_exercises_0.pdf.

[8] Perciavalle, Valentina & Blandini, Marta & Fecarotta, Paola & Buscemi, Andrea & Di Corrado, Donatella & Bertolo, Luana & Fichera, Fulvia & Coco, Marinella. (2017). The role of deep breathing on stress. *Neurological Sciences*. 38. 451-458. 10.1007/s10072-016-2790-8.

[9] Xio Ma X, Yue ZQ, Gong ZQ, Zhang, H., Duan, N-Y., Shi, Y-T., Wei, G-X. And Li, Y-F. The Effect of Diaphragmatic Breathing on Attention, Negative Affect and Stress in Healthy Adults. *Front. Psychol*. 2017;8: 874. Published 2017 Jun 6. doi:10.3389/fpsyg.2017.00874.

[10] Singh S, Katwal B, Panta PP, Slow and Deep Breathing Exercise (Pranayama) For a Stress Free Life amongst Medical Students. *International Journal of Research & Review*. 2017; 67 Vol. 4; Issue: 7:67-71.

[11] https://www.webmd.com/balance/stress-management/stress-relief-breathing-techniques.

[12] https://www.health.harvard.edu/mind-and-mood/relaxation-techniques-breath-control-helps-quell-errant-stress-response.

[13] Hayama Y, Inoue T (2012) The effects of deep breathing on 'tensione-anxiety' and fatigue in cancer patients undergoing adjuvant chemotherapy. *Complement. Ther. Clin. Pract.* 18:94-98.

[14] Abdullah MA, Van der Molen HT, Alauja AH, De Boer BJ (2014) Stress management in dental students: a systematic review. *Adv. Med. Educ. Pract.* 5:176. doi: 10.2147/AMEP.S46211 doi:10.1016/j.ctcp.2011.10.001.

Chapter 8

Aspirin (Acetylsalicylic Acid) in Neurosurgical Patients: Benefits and Risks for Cranial and Spinal Surgeries

Giorgio Mantovani, MD,
Pasquale De Bonis, MD, PhD
and Alba Scerrati*, MD
Department of Translational Medicine, University of Ferrara, Ferrara, Italy;
Department of Neurosurgery, Sant'Anna University Hospital, Ferrara, Italy

Abstract

Aspirin has always represented a sword of Damocles for surgeons, especially for neurosurgeons. On one hand, its discontinuation could be dangerous for patients with a high thromboembolic risk; on the other hand, its antiplatelets effects could significantly increase the risk of intra or post-procedural bleedings.

In this chapter we will review the main evidence in literature in order to better understand and define the risks for patients undergoing neurosurgical procedures and taking aspirin.

We will describe most common neurosurgical procedures, elective or in emergency, summarizing the most important and recent literature evidence about the topic.

We will also try to collect and describe data not only about the hemorrhagic risk, but also about the thrombo-embolic one.

We hope this chapter will constitute a practical guide for everyday practice in neurosurgery.

---

* Corresponding Author's Email: scrlba@unife.it.

In: Horizons in Neuroscience Research. Volume 48
Editors: Andres Costa and Eugenio Villalba
ISBN: 979-8-88697-230-6
© 2022 Nova Science Publishers, Inc.

Keywords: aspirin, acetylsalicylic acid, neurosurgery, cranial surgery, spinal surgery, bleeding risk, thromboembolic risk, cardiovascular risk, cerebral hemorrhage, traumatic brain injury

Introduction: Neurosurgery and Antithrombotics

Aspirin (aka Acetil-Salicilic Acid, ASA) management is a daily well-known dilemma for every neurosurgeon, both in elective and emergency settings. Indications for low-dose ASA (75 to 100 mg, but most commonly 81 mg) have expanded through the last decades, including but not limited, to primary prevention in high cardio/cerebro-vascular risk patients, secondary prevention in ischemic myocardial infarction, TIA and stroke, central or peripheral vascular disease. Meta-analysis on large population demonstrate that aspirin is effective in reducing myocardial infarction and major vascular events (Collaboration et al. 2009). The Antithrombotic Trialists' Collaboration in 2002 reported: "*reduced [...] outcome of any serious vascular event by about 1/4; non-fatal myocardial infarction by 1/3, non-fatal stroke by 1/4, and vascular mortality by 1/6, with antiplatelet therapy, of which aspirin was the most studied*" (Antithrombotic Trialists' Collaboration 2002). But its use in the surgical patient raises some concerns.

On one hand, ASA is believed to increase the hemorrhagic complications rate among neurosurgical patients, in which a sudden occupying lesion such as a hematoma could lead to tremendous consequences. For this reason, it should be stopped several days before the surgery (classically 5 to 7).

On the other hand, stopping a chronic ASA therapy could expose the patient to an increased risk for ischemic or thromboembolic acute events. In fact, myocardial infarction is the most common major vascular complication that occurs after noncardiac surgery (Devereaux et al. 2014). For this reason, in these kind of patients, ASA should be continued.

Other fields of non-cardiac surgery (*in primis* thoracic and abdominal) already investigated the issue and collected high-level evidence about the management of ASA in the perioperative period.

A large meta-analysis on 49.590 patients concluded that the risk of bleeding complications with aspirin therapy was increased by 50%, but that aspirin did not lead to greater severity of bleeding complications (Burger et al. 2005).

The POISE-2 trial (Devereaux et al. 2014) randomized 10.010 patients undergoing non-cardiac surgery to aspirin or placebo in the perioperative period, and concluded that aspirin did not significantly reduce mortality or nonfatal myocardial infarction but did increase the risk of major bleeding. It is uncertain whether patients with a low perioperative bleeding risk and a high risk of thrombo-embolic events could benefit from low-dose aspirin.

Indeed, and this is our point, neurosurgical patients are routinely excluded from these studies. one of the exclusion criteria of POISE-2 trial was a patient "*undergoing intracranial surgery, carotid endarterectomy, or retinal surgery.*" ESC/ESA 2014 Guidelines on non-cardiac surgery generally stated that "*For patients undergoing spinal surgery or certain neurosurgical or ophthalmological operations, it is recommended that aspirin be discontinued for at least seven days*" ("2014 ESC/ESA Guidelines on Non-Cardiac Surgery: Cardiovascular Assessment and Management: The Joint Task Force on Non-Cardiac Surgery: Cardiovascular Assessment and Management of the European Society of Cardiology (ESC) and the European Society of Anaesthesiology (ESA)" 2014).

ASA (and more generally antiplatelet drugs) management in neurosurgical patients is still a controversial and debated argument, since a clear and shared recommendation, based on high-quality scientific evidence, lacks. Literature mainly provides fragmented data, indirectly derived from studies not specifically designed for the scope. Reviews and meta-analysis rarely conclude with clear indications. Perhaps the only clear and evident principle is that a general and common rule doesn't exists, and it's not possible to manage all the situations in the same way. Clinical management of aspirin therapy has to be driven by the accurate *in toto* evaluation of the patient physiology and pathology, balancing risk and benefit.

In this chapter we provide a brief description of the main neurosurgical procedures, both elective or emergent, and the main current literature about aspirin management in these settings, in order to compose a practical basis for everyday clinical decisions.

Intracerebral Hemorrhages

Spontaneous

Intracerebral hemorrhage (ICH) of spontaneous (non- traumatic) origin has an estimated annual incidence of 12 to 15 per 100 000 in the USA, with a 30-day mortality approximately of 40–50% (Zahuranec et al. 2006), and many survivors remain severely disabled for the rest of life (Mendelow et al. 2013). ICH accounts for 11-22% of strokes and half of all stroke deaths (Feigin et al. 2015). Clinical manifestations of a lobar non traumatic ICH (the most frequent case) range from none to rapid death, based on localization and size of the hematoma.

There are some evidences that people assuming aspirin have an increased risk of developing an ICH (Collaboration et al. 2009) and a worst prognosis after the event compared with patients not taking any antithrombotics (Thompson et al. 2010). On the other side, in the setting of a high-income country, more than a quarter of patients with a lobar ICH assumes aspirin (Lovelock et al. 2007).

Most of cases don't require surgical intervention, and can be treated conservatively with medical therapy (Hemphill et al. 2015). Indications to surgery mainly regard clinical deterioration and midline shift (Hemphill et al. 2015); and surgery itself is intended as a life-saving procedure, seeing that its efficacy in achieving a better neurological outcome (compared to medical management) is unclear (Hemphill et al. 2015).

The effect of antiplatelet therapy on the onset and course of an ICH is still to determine, since different trials found conflicting results, and often were not specifically designed for aspirin.

Antiplatelet agent use was not associated with ICH expansion or clinical outcome (Sansing et al. 2009), but, on the other hand, altered platelet function measured by laboratory assessment has been linked to early clot growth and 3-months outcome (Naidech et al. 2009).

Platelet transfusion is effective in restoring platelet function (Naidech et al. 2012) and, in patient with high risk of clot growth, is associated with smaller final hemorrhage if administered within 12 hours from symptom onset. Thus, platelet transfusion cannot be recommended for routine use in ICH patients: a prospective RCT (PATCH) (Baharoglu et al. 2016)) demonstrated that platelet transfusion in people using antiplatelet therapy with an acute spontaneous primary ICH is associated with a worst outcome in terms of death or dependence at three months.

Traumatic

Traumatic Brain Injury (TBI) incidence is estimated at 235 per 100,000 people every year (Greuter et al. 2019), of which 80% are considered mild (MTIB; GCS 14-15). TBI is the most common single system injury resulting in death worldwide (Moore, Pasquale, & Badellino 2012), and it affects especially young adult and people older than 65.

2-3% of MTBI will subsequently deteriorate because of ischemic-hemorrhagic complications, resulting in severe neurological deficit (Moore, Pasquale, & Badellino 2012). Anticoagulation and antiplatelet therapies have been often advocated as main risk factors for TBI progression, combined with the classic elements of an aging brain: atrophy with larger spaces for blood to accumulate, reduced compliance of the intracranial content, general sensory-motor impairment in maintaining posture and preventing trauma.

Clinical management of a MTBI patient taking aspirin, and more in general antiplatelet drugs, is often complicated both on diagnostic and therapeutic side. One of the most known tools to decide if a patient needs a head CT scan for MTBI is the Canadian CT Head rule (Stiell et al. 2001). But, interestingly, aspirin (nor other therapy) isn't considered one of the decisional items, so this *clinical decision rule* can't provide help for this specific subtype of patients.

Instead, several guidelines on MTBI recommend an initial CT scan, upon arrival at the ED, in patients older than 65 *and* assuming antiplatelet (the Scandinavian Neurotrauma Committee (SNC) et al. 2013). Other guidelines, such as NICE ("Head Injury: Assessment and Early Management" 2019) or CDC ("Updated Mild Traumatic Brain Injury Guideline for Adults | Concussion | Traumatic Brain Injury | CDC Injury Center" 2021) doesn't include antiplatelet therapy in their flowcharts.

Overall, effect of antiplatelet on TBI patients prognosis is unclear: Peck et al. found a higher in-hospital mortality rate (Peck et al. 2014), but results are controversial and correlation specifically with antiplatelet is not clear (Narum et al. 2016). Conversely, Cull et al. (2015) found no difference in ICH, need for neurosurgical intervention or in hospital-mortality between patients taking antiplatelet therapy compared to standard population in a retrospective case-control study.

Since TBI is a dynamic and developing process, patient monitoring is crucial to promptly detect complications. Radiological monitoring with seriated CT scans has a significant cost burden, more cost-effective than treatments for a missed ICH or prolonged inpatient stay (Stein, Burnett, & Glick 2006). Scantling et al. (2017) demonstrated that a scheduled CT scan for elderly patients taking antiplatelet doesn't give clinical benefits, meaning that clinical observation is superior to radiological surveillance. Those cases in which a new ICH was observed at the scheduled CT didn't require any significant change in management. Interestingly, the majority of patients in this study was assuming aspirin (176/231).

Spektor et al. (2003) found that patients > 60 years old taking low-dose aspirin have no increased risk for ICH after MTBI compared to same-age patients without aspirin. At the multivariate analysis, they found that the most important predictor for ICH and the possible need for surgery was the clinical presentation at the emergency department. After a retrospective study on 793 patients, Antoni et al. (2019) furthermore concluded that in-hospital observation for head trauma patients using aspirin alone is not necessary due to the rarity of clinically relevant delayed ICH.

As previously stated, some patients will deteriorate clinically, thus requiring a surgical treatment. Moore et al. (Cull et al. 2015) found an increased overall risk for neurosurgical intervention and mortality in patients on antiplatelet at the moment of trauma, especially for those older than 65 year. Majority of patients were on Coumadin treatment, rather than aspirin.

Amongst the ones who underwent surgery, there were some evidences that aspirin doesn't play a significant prognostic role.

Greuter et al. (2019) conducted a prospective study on 143 patients undergoing craniotomy for TBI, examining association between post-operative bleedings complications and antiplatelet. They reported that antiplatelet group had a significant higher mean age, suffered more often from acute subdural hematoma (aSDH), showed larger hematoma volumes and larger extent of midline shift on preoperative imaging. Also, they determined that patients with hemorrhagic complications had a poorer prognosis, but, notably, antiplatelet therapy was not significantly associated with post-operative bleedings. They concluded that preoperative antiplatelet intake doesn't influence the rate of postoperative bleeding, outcome, or mortality in patients undergoing craniotomy due to TBI (Greuter et al. 2019).

Sturiale et al. (2012) didn't find associations between antiplatelet preoperative therapy and increasing in traumatic contusions size after decompressive craniectomy for refractory intracranial hypertension.

Han et al. (2016) stated that pre-TBI antiplatelet therapy (12/19 patients on antiplatelet were assuming aspirin) doesn't influence the rate of hemorrhagic complications and reoperation after decompressive craniectomy. Thus, they suggest that surgery shouldn't be delayed because of this therapy.

Acute Subdural Hematoma

Acute SDH (aSDH) complicates approximately 11% of mild to moderate TBIs and 20% of the severe ones (Al-Mufti & Mayer 2017), and it is more common in older patients (Bullock et al. 2006). A large majority of patients can be treated conservatively with good outcome, but from 6-10% will require evacuation surgery for raised intracranial pressure or SDH progression (Bajsarowicz et al. 2015).

Literature about aSDH and aspirin is particularly controversial, both on the surgical aspect (by mean if aspirin intake increases the necessity for surgical evacuation) and prognostic one (by mean if patients on aspirin have a worst general outcome).

Panczykowski et al. (Panczykowski & Okonkwo 2011) conducted a retrospective cohort study on 300 subjects and they concluded that premorbid antithrombotic therapy is not a significant risk factor for recurrence of aSDH necessitating additional evacuation. Moreover, history of antithrombotic assumption doesn't predict a major overall mortality. While premorbid use may predispose the patient to a SDH, the oral antithrombotic does not increase the risk of morbidity or mortality following surgical intervention. Among antiplatelets, aspirin was the more common (27%).

Bajsarowicz et al. (2015) stated that blood thinners (not specified) are not a significant risk factor for aSDH clinical deterioration, thus requiring surgery in an otherwise medically managed case.

Robinson et al. (2021) performed a case-control study (n=305) analyzing data from patients with an early (<72 h from injury) or delayed (>72 h from injury) aSDH expansion compared to those with stable aSDH. All were initially clinically managed. They found that antiplatelet use (not specifically aspirin) is not a risk factor for early expansion, neither its resumption is a risk factors for delayed ones.

On the other hand, Baraniskin et al. (2014) found that antiplatelet therapy is independently associated with recurrence of aSDH and in-hospital death.

Akamatsu et al. (2017) determined also that antiplatelet is associated with delayed aSDH evacuation, thus recommending careful monitoring of hematoma progression in those patients, for more than a week.

Interestingly, it is not possible in these trials to separate data on aspirin-only patients, and this aspect could explain such heterogeneity in similarly designed studies.

Chronic Subdural Hematoma

Chronic Subdural Hematoma (cSDH) is among the most common neurosurgical entities, daily present in clinical practice. Described for the first time in 1657 by Johannes Wepfer, its incidence is estimated nowadays in 1–5.3 in every 100,000 individuals (Tamura et al. 2021), more common in older population with (but not necessarily) a previous history of mTBI.

Literature regarding cSDH is vast and articulate, and some interesting data specifically regarding aspirin emerge.

Intuitively, it was previously believed that aspirin is a major risk factor for cSDH development, by facilitating blood extravasation after minimal vessel injury. De Bonis et al. (2013) recently gave evidence of this relationship in a large retrospective study: anticoagulant and antiplatelet therapies (18.3% patients on Cox inhibitors) have a significant association with an increased risk of developing CSDH.

Perioperative management of aspirin in cSDH patients still lacks guidelines regarding stopping, resumption, prognosis.

Kamenova et al. demonstrated in a series of studies specifically on this topic that:

- There is a comparable recurrence rates with and without discontinuation of aspirin in patients undergoing burr-hole drainage for cSDH (Kamenova et al. 2017). This evidence is confirmed by Scerrati et al. (2019) who showed that timing of aspirin discontinuation before surgery doesn't influence the clinical outcome. Also Baraniskin (Baraniskin et al. 2014) didn't find association between antiplatelet and recurrence rate of cSDH or in-hospital mortality. Notably, Raghavan et al. (2020) found a significant association between aspirin and increased 30-day mortality for patients treated with craniotomy (and not for burr-hole craniostomy) for cSDH.
- Early resumption of aspirin after burr-hole surgery is not associated with a higher recurrence rate compared with later resumption (Kamenova, Lutz, et al. 2016). Specifically: aspirin resumption is associated with a tendency toward a higher recurrence rate before post-op day 42 (not statistically significant) but there is no difference in the time this resumption takes place. The authors suggest that before aspirin treatment is resumed, its indication should be carefully

evaluated. If there are no clear indications for primary or secondary prevention of major cardiovascular events, aspirin should not be resumed. Finally, considering these results, aspirin could be safely resumed earlier for secondary prevention cases, in which it has demonstrated more clearly its efficacy. Phan et al. (2018), in their meta-analysis, confirmed this findings and stated that in selected patients antiplatelet therapy could be early resumed without additional hemorrhagic risk.

Intracranial Tumors

Postoperative intracranial hemorrhages can have tremendous consequences, as said earlier. These kinds of hemorrhages could also occur post-operatively after surgery for tumor resection. So, antithrombotic therapy in this setting is feared by every neurosurgeon. In 2006 a survey conducted in German neurosurgical facilities (M. C. Korinth 2006) showed that 75% of surgeons felt aspirin as a significant risk factor for post-craniotomy bleedings and 70.3% of them used some counteracting measures. Palmer et al. (Palmer, Sparrow, & Iannotti 1994) previously found that antithrombotic (aspirin, dipyridamole and non-steroidal anti-inflammatory) was the risk factor for bleedings in 43% of his patients.

Literature about the specific topic is sparse and of low-quality considering the ethical difficulty in conducting this kind of RCT. Main data come from retrospective studies on patients who couldn't interrupt aspirin preoperatively due to absolute cardiovascular contraindications. The obvious bias is that, in these cases, the risk of interrupting aspirin with a high grade of presumption overthrow the benefits, and this in conclusion doesn't completely clarify the decisional process for patients at intermediate risk.

To date, the largest retrospective study is from Hanalioglu et al. (2019). They collected data from 1291 patients treated with elective craniotomy for brain tumor. Of them, 1068 did not take aspirin, 104 stopped it before surgery and 119 never stopped it because of high cardiovascular risk. The analysis didn't find association between aspirin and blood loss, increased hemorrhagic or thromboembolic complications rate. The authors conclude that in patients at high cardiovascular risk, aspirin could be safely continued in the perioperative period for elective craniotomy for tumor surgery, together with a careful surgical hemostasis technique and good post-operative vital parameters control.

Similarly, Rahman et al. (2015) analyzed data from 452 patients, of which 28 never interrupt aspirin. They concluded that aspirin assumption is not a risk factor for perioperative complications, namely bleeding complications, need for reoperation, or thrombotic ones.

In a case series of 15 patients, Ogawa at al (Ogawa & Tominaga 2015) found that there were no differences in intraoperative bleeding and operative time between patients on antithrombotic (aspirin was the commonest) therapy and controls treated with trans-sphenoidal endoscopic surgeries.

Spinal Surgery

The relationship between aspirin and spinal surgery has been more investigated, in comparison with other neurosurgical fields, even if some conflictual results emerge. Most of spinal procedures require muscular detachment, bone removal and screw placement, all of these potentially implying a considerable amount of blood loss. So, here the question becomes: is aspirin associated with and increased blood loss? The incidence of major blood loss (defined as greater than 25% of the patient's total blood volume) in spine surgery for fusion is estimated to be between 16% and 81% (Pauyo et al. 2017). Moreover, similarly to the brain, hematoma collection in the closed epidural space could lead to severe neurological deficits, up to para/tetraplegia.

A 2006 survey on 210 German neurosurgery facilities explored the perception surgeons had about spinal patients under aspirin therapy (Marcus C. Korinth, Gilsbach, & Weinzierl 2007). 66.2% of responders felt that those patients were at higher risk of hemorrhagic complications, and 51.4% reported having personal experience of such problems. The majority (65.5%) used some counteracting therapy with specific drugs, variously described.

Park et al. (Park, Kwon, & Woo 2014) retrospectively analyzed data from 100 patients who underwent surgery for postero-lateral lumbar fusion in 2014. They found that preoperative aspirin and NSAIDs therapy was a significant risk factor for blood loss when two or more levels were involved, even if the drug was interrupted 7 days earlier. However, no differences were observed between groups for epidural hematomas and infections.

On the other hand, Sigari et al. (Akhavan-Sigari, Rohde, & Abili 2014) found that, in 100 patients in which antithrombotic therapy (aspirin and clopidogrel) prosecution was medically necessary, there was no significant difference in postoperative spinal bleeding.

Some recent systematic reviews and meta-analysis concluded similarly. Zhang et al. (2017) stating that patients undergoing spinal surgery without stopping aspirin don't have an increased risk for bleeding and neither for increased operative time and need for postoperative blood transfusion.

Cheng et al. (Cheng, Poon, & Demetriades 2018) also reported that there is no strong evidence demonstrating a difference in intraoperative blood loss, operation time, and postoperative complications, irrespective of aspirin discontinuation. However, meta-analysis wasn't possible due to the high risk of biases, caused by the great heterogeneity of the selected studies.

Goes et al. (2017) found no differences for aspirin patients in peri-operative complications, namely operation time, blood loss (perioperative blood loss and postoperative drainage), number of transfusions and postoperative complications in the first 30 days such as surgical site infections, stroke, postoperative significant hematomas (requiring surgery), ischemic events (including MI), transient ischemic attacks, and venous thrombo-embolism. Due to the strict criteria, they included only three surgical series.

The 2017 "*Canadian Consensus for the Prevention of Blood Loss in Spine Surgery* (Pauyo et al. 2017)" reported that the most important predictive factors for blood loss were treatment of spine tumors and prolonged operative time greater than 5 h. In the other hand, an accurate hemostasis is the most important factor to prevent a significant blood loss.

A double-blind RCT (Fuhrman 2021) is currently ongoing about the association between intraoperative blood loss and aspirin, and the investigator hypothesizes that there will be no significant difference. This study will provide, hopefully, high quality evidence data.

Miscellaneous

Kamenova et al. (Kamenova, Croci, et al. 2016) analyzed data from 172 consecutive patients treated with ventriculo-peritoneal shunt for hydrocephalus. Of them, 40 (23.3%) were on aspirin. They found no evidence for an increased risk of bleedings, postoperative cardiovascular events, hematological findings, morbidity, and mortality. A subgroup analysis showed that, among the ones who stopped aspirin before the procedure, the hemorrhagic complications were not linked to the time of withdrawal (more or less 7 days).

Table 1. Comparison of studies reporting higher risk of bleeding vs same risk of bleeding in patients taking aspirin

	Studies reporting higher risk of bleeding	Studies reporting same risks of bleeding
Intracerebral hemorrhage	Altered platelet function have been linked to early clot growth and 3-months outcome. Retrospective observational – 67 patients (Naidech et al. 2009)	Antiplatelet agent use was not associated with ICH expansion or clinical outcome. Retrospective observational – 282 patients (Sansing et al. 2009)
	Higher in-hospital mortality rate in ICH patients assuming antiplatelets. Retrospective observational - 353 patients (Peck et al. 2014)	No difference in ICH, need for neurosurgical intervention or in hospital-mortality between patients with antiplatelet therapy compared to standard population. Retrospective observational – 1547 patients (Cull et al. 2015)
	Increased overall risk for neurosurgical intervention and mortality in patients on antiplatelet (Coumadin mainly) at the moment of trauma. Retrospective observational – 1547 patients (Cull et al. 2015)	Patients > 60 years old taking low-dose aspirin have no increased risk for ICH after MTBI compared to same-age patients without aspirin. Retrospective observational – 231 patients (Spektor et al. 2003)
		In-hospital observation for head trauma patients using aspirin alone is not necessary due to the rarity of clinically relevant delayed ICH Retrospective observational -793 patients (Antoni et al. 2019)
		Preoperative antiplatelet intake doesn't influence the rate of postoperative bleeding, outcome, or mortality in patients undergoing craniotomy due to TBI Retrospective observational - 143 patients (Greuter et al. 2019)
		No association between antiplatelet preoperative therapy and increasing in traumatic contusions size after decompressive craniectomy for refractory intracranial hypertension. Retrospective observational – 57 patients (Sturiale et al. 2012)
		Pre-TBI antiplatelet therapy doesn't influence the rate of hemorrhagic complications and reoperation after decompressive craniectomy. Retrospective observational - 90 patients (Han et al. 2016)

	Studies reporting higher risk of bleeding	Studies reporting same risks of bleeding
Acute Subdural hematoma	Antiplatelet therapy is independently associated with recurrence of aSDH and in-hospital death. Retrospective observational – 476 patients (Baraniskin et al. 2014)	Premorbid antithrombotic therapy is not a significant risk factor for recurrence of aSDH necessitating additional evacuation. Retrospective observational - 300 patients (Panczykowski & Okonkwo 2011)
	Antiplatelet is associated with delayed aSDH evacuation. Retrospective observational – 64 patients (Akamatsu et al. 2017)	Blood thinners are not a significant risk factor for aSDH clinical deterioration. Retrospective observational. (Bajsarowicz et al. 2015)
		Antiplatelet use (not specifically aspirin) is not a risk factor for early expansion, neither its resumption is a risk factors for delayed ones. Retrospective observational - 305 patients (Robinson et al. 2021)
Chronic subdural hematoma	Anticoagulant and antiplatelet therapies association with an increased risk of developing CSDH. Retrospective observational -1380 patients (Bonis et al. 2013)	Comparable recurrence rates with and without discontinuation of aspirin in patients undergoing burr-hole drainage for cSDH. Retrospective observational - 963 patients (Kamenova et al. 2017)
	Significant association between aspirin and increased 30-day mortality for patients treated with craniotomy for cSDH. Retrospective observational – 299 patients (Raghavan et al. 2020)	Timing of aspirin discontinuation before surgery doesn't influence the clinical outcome. Retrospective observational -164 patients (Scerrati et al. 2019)
		No association between antiplatelet and recurrence rate of cSDH or in-hospital mortality. Retrospective observational – 476 patients (Baraniskin et al. 2014)
		Early resumption of aspirin after burr-hole surgery is not associated with a higher recurrence rate compared with later resumption. Retrospective observational – 140 patients (Kamenova, Lutz, et al. 2016)
		In selected patients antiplatelet therapy could be early resumed without additional hemorrhagic or thromboembolic risk. Meta-analysis (Phan et al. 2018)

Table 1. (Continued)

	Studies reporting higher risk of bleeding	Studies reporting same risks of bleeding
Intracranial tumors	Antithrombotic is a risk factor for bleedings in 43% of patients. Retrospective observational – 69 patients (Palmer, Sparrow, & Iannotti 1994)	No association between aspirin and blood loss, increased hemorrhagic or thromboembolic complications rate. Retrospective observational - 1291 patients (Hanalioglu et al. 2019)
		Aspirin assumption is not a risk factor for perioperative complications. Retrospective observational - 452 patients. (Rahman et al. 2015)
		No differences in intraoperative bleeding and operative time in patients treated with trans-sphenoidal endoscopic surgeries. Case series – 15 patients. (Ogawa & Tominaga 2015)
Spinal surgery	Preoperative aspirin and NSAIDs therapy is a significant risk factor for blood loss when two or more levels are involved. Retrospective observational - 100 patients. (Park, Kwon, & Woo 2014)	No significant difference in postoperative spinal bleeding for patients in which antithrombotic therapy (aspirin and clopidogrel) prosecution is medically necessary. Retrospective observational - 100 patients. (Akhavan-Sigari, Rohde, & Abili 2014)
		No increased risk for bleeding and neither for increased operative time and need for postoperative blood transfusion in patients taking aspirin. Meta-analysis. (Zhang et al. 2017)
		No strong evidence demonstrating a difference in intraoperative blood loss, operation time, and postoperative complications, irrespective of aspirin discontinuation. Systemic review (Cheng, Poon, & Demetriades 2018)
		No differences for aspirin patients in peri-operative complications. Meta-analysis. (Goes et al. 2017)
Miscellaneous		No evidence for an increased risk of bleedings, postoperative cardiovascular events, hematological findings, morbidity, and mortality in patients taking aspirin for ventriculo-peritoneal shunt. Retrospective observational - 172 patients. (Kamenova, Croci, et al. 2016)

Table 1 shows comparison of studies reporting higher risk of bleeding VS same risk of bleeding in patients taking aspirin.

Conclusion

Management of ASA in neurosurgical patients still present many open questions and is still entrusted mainly to the surgeon experience's rather than to robust guidelines.

Moreover, most of the studies mainly investigated the hemorrhagic complications, but still the thromboembolic risk results very underestimated.

Further studies, evaluating both risks (hemorrhagic and thrombo-embolic) are required in order to guarantee a better evidence based practice in this particular field.

References

"2014 ESC/ESA Guidelines on Non-Cardiac Surgery: Cardiovascular Assessment and Management: The Joint Task Force on Non-Cardiac Surgery: Cardiovascular Assessment and Management of the European Society of Cardiology (ESC) and the European Society of Anaesthesiology (ESA)". 2014. *European Heart Journal* 35 (35): 2383–2431. https://doi.org/10.1093/eurheartj/ehu282.

Akamatsu, Yosuke, Tohru Sasaki, Masayuki Kanamori, Shinsuke Suzuki, Hiroshi Uenohara, & Teiji Tominaga. 2017. "[Factors Contributing to Surgical Intervention for Subacute Subdural Hematoma Enlargement in Patients with Mild Head Injuries]". *No Shinkei Geka. Neurological Surgery* 45 (9): 771–79. https://doi.org/10.11477/mf.1436203591.

Akhavan-Sigari, Reza, Veit Rohde, & Mehdi Abili. 2014. "Continuation of medically necessary platelet aggregation inhibitors - acetylsalicylic acid and clopidogrel - during surgery for spinal degenerative disorders: Results in 100 patients". *Surgical Neurology International* 5 (Suppl 7): S376–79. https://doi.org/10.4103/2152-7806.139675.

Al-Mufti, Fawaz, & Stephan A. Mayer. 2017. "Neurocritical Care of Acute Subdural Hemorrhage". *Neurosurgery Clinics of North America*, Subdural Hematomas, 28 (2): 267–78. https://doi.org/10.1016/j.nec.2016.11.009.

Antithrombotic Trialists' Collaboration. 2002. "Collaborative Meta-Analysis of Randomised Trials of Antiplatelet Therapy for Prevention of Death, Myocardial Infarction, and Stroke in High Risk Patients". *BMJ (Clinical Research Ed.)* 324 (7329): 71–86. https://doi.org/10.1136/bmj.324.7329.71.

Antoni, Anna, Elisabeth Schwendenwein, Harald Binder, Martin Schauperl, Philip Datler, & Stefan Hajdu. 2019. "Delayed Intracranial Hemorrhage in Patients with Head

Trauma and Antithrombotic Therapy". *Journal of Clinical Medicine* 8 (11): 1780. https://doi.org/10.3390/jcm8111780.

Baharoglu, M. Irem, Charlotte Cordonnier, Rustam Al-Shahi Salman, Koen de Gans, Maria M. Koopman, Anneke Brand, Charles B. Majoie, Ludo F Beenen, Henk A Marquering, Marinus Vermeulen, Paul J Nederkoorn, Rob J de Haan, Yvo B Roos, PATCH Investigators. 2016. "Platelet Transfusion versus Standard Care after Acute Stroke Due to Spontaneous Cerebral Haemorrhage Associated with Antiplatelet Therapy (PATCH): A Randomised, Open-Label, Phase 3 Trial". *Lancet (London, England)* 387 (10038): 2605–13. https://doi.org/10.1016/S0140-6736 (16)30392-0.

Bajsarowicz, Paul, Ipshita Prakash, Julie Lamoureux, Rajeet Singh Saluja, Mitra Feyz, Mohammad Maleki, & Judith Marcoux. 2015. "Nonsurgical Acute Traumatic Subdural Hematoma: What Is the Risk?" *Journal of Neurosurgery* 123 (5): 1176–83. https://doi. org/10.3171/2014.10.JNS141728.

Baraniskin, Alexander, Carla Steffens, Albrecht Harders, Wolff Schmiegel, Roland Schroers, & Peter Spangenberg. 2014. "Impact of Pre-Hospital Antithrombotic Medication on the Outcome of Chronic and Acute Subdural Hematoma". *Journal of Neurological Surgery Part A: Central European Neurosurgery* 75 (1): 31–36. https://doi.org/10.1055/s-0032-1325629.

Bonis, Pasquale De, Gianluca Trevisi, Chiara de Waure, Antonella Sferrazza, Massimo Volpe, Angelo Pompucci, Carmelo Anile, & Annunziato Mangiola. 2013. "Antiplatelet/ Anticoagulant Agents and Chronic Subdural Hematoma in the Elderly". *PLOS ONE* 8 (7): e68732. https://doi.org/10.1371/journal.pone.0068732.

Bullock, M. Ross, Randall Chesnut, Jamshid Ghajar, David Gordon, Roger Hartl, David W. Newell, Franco Servadei, Beverly C. Walters, Jack Wilberger, & Surgical Management of Traumatic Brain Injury Author Group. 2006. "Surgical Management of Traumatic Parenchymal Lesions". *Neurosurgery* 58 (3 Suppl): S25-46; discussion Si-iv. https://doi.org/10.1227/01.NEU.0000210365.36914.E3.

Burger, W., J.-M. Chemnitius, G. D. Kneissl, & G. Rücker. 2005. "Low-Dose Aspirin for Secondary Cardiovascular Prevention - Cardiovascular Risks after Its Perioperative Withdrawal versus Bleeding Risks with Its Continuation - Review and Meta-Analysis". *Journal of Internal Medicine* 257 (5): 399–414. https://doi.org/10.1111/ j.1365-2796.2005.01477.x.

Cheng, Ann, Michael T. C. Poon, & Andreas K. Demetriades. 2018. "Aspirin Therapy Discontinuation and Intraoperative Blood Loss in Spinal Surgery: A Systematic Review". *Neurosurgical Review* 41 (4): 1029–36. https://doi.org/10.1007/s10143-018-0945-1.

Collaboration, Antithrombotic Trialists' (ATT), Colin Baigent, Lisa Blackwell, Rory Collins, Jonathan Emberson, Jon Godwin, Richard Peto, Julie Buring, Charles Hennekens, Patricia Kearney, Tom Meade, Carlo Patrono, Maria Carla Roncaglioni, & Alberto Zanchetti. 2009. "Aspirin in the Primary and Secondary Prevention of Vascular Disease: Collaborative Meta-Analysis of Individual Participant Data from Randomised Trials." *Lancet* 373 (9678): 1849–60.

Cull, J. D., Sakai, L. M., Sabir, I., Johnson, B., Tully, A., Nagy, K., Dennis, A., Starr, F. L., Joseph, K., Wiley, D., Moore, H. R., Oliphant, U. J., & Bokhari, F. 2015.

"Outcomes in Traumatic Brain Injury for Patients Presenting on Antiplatelet Therapy". *The American Surgeon* 81 (2): 128–32.

Devereaux, P. J., Mrkobrada, M., Sessler, D. I., Leslie, K., Alonso-Coello, P., Kurz, A., Villar, J. C., Sigamani, A., Biccard, B. M., Meyhoff, C. S., Parlow, J. L., Guyatt, G., Robinson, A., Garg, A. X., Rodseth, R. N., Botto, F., Lurati Buse, G., Xavier, D., Chan, M. T. V., & Yusuf, S. 2014. "Aspirin in Patients Undergoing Noncardiac Surgery". *New England Journal of Medicine* 370 (16): 1494–1503. https://doi.org/10.1056/NEJMoa1401105.

Feigin, Valery L, Rita V Krishnamurthi, Priya Parmar, Bo Norrving, George A Mensah, Derrick A Bennett, Suzanne Barker-Collo, Andrew E Moran, Ralph L Sacco, Thomas Truelsen, Stephen Davis, Jeyaraj Durai Pandian, Mohsen Naghavi, Mohammad H Forouzanfar, Grant Nguyen, Catherine O Johnson, Theo Vos, Atte Meretoja, Christopher J L Murray, Gregory A Roth, GBD 2013 Writing Group; GBD 2013 Stroke Panel Experts Group. 2015. "Update on the Global Burden of Ischemic and Hemorrhagic Stroke in 1990-2013: The GBD 2013 Study". *Neuroepidemiology* 45 (3): 161–76. https://doi.org/10.1159/000441085.

Fuhrman, Heather. 2021. "*Association Between Perioperative Bleeding and Aspirin Use in Spine Surgery: A Randomized, Controlled Trial*". Clinical trial registration NCT02807441. clinicaltrials.gov. https://clinicaltrials.gov/ct2/show/NCT02807441.

Goes, Rik, Ivo S. Muskens, Timothy R. Smith, Rania A. Mekary, Marike L. D. Broekman, & Wouter A. Moojen. 2017. "Risk of Aspirin Continuation in Spinal Surgery: A Systematic Review and Meta-Analysis". *The Spine Journal: Official Journal of the North American Spine Society* 17 (12): 1939–46. https://doi.org/10.1016/j.spinee.2017.08.238.

Greuter, Ladina, Muriel Ullmann, Luigi Mariani, Raphael Guzman, & Jehuda Soleman. 2019. "Effect of Preoperative Antiplatelet or Anticoagulation Therapy on Hemorrhagic Complications in Patients with Traumatic Brain Injury Undergoing Craniotomy or Craniectomy". *Neurosurgical Focus* 47 (5): E3. https://doi.org/10.3171/2019.8. FOCUS19546.

Han, Hokyun, Eun Jung Koh, Hyunho Choi, Byong-Cheol Kim, Seung Yeob Yang, & Keun-Tae Cho. 2016. "The Effect of Preoperative Antiplatelet Therapy on Hemorrhagic Complications after Decompressive Craniectomy in Patients with Traumatic Brain Injury". *Korean Journal of Neurotrauma* 12 (2): 61. https://doi.org/10.13004/kjnt. 2016.12.2.61.

Hanalioglu, Sahin, Balkan Sahin, Omer Selcuk Sahin, Abdulbaki Kozan, Melih Ucer, Ulas Cikla, Steven L. Goodman, & Mustafa K. Baskaya. 2019. "Effect of Perioperative Aspirin Use on Hemorrhagic Complications in Elective Craniotomy for Brain Tumors: Results of a Single-Center, Retrospective Cohort Study". *Journal of Neurosurgery* 132 (5): 1529–38. https://doi.org/10.3171/2018.12.JNS182483.

"Head Injury: Assessment and Early Management". 2019. *Head Injury*, 49.

Hemphill, J. C., Greenberg, S. M., Anderson, C. S., Becker, K., Bendok, B. R., Cushman, M., Fung, G. L., Goldstein, J. N., Macdonald, R. L., Mitchell, P. H., Scott, P. A., Selim, M. H., & Woo, D. 2015. "Guidelines for the Management of Spontaneous Intracerebral Hemorrhage". *Stroke* 46 (7): 2032–60. https://doi.org/10.1161/STR.0000000000000069.

Kamenova, Maria, Davide Croci, Raphael Guzman, Luigi Mariani, & Jehuda Soleman. 2016. "Low-Dose Acetylsalicylic Acid and Bleeding Risks with Ventriculoperitoneal Shunt Placement". *Neurosurgical Focus* 41 (3): E4. https://doi.org/10.3171/2016.6.FOCUS16173.

Kamenova, Maria, Katharina Lutz, Sabine Schaedelin, Javier Fandino, Luigi Mariani, & Jehuda Soleman. 2016. "Does Early Resumption of Low-Dose Aspirin After Evacuation of Chronic Subdural Hematoma With Burr-Hole Drainage Lead to Higher Recurrence Rates?" *Neurosurgery* 79 (5): 715–21. https://doi.org/10.1227/NEU.0000000000001393.

Kamenova, Maria, Edin Nevzati, Katharina Lutz, Armando Dolp, Javier Fandino, Luigi Mariani, & Jehuda Soleman. 2017. "Burr-Hole Drainage for Chronic Subdural Hematoma Under Low-Dose Acetylsalicylic Acid: A Comparative Risk Analysis Study". *World Neurosurgery* 100 (aprile): 594–600. https://doi.org/10.1016/j.wneu.2017.01.065.

Korinth, M. C. 2006. "Low-Dose Aspirin before Intracranial Surgery--Results of a Survey among Neurosurgeons in Germany". *Acta Neurochirurgica* 148 (11): 1189–96; discussion 1196. https://doi.org/10.1007/s00701-006-0868-4.

Korinth, Marcus C., Joachim M. Gilsbach, & Martin R. Weinzierl. 2007. "Low-Dose Aspirin before Spinal Surgery: Results of a Survey among Neurosurgeons in Germany". *European Spine Journal: Official Publication of the European Spine Society, the European Spinal Deformity Society, and the European Section of the Cervical Spine Research Society* 16 (3): 365–72. https://doi.org/10.1007/s00586-006-0216-7.

Lovelock, C. E., A. J. Molyneux, P. M. Rothwell, & Oxford Vascular Study. 2007. "Change in Incidence and Aetiology of Intracerebral Haemorrhage in Oxfordshire, UK, between 1981 and 2006: A Population-Based Study". *The Lancet. Neurology* 6 (6): 487–93. https://doi.org/10.1016/S1474-4422 (07)70107-2.

Mendelow, A. David, Barbara A. Gregson, Elise N. Rowan, Gordon D. Murray, Anil Gholkar, & Patrick M. Mitchell. 2013. "Early Surgery versus Initial Conservative Treatment in Patients with Spontaneous Supratentorial Lobar Intracerebral Haematomas (STICH II): A Randomised Trial". *The Lancet* 382 (9890): 397–408. https://doi.org/10.1016/S0140-6736 (13)60986-1.

Moore, Margaret M., Michael D. Pasquale, & Michael Badellino. 2012. "Impact of Age and Anticoagulation: Need for Neurosurgical Intervention in Trauma Patients with Mild Traumatic Brain Injury". *Journal of Trauma and Acute Care Surgery* 73 (1): 126–30. https://doi.org/10.1097/TA.0b013e31824b01af.

Naidech, Andrew M., Borko Jovanovic, Storm Liebling, Rajeev K. Garg, Sarice L. Bassin, Bernard R. Bendok, Richard A. Bernstein, Mark J. Alberts, & H. Hunt Batjer. 2009. "Reduced Platelet Activity Is Associated With Early Clot Growth and Worse 3-Month Outcome After Intracerebral Hemorrhage". *Stroke* 40 (7): 2398–2401. https://doi.org/10.1161/STROKEAHA.109.550939.

Naidech, Andrew M., Storm M. Liebling, Neil F. Rosenberg, Paul F. Lindholm, Richard A. Bernstein, H. Hunt Batjer, Mark J. Alberts, & Hau C. Kwaan. 2012. "Early Platelet Transfusion Improves Platelet Activity and May Improve Outcomes After

Intracerebral Hemorrhage". *Neurocritical Care* 16 (1): 82–87. https://doi.org/10.1007/s12028-011-9619-3.

Narum, Sigrid, Odd Brørs, Olav Stokland, & Marianne K. Kringen. 2016. "Mortality among head trauma patients taking preinjury antithrombotic agents: a retrospective cohort analysis from a Level 1 trauma centre". *BMC Emergency Medicine* 16 (1): 29. https://doi.org/10.1186/s12873-016-0094-1.

Ogawa, Yoshikazu, & Teiji Tominaga. 2015. "Sellar and Parasellar Tumor Removal without Discontinuing Antithrombotic Therapy". *Journal of Neurosurgery* 123 (3): 794–98. https://doi.org/10.3171/2014.9.JNS141088.

Palmer, J. D., O. C. Sparrow, & F. Iannotti. 1994. "Postoperative Hematoma: A 5-Year Survey and Identification of Avoidable Risk Factors". *Neurosurgery* 35 (6): 1061–64; discussion 1064-1065. https://doi.org/10.1227/00006123-199412000-00007.

Panczykowski, David M., & David O. Okonkwo. 2011. "Premorbid Oral Antithrombotic Therapy and Risk for Reaccumulation, Reoperation, and Mortality in Acute Subdural Hematomas: Clinical Article". *Journal of Neurosurgery* 114 (1): 47–52. https://doi.org/10.3171/2010.7.JNS10446.

Park, Heui-Jeon, Ki-Youn Kwon, & Ju-Hyung Woo. 2014. "Comparison of Blood Loss According to Use of Aspirin in Lumbar Fusion Patients". *European Spine Journal* 23 (8): 1777–82. https://doi.org/10.1007/s00586-014-3294-y.

Pauyo, Thierry, Neil Verma, Yousef Marwan, Ahmed Aoude, Morsi Khashan, & Michael H. Weber. 2017. "Canadian Consensus for the Prevention of Blood Loss in Spine Surgery". *Spine* 42 (1): E50. https://doi.org/10.1097/BRS.0000000000001686.

Peck, Kimberly A., Richard Y. Calvo, Mark S. Schechter, C. Beth Sise, Jessica E. Kahl, Meghan C. Shackford, Steven R. Shackford, Michael J. Sise, & Donald J. Blaskiewicz. 2014. "The Impact of Preinjury Anticoagulants and Prescription Antiplatelet Agents on Outcomes in Older Patients with Traumatic Brain Injury". *The Journal of Trauma and Acute Care Surgery* 76 (2): 431–36. https://doi.org/10.1097/TA.0000000000000107.

Phan, Kevin, David Abi-Hanna, Jack Kerferd, Victor M. Lu, Adam A. Dmytriw, Yam-Ting Ho, Jacob Fairhall, Rajesh Reddy, & Peter Wilson. 2018. "Resumption of Antithrombotic Agents in Chronic Subdural Hematoma: A Systematic Review and Meta-Analysis". *World Neurosurgery* 109 (gennaio): e792–99. https://doi.org/10.1016/j.wneu.2017.10.091.

Raghavan, A., Smith, G., Onyewadume, L., Peck, M. R., Herring, E., Pace, J., Rogers, M., Momotaz, H., Hoffer, S. A., Hu, Y., Liu, H., Tatsuoka, C., Sajatovic, M., & Sloan, A. E. 2020. "Morbidity and Mortality After Burr Hole Craniostomy Versus Craniotomy for Chronic Subdural Hematoma Evacuation: A Single-Center Experience". *World Neurosurgery* 134 (febbraio): e196–203. https://doi.org/10.1016/j.wneu.2019.10.023.

Rahman, Maryam, Lauren L. Donnangelo, Dan Neal, Kiran Mogali, Matthew Decker, & Mustafa M. Ahmed. 2015. "Effects of Perioperative Acetyl Salicylic Acid on Clinical Outcomes in Patients Undergoing Craniotomy for Brain Tumor". *World Neurosurgery* 84 (1): 41–47. https://doi.org/10.1016/j.wneu.2015.02.016.

Robinson, David, Logan Pyle, Brandon Foreman, Laura B. Ngwenya, Opeolu Adeoye, & Daniel Woo, Natalie Kreitzer. 2021. "Factors Associated with Early versus Delayed

Expansion of Acute Subdural Hematomas Initially Managed Conservatively". *Journal of Neurotrauma* 38 (7): 903–10. https://doi.org/10.1089/neu.2020.7192.

Sansing, L. H., S. R. Messe, B. L. Cucchiara, S. N. Cohen, P. D. Lyden, S. E. Kasner, & CHANT Investigators. 2009. "Prior Antiplatelet Use Does Not Affect Hemorrhage Growth or Outcome after ICH". *Neurology* 72 (16): 1397–1402. https://doi.org/10.1212/01.wnl.0000342709.31341.88.

Scantling, D., C. Fischer, R. Gruner, A. Teichman, B. McCracken, & J. Eakins. 2017. "The Role of Delayed Head CT in Evaluation of Elderly Blunt Head Trauma Victims Taking Antithrombotic Therapy". *European Journal of Trauma and Emergency Surgery* 43 (6): 741–46. https://doi.org/10.1007/s00068-017-0793-7.

Scerrati, A., Germanò, A., Trevisi, G., Visani, J., Lofrese, G., D'Angelo, L., Raffa, G., Fazzari, E., Mangiola, A., Cavallo, M. A., & De Bonis, P. 2019. "Timing of Low-Dose Aspirin Discontinuation and the Influence on Clinical Outcome of Patients Undergoing Surgery for Chronic Subdural Hematoma". *World Neurosurgery* 129 (settembre): e695–99. https://doi.org/10.1016/j.wneu.2019.05.252.

Spektor, Sergey, Samuel Agus, Vladimir Merkin, & Shlomo Constantini. 2003. "Low-Dose Aspirin Prophylaxis and Risk of Intracranial Hemorrhage in Patients Older than 60 Years of Age with Mild or Moderate Head Injury: A Prospective Study". *Journal of Neurosurgery* 99 (4): 661–65. https://doi.org/10.3171/jns.2003.99.4.0661.

Stein, Sherman C., Mark G. Burnett, & Henry A. Glick. 2006. "Indications for CT Scanning in Mild Traumatic Brain Injury: A Cost-Effectiveness Study". *The Journal of Trauma* 61 (3): 558–66. https://doi.org/10.1097/01.ta.0000233766.60315.5e.

Stiell, I. G., Wells, G. A., Vandemheen, K., Clement, C., Lesiuk, H., Laupacis, A., McKnight, R. D., Verbeek, R., Brison, R., Cass, D., Eisenhauer, M. A., Greenberg, G. H., & Worthington, J. 2001. "The Canadian CT Head Rule for Patients with Minor Head Injury". *The Lancet* 357 (9266): 1391–96. https://doi.org/10.1016/S0140-6736(00)04561-X.

Sturiale, C. L., De Bonis, P., Rigante, L., Calandrelli, R., D'Arrigo, S., Pompucci, A., Mangiola, A., D'Apolito, G., Colosimo, C., & Anile, C. 2012. "Do Traumatic Brain Contusions Increase in Size after Decompressive Craniectomy?" *Journal of Neurotrauma* 29 (18): 2723–26.

Tamura, Ryota, Mizuto Sato, Kazunari Yoshida, & Masahiro Toda. 2021. "History and Current Progress of Chronic Subdural Hematoma". *Journal of the Neurological Sciences* 429 (ottobre): 118066. https://doi.org/10.1016/j.jns.2021.118066.

The Scandinavian Neurotrauma Committee (SNC), Johan Undén, Tor Ingebrigtsen, & Bertil Romner. 2013. "Scandinavian Guidelines for Initial Management of Minimal, Mild and Moderate Head Injuries in Adults: An Evidence and Consensus-Based Update". *BMC Medicine* 11 (1): 50. https://doi.org/10.1186/1741-7015-11-50.

Thompson, B. B., Bejot, Y., Caso, V., Castillo, J., Christensen, H., Flaherty, M. L., Foerch, C., Ghandehari, K., Giroud, M., Greenberg, S. M., Hallevi, H., Hemphill, J. C., Heuschmann, P., Juvela, S., Kimura, K., Myint, P. K., Nagakane, Y., Naritomi, H., Passero, S., & Smith, E. E. 2010. "Prior Antiplatelet Therapy and Outcome Following Intracerebral Hemorrhage: A Systematic Review". *Neurology* 75 (15): 1333–42. https://doi.org/10.1212/WNL.0b013e3181f735e5.

"*Updated Mild Traumatic Brain Injury Guideline for Adults | Concussion | Traumatic Brain Injury | CDC Injury Center*". 2021. 11 maggio 2021. https://www.cdc.gov/traumaticbraininjury/mtbi_guideline.html.

Zahuranec, D. B., N. R. Gonzales, D. L. Brown, L. D. Lisabeth, P. J. Longwell, S. V. Eden, M. A. Smith, N. M. Garcia, J. T. Hoff, & L. B. Morgenstern. 2006. "Presentation of Intracerebral Haemorrhage in a Community". *Journal of Neurology, Neurosurgery & Psychiatry* 77 (3): 340–44. https://doi.org/10.1136/jnnp.2005.077164.

Zhang, Chenggui, Guodong Wang, Xiaoyang Liu, Yang Li, & Jianmin Sun. 2017. "Safety of Continuing Aspirin Therapy during Spinal Surgery: A Systematic Review and Meta-Analysis". *Medicine* 96 (46): e8603. https://doi.org/10.1097/MD.0000000000008603.

Biographical Sketch

Alba Scerrati

Affiliation: University of Ferrara

Education: Medical Doctor and Researcher

Business Address: Via Aldo Moro, 8, 44124, Ferrara, Italy

Research and Professional Experience: Neurosurgeon specialized in neuroncology, neurovascular surgery and brain trauma.

Publications from the Last 3 Years:

1. Sturiale CL, Scerrati A, Ricciardi L, Rustemi O, Auricchio AM, Norri N, Piazza A, Ranieri F, Tomatis A, Albanese A, Di Egidio V, Farneti M, Mangiola A, Marchese E, Raco A, Volpin L, Trevisi G. Clipping versus coiling for treatment of middle cerebral artery aneurysms: a retrospective Italian multicenter experience. *Neurosurg Rev.* 2022 Jun 4. doi: 10.1007/s10143-022-01822-3. Epub ahead of print. PMID: 35665868.
2. Vigo V, Tassinari A, Scerrati A, Cavallo MA, Rodriguez-Rubio R, Fernandez-Miranda JC, De Bonis P. Ideal trajectory for frontal ventriculostomy: Radiological study and anatomical study. *Clin Neurol Neurosurg.* 2022 Jun;217:107264. doi: 10.1016/j.clineuro.2022.107264. Epub 2022 Apr 26. PMID: 35526512.
3. Trevisi G, Caccavella VM, Scerrati A, Signorelli F, Salamone GG, Orsini K, Fasciani C, D'Arrigo S, Auricchio AM, D'Onofrio G, Salomi F,

Albanese A, De Bonis P, Mangiola A, Sturiale CL. Machine learning model prediction of 6-month functional outcome in elderly patients with intracerebral hemorrhage. *Neurosurg Rev*. 2022 May 6. doi: 10.1007/s10143-022-01802-7. Epub ahead of print. PMID: 35522333.

4. Sacco C, Olivi S, Visani J, Donati R, Veronesi V, Mencarani C, Capone C, Bizzocchi G, Kiekens C, De Bonis P, Scerrati A, Staffa G. Functional outcome after transfer of brachialis on anterior interosseous and supinator on posterior interosseous nerves: A preliminary report. *Microsurgery*. 2022 Apr 28. doi: 10.1002/micr.30891. Epub ahead of print. PMID: 35484858.
5. Trevisi G, Scerrati A, Rustemi O, Ricciardi L, Raneri F, Tomatis A, Piazza A, Auricchio AM, Stifano V, Dughiero M, DE Bonis P, Mangiola A, Sturiale CL. The role of the craniotomy size in the surgical evacuation of acute subdural hematomas in elderly patients: a retrospective multicentric study. *J Neurosurg Sci*. 2022 Apr 5. doi: 10.23736/S0390-5616.22.05648-X. Epub ahead of print. PMID: 35380204.
6. Fontanella MM, Zanin L, Panciani P, Belotti F, Doglietto F, Cremonesi A, Migliorati K, Roca E, De Maria L, Franzin A, Vivaldi O, Griva F, Narducci A, Draghi R, Calbucci F, Borghesi I, Crobeddu E, Cossandi C, Fioravanti A, Arias JA, Scerrati A, De Bonis P, Locatelli D, Agosti E, Veiceschi P, Ceraudo M, Zona G, Gasparotti R, Terzi di Bergamo L, Rigamonti D. Preliminary Validation of FoRCaSco: A New Grading System for Cerebral and Cerebellar Cavernomas. *World Neurosurg*. 2022 Jun;162:e597-e604. doi: 10.1016/j.wneu.2022.03.070. Epub 2022. Mar 18. PMID: 35314403.
7. Ricciardi L, Sturiale CL, Scerrati A, Stifano V, Somma T, Ius T, Trungu S, Acqui M, Raco A, Miscusi M, Della Pepa GM. 5-Aminolevulinic Acid False-Positive Rates in Newly Diagnosed and Recurrent Glioblastoma: Do Pseudoprogression and Radionecrosis Play a Role? A Meta-Analysis. *Front Oncol*. 2022 Feb 17;12:848036. doi: 10.3389/fonc.2022.848036. PMID: 35252015; PMCID: PMC8891510.
8. Staartjes VE, Stumpo V, Ricciardi L, Maldaner N, Eversdijk HAJ, Vieli M, Ciobanu-Caraus O, Raco A, Miscusi M, Perna A, Proietti L, Lofrese G, Dughiero M, Cultrera F, Nicassio N, An SB, Ha Y, Amelot A, Alcobendas I, Viñuela-Prieto JM, Gandía-González ML, Girod PP, Lener S, Kögl N, Abramovic A, Safa NA, Laux CJ, Farshad M, O'Riordan D, Loibl M, Mannion AF, Scerrati A, Molliqaj G, Tessitore E, Schröder ML, Vandertop WP, Stienen MN, Regli L, Serra C. FUSE-ML: development and external validation of a clinical prediction model for mid-term

outcomes after lumbar spinal fusion for degenerative disease. *Eur Spine J.* 2022 Feb 21. doi: 10.1007/s00586-022-07135-9. Epub ahead of print. PMID: 35188587.

9. Zamboni P, Scerrati A, Sessa F, Pomara C, Mannucci PM. Vaccine-induced immune thrombotic thrombocytopenia with atypical vein thrombosis: Implications for clinical practice. *Phlebology.* 2022 Apr;37 (3):180-187. doi: 10.1177/02683555211068948. Epub 2022 Jan 23. PMID: 35068258.
10. Montemurro N, Scerrati A, Ricciardi L, Trevisi G. The Exoscope in Neurosurgery: An Overview of the Current Literature of Intraoperative Use in Brain and Spine Surgery. *J Clin Med.* 2021 Dec 31;11 (1):223. doi: 10.3390/jcm11010223. PMID: 35011964; PMCID: PMC8745525.
11. Scerrati A, Trevisi G, Sturiale CL, Salomi F, De Bonis P, Saletti A, Mangiola A, Tomatis A, Di Egidio V, Vigo V, Pedicelli A, Valente I, Rustemi O, Beggio G, Iannucci G, Milonia L, Ricciardi L, Cervo A, Pero G, Piano M. Radiological outcomes for endovascular treatment of posterior communicating artery aneurysms: a retrospective multicenter study of the occlusion rate. *J Integr Neurosci.* 2021 Dec 30;20 (4):919-931. doi: 10.31083/j.jin2004093. PMID: 34997715.
12. Alexandre AM, Sturiale CL, Bartolo A, Romi A, Scerrati A, Flacco ME, D'Argento F, Scarcia L, Garignano G, Valente I, Lozupone E, Pedicelli A. Endovascular Treatment of Cavernous Sinus Dural Arteriovenous Fistulas. Institutional Series, Systematic Review and Meta-Analysis. *Clin Neuroradiol.* 2021 Dec 15. doi: 10.1007/s00062-021-01107-0. Epub ahead of print. PMID: 34910224.
13. Ricciardi L, Piazza A, Capobianco M, Della Pepa GM, Miscusi M, Raco A, Scerrati A, Somma T, Lofrese G, Sturiale CL. Lumbar interbody fusion using oblique (OLIF) and lateral (LLIF) approaches for degenerative spine disorders: a meta-analysis of the comparative studies. *Eur J Orthop Surg Traumatol.* 2021 Nov 26. doi: 10.1007/s00590-021-03172-0. Epub ahead of print. PMID: 34825987.
14. Scerrati A, Travaglini F, Gelmi CAE, Lombardo A, De Bonis P, Cavallo MA, Zamboni P. Patient specific Polymethyl methacrylate customised cranioplasty using 3D printed silicone moulds: Technical note. *Int J Med Robot.* 2022 Apr;18 (2):e2353. doi: 10.1002/rcs.2353. Epub 2021 Nov 24. PMID: 34786816.
15. Mongardi L, Visani J, Mantovani G, Vitali C, Ricciardi L, Giordano F, Cavallo MA, Lofrese G, D'andrea M, Roblot P, De Bonis P, Scerrati A. Long term results of Dorsal Root Entry Zone (DREZ) lesions for the

treatment of intractable pain: A systematic review of the literature on 1242 cases. *Clin Neurol Neurosurg.* 2021 Nov;210:107004. doi: 10.1016/j.clineuro.2021.107004. Epub 2021 Oct 24. PMID: 34739884.

16. Neri M, Braccia A, Panteghini C, Garavaglia B, Gualandi F, Cavallo MA, Scerrati A, Ferlini A, Sensi M. Parkinson's disease-dementia in trans LRP10 and GBA variants: Response to deep brain stimulation. *Parkinsonism Relat Disord.* 2021 Nov;92:72-75. doi: 10.1016/j.parkreldis.2021.10.020. Epub 2021 Oct 24. PMID: 34710740.
17. Scerrati A, De Bonis P, Zamboni P, Dones F, Fontanella M, Cenzato M, Visani J, Bianchi F, Zanin L, Cavallo MA, Sturiale CL. A New Insight in Nonaneurysmal Subarachnoid Hemorrhage: the Potential Role of the Internal Jugular Veins. *J Neurol Surg A Cent Eur Neurosurg.* 2021 Oct 22. doi: 10.1055/s-0041-1733895. Epub ahead of print. PMID: 34687035.
18. Guarino S, Marchese E, Ponticelli GS, Scerrati A, Tagliaferri V, Trovalusci F. Additive Manufacturing for Neurosurgery: Digital Light Processing of Individualized Patient-Specific Cerebral Aneurysms. *Materials* (Basel). 2021 Oct 14;14 (20):6057. doi: 10.3390/ma14206057. PMID: 34683649; PMCID: PMC8539393.
19. Lofrese G, Visani J, Cultrera F, De Bonis P, Tosatto L, Scerrati A. Anterior Dural Tear in Thoracic and Lumbar Spinal Fractures: Single-Center Experience with Coating Technique and Literature *Review of the Available Strategies.* Life (Basel). 2021 Aug 25;11 (9):875. doi: 10.3390/life11090875. PMID: 34575024; PMCID: PMC8465010.
20. Lofrese G, Ricciardi L, De Bonis P, Cultrera F, Cappuccio M, Scerrati A, Martucci A, Musio A, Tosatto L, De Iure F. Use of the SpineJack direct reduction for treating type A2, A3 and A4 fractures of the thoracolumbar spine: a retrospective case series. *J Neurointerv Surg.* 2021 Aug 25: neurintsurg-2021-017682. doi: 10.1136/neurintsurg-2021-017682. Epub ahead of print. PMID: 34433644.
21. Rubbini M, Greco P, Manservigi M, Martinello R, Gasbarro V, Piccolo E, Occhionorelli S, Lacavalla D, Massari L, Caruso G, Caldaria A, Perri P, Salgari N, Cavallesco GN, Anania G, Chiozza M, Carcoforo P, Maruca AM, Cavallo MA, Scerrati A, Capone G, Feo CV, Fabbri N, Fazzin M, Forini ME. Impact of COVID-19 on surgical activities and personnel: lessons for the future. *Minerva Surg.* 2022 Feb;77 (1):14-21. doi: 10.23736/S2724-5691.21.08919-X. Epub 2021 Aug 2. PMID: 34338460.
22. Ricciardi L, Acqui M, Pucci R, Napoli C, Scerrati A. Transient Trigeminal Neuralgia Recurrence During Coronavirus disease-19 in Carbamazepine

Responders Patients. *J Craniofac Surg*. 2021 Nov-Dec 01;32 (8):e834. doi: 10.1097/SCS.0000000000007893. PMID: 34292248.

23. Visani J, Mongardi L, Cultrera F, Bonis P, Lofrese G, Ricciardi L, Scerrati A. Surgical treatment of metastatic pheochromocytomas of the spine: a systematic review. *J Integr Neurosci*. 2021 Jun 30;20 (2):499-507. doi: 10.31083/j.jin2002053. PMID: 34258952.
24. Scerrati A, Germano' A, Montano N, Visani J, Cacciola F, Raffa G, Ghetti I, Pignotti F, Cavallo MA, Olivi A, de Bonis P. Factors affecting functional outcome after anterior cervical discectomy and fusion: A multicenter study. *J Craniovertebr Junction Spine*. 2021 Apr-Jun;12 (2):144-148. doi: 10.4103/jcvjs.jcvjs_1_21. Epub 2021 Jun 10. PMID: 34194160; PMCID: PMC8214232.
25. Piazza A, Ricciardi L, Trungu S, Forcato S, di Bartolomeo A, Scerrati A, Miscusi M, Raco A. The Lone Star Retractor System in Neurosurgery. *World Neurosurg*. 2021 Sep;153:36-40. doi: 10.1016/j.wneu.2021.06.097. Epub 2021 Jun 26. PMID: 34186216.
26. Ius T, Tel A, Minniti G, Somma T, Solari D, Longhi M, De Bonis P, Scerrati A, Caccese M, Barresi V, Fiorentino A, Gorgoglione L, Lombardi G, Robiony M. Advances in Multidisciplinary Management of Skull Base Meningiomas. *Cancers* (Basel). 2021 May 28;13 (11):2664. doi: 10.3390/cancers13112664. PMID: 34071391; PMCID: PMC8198762.
27. Ricciardi L, Scerrati A, Bonis P, Miscusi M, Trungu S, Visocchi M, Papacci F, Raco A, Proietti L, Pompucci A, Olivi A, Montano N. Long-term Radiologic and Clinical Outcomes after Three-level Contiguous Anterior Cervical Diskectomy and Fusion without Plating: A Multicentric Retrospective Study. *J Neurol Surg A Cent Eur Neurosurg*. 2021 Nov;82 (6):556-561. doi: 10.1055/s-0041-1726112. Epub 2021 May 19. PMID: 34010980.
28. Scerrati A, Norri N, Mongardi L, Dones F, Ricciardi L, Trevisi G, Menegatti E, Zamboni P, Cavallo MA, De Bonis P. Styloidogenic-cervical spondylotic internal jugular venous compression, a vascular disease related to several clinical neurological manifestations: diagnosis and treatment-a comprehensive literature review. *Ann Transl Med*. 2021 Apr;9 (8):718. doi: 10.21037/atm-20-7698. PMID: 33987416; PMCID: PMC8106058.
29. Ricciardi L, Della Pepa GM, Scerrati A, Sturiale CL. Should younger researchers pursue citations or innovations? *J Neurosurg Sci*. 2022 Feb;66 (1):71. doi: 10.23736/S0390-5616.21.05357-1. Epub 2021 Apr 16. PMID: 33870674.

30. Scerrati A, Cavallo MA, De Bonis P. Letter: "Awake intraoperative mapping to identify cortical regions related to music performance: Technical note". *J Clin Neurosci.* 2021 Apr;86:18-19. doi: 10.1016/ j.jocn.2020.12.027. Epub 2021 Jan 25. PMID: 33775323.
31. Scerrati A, DE Bonis P. Perioperative interruption of antiplatelet medications for elective extradural non-instrumented spine surgery: is it really necessary? *J Neurosurg Sci.* 2021 Oct;65 (5):542-543. doi: 10. 23736/S0390-5616.21.05272-3. Epub 2021 Mar 11. PMID: 33709664.
32. Scerrati A, Menegatti E, Zamboni M, Malagoni AM, Tessari M, Galeotti R, Zamboni P. Internal Jugular Vein Thrombosis: Etiology, Symptomatology, Diagnosis and Current Treatment. *Diagnostics* (Basel). 2021 Feb 23;11 (2):378. doi: 10.3390/diagnostics11020378. PMID: 33672254; PMCID: PMC7926529.
33. Scerrati A, Pangallo G, Dughiero M, Mongardi L, Ricciardi L, Lofrese G, Dones F, Cavallo MA, De Bonis P. Influence of nutritional status on the clinical outcome of patients with chronic subdural hematoma: a prospective multicenter clinical study. *Nutr Neurosci.* 2021 Mar 5:1-8. doi: 10.1080/1028415X.2021.1895480. Epub ahead of print. PMID: 33666524.
34. Lofrese G, Scerrati A, Balsano M, Bassani R, Cappuccio M, Cavallo MA, Cofano F, Cultrera F, De Iure F, Biase FD, Donati R, Garbossa D, Menegatti M, Olivi A, Palandri G, Raco A, Ricciardi L, Spena G, Tosatto L, Visani J, Visocchi M, Zona G, De Bonis P. Surgical Treatment of Diffuse Idiopathic Skeletal Hyperostosis (DISH) Involving the Cervical Spine: Technical Nuances and Outcome of a Multicenter Experience. *Global Spine J.* 2021 Feb 16:2192568220988272. doi: 10.1177/219 2568220988272. Epub ahead of print. PMID: 33590802.
35. Ricciardi L, Trungu S, Scerrati A, Mongardi L, Flacco ME, Raco A, Miscusi M, De Bonis P, Sturiale CL. Surgical treatment of intracranial blister aneurysms: A systematic review. *Clin Neurol Neurosurg.* 2021 Mar;202:106550. doi: 10.1016/j.clineuro.2021.106550. Epub 2021 Feb 6. PMID: 33588360.
36. De Bonis P, Cavallo MA, Sturiale CL, Martellucci C, Flacco ME, Dughiero M, Auricchio AM, Ricciardi L, Raco A, Bortolotti C, Tosatto L, D'Andrea M, Ruggiero M, Mongardi L, Zona G, Fiaschi P, Cofano F, Garbossa D, Scerrati A. Incidence of hemorrhagic cerebrovascular disease due to vascular malformations during the COVID-19 national quarantine in Italy. *Clin Neurol Neurosurg.* 2021 Mar;202:106503. doi: 10.1016/ j.clineuro.2021.106503. Epub 2021 Jan 19. PMID: 33493878.

37. Scerrati A, Visani J, Flacco ME, Ricciardi L, Trungu S, Raco A, Dones F, De Bonis P, Sturiale CL. Endovascular Treatment of Ruptured Intracranial Blister Aneurysms: A Systematic Review and Meta-analysis. *AJNR Am J Neuroradiol.* 2021 Mar;42 (3):538-545. doi: 10.3174/ajnr.A6924. Epub 2020 Dec 24. PMID: 33361375; PMCID: PMC 7959417.
38. Mongardi L, Visani J, Mantovani G, Olivetti ME, Scerrati A, Cultrera F, Ricciardi L, De Bonis P, Cavallo MA, Lofrese G. Ct guided reference markers for spinal dorsal lesions: A safe and valuable tool impacting intraoperative localization time. *J Clin Neurosci.* 2021 Feb;84:97-101. doi: 10.1016/j.jocn.2020.11.039. Epub 2020 Dec 25. PMID: 33358493.
39. De Bonis P, Musio A, Mongardi L, Lofrese G, La Marca F, Visani J, Cavallo MA, Scerrati A. Transpars approach for L5-S1 foraminal and extra-foraminal lumbar disc herniations: technical note. *J Neurosurg Sci.* 2020 Dec 9. doi: 10.23736/S0390-5616.20.05165-6. Epub ahead of print. PMID: 33297610.
40. Mongardi L, Dones F, Mantovani G, De Bonis P, Rustemi O, Ricciardi L, Cavallo MA, Scerrati A. Low-Dose Acetylsalicylic Acid in Chronic Subdural Hematomas: A Neurosurgeon's Sword of Damocles. *Front Neurol.* 2020 Sep 29;11:550084. doi: 10.3389/fneur.2020.550084. PMID: 33133003; PMCID: PMC7550681.
41. Mongardi L, Rispoli V, Scerrati A, Giordano F, Capone JG, Vaudano AE, De Bonis P, Morgante F, Picillo M, Cavallo MA, Sensi M. Deep brain stimulation of the ventralis oralis anterior thalamic nucleus is effective for dystonic tremor. *Parkinsonism Relat Disord.* 2020 Dec;81:8-11. doi: 10.1016/j.parkreldis.2020.09.040. Epub 2020 Sep 29. PMID: 33035802.
42. Ricciardi L, Trungu S, Scerrati A, De Bonis P, Rustemi O, Mazzetto M, Lofrese G, Cultrera F, Barrey CY, Di Bartolomeo A, Piazza A, Miscusi M, Raco A. Odontoid screw placement for Anderson type II odontoid fractures: how do duration from injury to surgery and clinical and radiological factors influence the union rate? A multicenter retrospective study. *J Neurosurg Spine*. 2020 Oct 2:1-5. doi: 10.3171/2020.6.SPINE20 318. Epub ahead of print. PMID: 33007754.
43. Trevisi G, Sturiale CL, Scerrati A, Rustemi O, Ricciardi L, Raneri F, Tomatis A, Piazza A, Auricchio AM, Stifano V, Romano C, De Bonis P, Mangiola A. Acute subdural hematoma in the elderly: outcome analysis in a retrospective multicentric series of 213 patients. *Neurosurg Focus.* 2020 Oct;49 (4):E21. doi: 10.3171/2020.7.FOCUS20437. PMID: 3300 2873.

44. Scerrati A, Visani J, Ricciardi L, Dones F, Rustemi O, Cavallo MA, De Bonis P. To drill or not to drill, that is the question: nonsurgical treatment of chronic subdural hematoma in the elderly. A systematic review. *Neurosurg Focus*. 2020 Oct;49 (4):E7. doi: 10.3171/2020.7.FOCUS 20237. PMID: 33002869.
45. Stienen MN, Freyschlag CF, Schaller K, Meling T; EANS Young Neurosurgeons and EANS Training Committee. Procedures performed during neurosurgery residency in Europe. *Acta Neurochir* (Wien). 2020 Oct;162 (10):2303-2311. doi: 10.1007/s00701-020-04513-4. Epub 2020 Aug 16. PMID: 32803372; PMCID: PMC7496021.
46. Lofrese G, Cultrera F, Visani J, Scerrati A, Mongardi L, Donati R, Tosatto L, De Bonis P. Chylothorax in spine fractures: A rarely reported complication? Literature review with an example case. *J Trauma Acute Care Surg*. 2020 Nov;89 (5):e140-e146. doi: 10.1097/TA.000000000000 2896. PMID: 32769951.
47. Scerrati A, De Bonis P, Zamboni P. Letter to the Editor Regarding "Styloidectomy and Venous Stenting for Treatment of Styloid-Induced Internal Jugular Vein Stenosis: A Case Report and Literature Review". *World Neurosurg*. 2020 Jul;139:697. doi: 10.1016/j.wneu.2020.04.021. PMID: 32689686.
48. De Bonis P, Mantovani G, Lofrese G, Cavallo MA, Valpiani G, Morotti C, Scerrati A. Transcranial Sonography versus CT for Postoperative Monitoring After Decompressive Craniectomy. *J Neuroimaging.* 2020 Nov;30 (6):800-807. doi: 10.1111/jon.12756. Epub 2020 Jul 18. PMID: 32681813.
49. De Bonis P, Musio A, Mantovani G, Pompucci A, Visani J, Lofrese G, Scerrati A. Simplified four-step retropharyngeal approach for the upper cervical spine: technical note. *Eur Spine J.* 2020 Nov;29 (11):2752-2757. doi: 10.1007/s00586-020-06521-5. Epub 2020 Jul 9. PMID: 32648083.
50. Scerrati A, Zamboni P, De Bonis P. Letter: C1 Transverse Process Resection for Management of Jugular Stenosis. *Oper Neurosurg* (Hagerstown). 2020 Sep 15;19 (4):E465. doi: 10.1093/ons/opaa200. PMID: 32629482.
51. Scerrati A, Labanti S, Lofrese G, Mongardi L, Cavallo MA, Ricciardi L, De Bonis P. Artists playing music while undergoing brain surgery: A look into the scientific evidence and the social media perspective. *Clin Neurol Neurosurg*. 2020 Sep;196:105911. doi: 10.1016/j.clineuro.2020.105911. Epub 2020 Jun 4. PMID: 32505870.

52. Scerrati A, Mongardi L, Cavallo MA, Labanti S, Simioni V, Ricciardi L, De Bonis P. Awake surgery for skills preservation during a sensory area tumor resection in a clarinet player. *Acta Neurol Belg*. 2021 Oct;121 (5):1235-1239. doi: 10.1007/s13760-020-01368-5. Epub 2020 May 5. PMID: 32372400.
53. Ricciardi L, Trungu S, Scerrati A, DE Bonis P, Miscusi M, Raco A. Neurosurgery at the time of COVID-19: how this pandemic infectious disease is influencing neurosurgical activities and patient management. *J Neurosurg Sci*. 2021 Apr;65 (2):216-217. doi: 10.23736/S0390-5616. 20.04976-0. Epub 2020 Apr 29. PMID: 32347683.
54. Scerrati A, Mongardi L, Visani J, Lofrese G, Cavallo MA, Fiorentino A, De Bonis P. The controversial role of Bevacizumab in the treatment of patients with intracranial meningioma: a comprehensive literature review. *Expert Rev Anticancer Ther*. 2020 Mar;20 (3):197-203. doi: 10.1080/ 14737140.2020.1736567. Epub 2020 Mar 6. PMID: 32116057.
55. De Bonis P, Chiccoli M, Visani J, Cavallo MA, Scerrati A. Functional outcome of patients with unstable single- level/ two- level lumbar stenosis treated with decompression plus divergent screws (cortical bone trajectory) or percutaneous convergent pedicle screws. *J Neurosurg Sci*. 2020 Feb 25. doi: 10.23736/S0390-5616.20.04893-6. Epub ahead of print. PMID: 32100520.
56. Musio A, Scerrati A, Pintye D, Salomi F, Cavallo MA, De Bonis P. Filthy operative rooms and other mistakes during movies on neurosurgical procedures: Fascinating and powerful neurosurgical scenarios presented, in different ways, to non-neurosurgical society. How many mistakes and stereotypes can be made in movies for people not daily involved in medical life? *Clin Neurol Neurosurg*. 2020 Apr;191:105695. doi: 10.1016/j.clineuro.2020.105695. Epub 2020 Feb 1. PMID: 32086118.
57. Lofrese G, Mongardi L, De Bonis P, Scerrati A, Nicassio N, Cultrera F. Spontaneous Repositioning of Isolated Blow-In Orbital Roof Fracture: Could Wait and See Be a Strategy in Asymptomatic Cases? *J Craniofac Surg*. 2020 May/Jun;31 (3):e263-e266. doi: 10.1097/SCS.000000000000 6231. PMID: 32049903.
58. Beggio G, Raneri F, Rustemi O, Scerrati A, Zambon G, Piacentino M. Techniques for pneumocephalus and brain shift reduction in DBS surgery: a review of the literature. *Neurosurg Rev*. 2020 Feb;43 (1):95-99. doi: 10.1007/s10143-019-01220-2. Epub 2020 Jan 2. PMID: 31897886.
59. Ricciardi L, Scerrati A, Olivi A, Sturiale CL, De Bonis P, Montano N. The role of cervical collar in functional restoration and fusion after

anterior cervical discectomy and fusion without plating on single or double levels: a systematic review and meta-analysis. *Eur Spine J.* 2020 May;29 (5):955-960. doi: 10.1007/s00586-019-06270-0. Epub 2020 Jan 1. PMID: 31894403.

60. Rustemi O, Raneri F, Scerrati A. Letter by Rustemi et al. Regarding Article, "Flow Diverters for Intracranial Aneurysms: The DIVERSION National Prospective Cohort Study." *Stroke.* 2020 Feb;51 (2):e35. doi: 10.1161/STROKEAHA.119.028244. Epub 2019 Dec 23. PMID: 31865 893.
61. Zamboni P, Scerrati A, Menegatti E, Galeotti R, Lapparelli M, Traina L, Tessari M, Ciorba A, De Bonis P, Pelucchi S. The eagle jugular syndrome. *BMC Neurol.* 2019 Dec 21;19 (1):333. doi: 10.1186/s12883-019-1572-3. PMID: 31864313; PMCID: PMC6925502.
62. Scerrati A, Trevisi G, De Bonis P, Mangiola A. Repeat head CT in mild traumatic brain injury is really necessary? *Am J Emerg Med.* 2020 Feb;38 (2):393-394. doi: 10.1016/j.ajem.2019.10.010. Epub 2019 Nov 18. PMID: 31785974.
63. Scerrati A, Visani J, Norri N, Cavallo M, Giganti M, De Bonis P. Effect of external cervical orthoses on clinical and radiological outcome of patients undergoing anterior cervical discectomy and fusion. *Acta Neurochir* (Wien). 2019 Oct;161 (10):2195-2200. doi: 10.1007/s00701-019-04046-5. Epub 2019 Aug 27. PMID: 31455994.
64. Scerrati A, Germanò A, Trevisi G, Visani J, Lofrese G, D'Angelo L, Raffa G, Fazzari E, Mangiola A, Cavallo MA, De Bonis P. Timing of Low-Dose Aspirin Discontinuation and the Influence on Clinical Outcome of Patients Undergoing Surgery for Chronic Subdural Hematoma. *World Neurosurg.* 2019 Sep;129:e695-e699. doi: 10.1016/j.wneu.2019.05.252. Epub 2019 Jun 11. PMID: 31279757.
65. Mongardi L, Mantovani G, Scerrati A, De Bonis P, Cavallo MA. Epilepsy and cranial hemangioma in Lowe syndrome. *Acta Neurol Belg.* 2020 Oct;120 (5):1199-1200. doi: 10.1007/s13760-019-01162-y. Epub 2019 Jun 12. PMID: 31190138.
66. De Bonis P, Menegatti E, Cavallo MA, Sisini F, Trapella G, Scerrati A, Zamboni P. JEDI (jugular entrapment, dilated ventricles, intracranial hypertension) syndrome: a new clinical entity? A case report. *Acta Neurochir* (Wien). 2019 Jul;161 (7):1367-1370. doi: 10.1007/s00701-019-03908-2. Epub 2019 Apr 25. PMID: 31025176.
67. Scerrati A, Sabatino G, Della Pepa GM, Albanese A, Marchese E, Puca A, Olivi A, Sturiale CL. Treatment and outcome of thrombosed

aneurysms of the middle cerebral artery: institutional experience and a systematic review. *Neurosurg Rev.* 2019 Sep;42 (3):649-661. doi: 10.1007/s10143-018-0984-7. Epub 2018 May 22. PMID: 29790066.

68. Scerrati A, Mangiola A, Rigoni F, Olei S, Santantonio M, Trevisi G, Anile C, Cavallo MA, DE Bonis P. Do antiplatelet and anticoagulant drugs modify outcome of patients treated for chronic subdural hematoma? Still a controversial issue. *J Neurosurg Sci.* 2021 Dec;65 (6):626-633. doi: 10.23736/S0390-5616.18.04311-4. Epub 2018 Apr 18. PMID: 29671291.
69. Della Pepa GM, Bianchi F, Scerrati A, Albanese A, Cotroneo E, Delitala A, Gigli R, La Rocca G, Marchese E, Pedicelli A, Puca A, Sabatino G, Olivi A, Sturiale CL. Secondary coiling after incomplete surgical clipping of cerebral aneurysms: a rescue strategy or a treatment option for complex cases? Institutional series and systematic review. *Neurosurg Rev.* 2019 Jun;42 (2):337-350. doi: 10.1007/s10143-018-0950-4. Epub 2018 Feb 7. PMID: 29417290.

Chapter 9

Inflammation and Stroke

Arsenio Fernández-Lopez[1,2,*], Oscar Balboa Arregui[3,†] and Javier Tejada[4,‡]

[1]Department of Molecular Biology, University of Leon, Leon, Spain
[2]Neural Therapies SL, Leon, Spain
[3]Department of Radiology, Hospital de Leon, Leon, Spain
[4]Department of Neurology, Hospital del Leon, Leon, Spain

Abstract

Inflammation plays crucial roles in the pathogenesis of atherosclerosis, which can result in thromboembolic events and different stroke subtypes such as large artery or cryptogenic ischemic stroke. Furthermore, both the blood flow withdrawal and the subsequent blood flow reperfusion that follows the ischemic events elicit inflammatory processes. This inflammatory response plays a dual role in stroke pathology: the initial response aims to fight the damaged tissue, while the continuous inflammatory activity after stroke exacerbates the neural damage. The inflammatory process involves a complex cellular and molecular response that includes not only the intrinsic cells in the brain (glia, neurons, vascular endothelium) but the involvement of the peripheral cells (macrophages, neutrophils, dendritic cells, lymphocytes) at different times after stroke eliciting, among other effects, a complicated sequence of cytokines that control the evolution of the inflammation and blood-brain barrier permeability. Different non-invasive imaging techniques such as computed tomography angiography, computed tomography perfusion, or magnetic resonance imaging, among others,

* Corresponding Author's Emails: aferl@unileon.es; a.f.lopez@neuraltherapies.com.
† Corresponding Author's Email: obalboa@saludcastillayleon.es.
‡ Corresponding Author's Email: jtejada@saludcastillayleon.es.

In: Horizons in Neuroscience Research. Volume 48
Editors: Andres Costa and Eugenio Villalba
ISBN: 979-8-88697-230-6
© 2022 Nova Science Publishers, Inc.

allow following the atherosclerotic plaque instability and the neuro-inflammatory progression.

Abbreviations

ALDH1A1	aldehyde dehydrogenase 1 family member L1
AMPA	α-amino-3-hydroxy-5-methyl-4-isoxazolepropionic acid
AQP	aquaporin
Arg1	arginase 1
ATP	adenosine triphosphate
BBB	blood-brain barrier
BCSFB	blood-cerebrospinal fluid barrier
C1q	complement component 1q
CAM	cell adhesion molecule
CBF	cerebral blood flow
CBV	cerebral blood volume
CC chemokines	chemokines with two N-terminal adjacent cysteines
CD	cluster of differentiation
CNS	central nervous system
COX-2	cyclooxygenase 2
cPLA2	cytosolic phospholipase A2
CRP	C-reactive protein
CSF	cerebrospinal fluid
CT	computed tomography
CTA	computed tomography angiography
CTP	computed tomography perfusion
CXC chemokines	chemokines with two N-terminal cysteines separated by an amino acid
DAMPs	danger-/damage-associated molecular patterns
DWI	diffusion-weighted imaging
EC	endothelial cell
ECM	extracellular matrix
FDG	^{18}F-fluorodeoxyglucose
FIZZ1	found in inflammatory zone
FLAIR	fluid-attenuated inversion recovery
FMZ	^{11}C-flumazenil

GFAP	glial fibrillary acidic protein
HClO	hypochlorous acid
HIF-1α	hypoxia-inducible factor-1α
HMGB1	high-mobility group box 1 protein
ICAM-1	intercellular cell adhesion molecule-1
IFN- γ	interferon gamma
IFN	interferon
IL	interleukin
IL-1ra	IL-1 receptor antagonist
iNOS	inducible nitric oxide synthase
LDL	low-density lipoprotein
MC	Central nervous system (CNS)-resident mast cell
MCAO	middle cerebral artery occlusion
MCP-1	monocyte chemotactic protein 1
MHCII	major histocompatibility complex
MMP	matrix metalloproteinase
MPO	myeloperoxidase
MRI	magnetic resonance imaging
Mrp	myeloid-related protein
MRS	magnetic resonance spectroscopy
MTT	mean transit time
NADPH	nicotinamide adenine dinucleotide phosphate
NaF	^{18}F--sodium fluoride (NaF)
NF-κB	nuclear factor kappa light chain enhancer of activated B cells
NK	natural killer
NMDA	N-methyl-D-aspartate
nNOS	neuronal nitric oxide synthase
NO	nitric oxide
NOS	nitric oxide synthases
Nrf2	nuclear factor erythroid 2-related factor 2
NSC	neural stem cell
OEF	oxygen extraction fraction
PAMPs	pathogen-associated molecular patterns
PDM	PWI/DWI mismatch
PET	positron emission tomography
PLA2	phospholipase A2
PPARγ	peroxisome proliferator-activated receptor γ
PRRs	pattern recognition receptors
PWI	perfusion-weighted imaging

RCD	regulated cell death
RNS	reactive nitrogen species
ROS	reactive oxygen species
S100B	S100 calcium-binding protein B
SNL	selective neuronal loss
STAT	signal transducers and activators of transcription
SVD	small vessel disease
TE	time to echo
TGF-ß	transforming growth factor ß
TIMP	tissue inhibitor of metalloproteinase (TIMP)
TLR	toll-like receptor
tNAA	N-acetyl aspartate
TNF	tumor necrosis factor
TNF-α	tumor necrosis factor α
TR	repetition time
Tregs	regulatory T cells
TTP	timc to peak
UTP	Uridine triphosphate
VCAM-1	vascular cell adhesion protein 1
VEGF	vascular endothelial growth factor
vWF	von Willebrand factor

Introduction

According to the Global Burden of Disease (GBD) Study 2016, stroke risk has increased from 1990 to 2016 and remains the second leading cause of death worldwide. Mortality is slightly lower for women than men, although the risks of this pathology are almost similar for both sexes. Stroke incidence is similar for men and women up to 55 years of age and increases in men at 55–75. Stroke is estimated to be the second leading cause of loss of quality of life, and it is expected to increase in the next few years. The incidence varies in different regions: East Asia has the highest incidence, Western Europe and North America present similar values, while sub-Saharan Africa has the lowest risk (GBD 2016; Gorelick 2019).

Stroke can be subdivided into two categories, namely ischemic and hemorrhagic. Thrombosis, embolism, or systemic hypo-perfusion lead to an ischemic stroke by restricting the blood flow to the brain, resulting in insufficient oxygen and glucose delivery to support cellular homeostasis

(Doyle et al. 2008). In contrast, hemorrhagic stroke occurs by rupture of a blood vessel in the central nervous system (CNS). This phenomenon can occur in the brain parenchyma (intracerebral hemorrhage) or into the subarachnoid space (subarachnoid hemorrhage) (Parmet et al. 2004; Montaño et al. 2021). This chapter only reviews the main inflammatory processes described for ischemic stroke. This type accounts for about 87% of stroke cases and has been the target of most drug trials (Rosamond et al. 2007).

Ischemic Stroke

Ischemic stroke occurs as a consequence of vessel occlusion in the CNS, usually due to an embolus or thrombus in a major artery, and is strongly related to atherosclerosis and inflammation (see Atherosclerosis and Stroke section). The region irrigated by the occluded vessel suffers a sudden interruption of blood flow, resulting in reduced oxygen and nutrients, a process called ischemia. The subsequent failure in body functions controlled by this region characterizes an ischemic stroke and appears seconds to minutes after the vessel occlusion. Tissue damage and cell death continue for minutes, hours, or days depending on factors such as the vulnerability of the area affected or the residual perfusion (Baron 1999; Mehta et al. 2007; Moskowitz et al. 2010). In physiological conditions, blood flows in the brain at 50–60 mL/100 g/min, and ischemia reduces this flow to different degrees into the irrigated area. Thus, regions with blood flow below 7 mL/100 g/min constitute the so-called ischemic core in the ischemic territory, which suffers irreversible damage (Baron 1999). In the ischemic core, the lack of energy results in intracellular ionic imbalance, mitochondrial failure, and activation of different enzymes that damage cell integrity. Neurons progress toward necrotic or regulated cell death (RCD), such as apoptosis or necroptosis, depending on the severity of the stress (Mehta et al. 2007; Anrather and Iadecola 2016). The region surrounding the ischemic core with a blood flow ranging from 7 to 17 mL/100 g/min remains metabolically active although electrically silent (Astrup et al. 1981). In this area, named penumbra (a term coined by Linday Simon), neurons will die in several hours if blood flow is not restored. Therefore, rescuing the penumbra as much and as early as possible is one of the therapeutic goals (Astrup et al. 1981; Moskowitz et al. 2010; Baron 2018; Davis and Donnan 2021). It must be highlighted that the penumbra changes over time and therefore is a dynamic and heterogeneous region that suffers delayed and progressive infarction (Carmichael 2016). Imaging stroke is crucial in the clinic to identify the damaged area and to treat patients, as well as for basic research (see Stroke Imaging section).

Inflammation in Stroke

The classical definition of inflammation comes from Celsus (first century AD), and is characterized by the presence of *calor* (warmth), *rubor* (redness), *tumor* (swelling), and *dolo*r (pain). Later, Galen (129–128 AD) added *function laesa* (loss of function). Functionally, inflammation represents a body's response to protect itself from endogenous signals released by damaged cells (sterile inflammation) or from invading pathogens (Rock et al. 2010). Transmigration of leukocytes from blood vessels to specific tissues after injury constitutes the main hallmark of inflammation (Perretti et al. 1997). However, the progressive advance in knowledge of inflammatory mechanisms has revealed the presence of complex signaling that courses along the inflammatory process and varies in different tissues and diseases (Anrather and Iadecola 2016; Netea et al. 2017; Drieu et al. 2018; Jayaraj 2019; Shi et al. 2019; Muhammad et al. 2021).

The inflammatory process that follows ischemia, known as the ischemic pathway, is described by some authors in acute, subacute, and late (chronic) phases (Iadecola and Anrather 2011; Khatri et al. 2012; Drieu et al. 2018; Kirdajova et al. 2020). However, differences in the onset and duration in describing these phases mirror differences in the study models and species. The early post-ischemic period (acute phase) occurs in the first hours after ischemia, and its main characteristics include an increase in regional cerebral blood flow (CBF; hyperemia), augmented blood-brain barrier (BBB) permeability, and loss of cerebral regulation (Kathri et al. 2012). This phase includes edema, reperfusion, and release of multiple signaling molecules that elicit and enhance the inflammatory pathway. This pathway is characterized essentially by activation of the cellular response, infiltration of leukocytes across the BBB, disruption of the BBB, and clearing of dead cells by macrophages (Liang et al. 2007; Amantea et al. 2008; Drieu et al. 2018). The second phase (subacute phase) occurs in the first days after stroke. Its main characteristic is the resolution of inflammation, where the inflamed tissues recover their homeostasis (Spite et al. 2010; Iadecola and Anrather 2011; Drieu et al. 2018). The resolution of inflammation includes the limitation of neutrophil tissue infiltration, the regulation of inflammatory mediators, the elimination of activated neutrophils, the return of macrophages to the non-activated state, and the initiation of the healing process (Serhan and Savill 2006; Headland and Norlin 2015). The third phase (late phase) includes tissue repair and glial scar formation and can remain for days or weeks after the stroke (Drieu et al. 2018).

The Acute Phase of Inflammation in Stroke

The occlusion of a blood vessel in the CNS elicits a complex cascade of events that activates cells from the CNS and the periphery and starts in the intravascular compartment as well as the CNS parenchyma (Iadecola and Anrather 2011). The occlusion results in the cessation of blood flow and hypoxia, which changes the shear stress conditions in the vessel and induces reactive oxygen species (ROS) production and the rapid activation of vascular endothelium and platelets, triggering the coagulation cascade and activating the complement system. This response leads to BBB disruption and leukocyte invasion (Huang et al. 2006; Iadecola and Anrather 2011; Anrather and Iadecola 2016; De Meyer et al. 2016). The brain parenchyma, in turn, also presents rapid inflammatory processes due to the damaged or dying cells, which release signaling molecules called danger/damage-associated molecular patterns (DAMPs). These molecules activate pattern recognition receptors (PRRs) located in CNS and peripheral cells (Gülke et al. 2018; Roh and Shohn 2018). Activated microglia releases cytokines that provide feedback to the inflammatory cascade, enhancing cytokine production in endothelial cells (ECs) and astrocytes (Anrather and Iadecola 2016).

Edema

Ischemia or hypoxia leads to a depletion in adenosine triphosphate (ATP), resulting in a loss of balance of ionic gradients, which drives sodium influx into the cells that, in turn, promotes Cl^- influx. Different types of membrane transporters increase intracellular osmolarity, resulting in water inflow through cell membrane channels such as aquaporins (AQPs), leading to cell swelling, a phenomenon known as cytotoxic edema (Papadopoulos et al. 2013; Dalby et al. 2020). Cytotoxic edema begins about 30 minutes after the vessel occlusion and remains for up to 24 hours after reperfusion (Liang et al. 2007; Dalby et al. 2020). However, cytotoxic edema itself does not produce brain swelling. Instead, the depletion of Na^+, Cl^-, and water in the extracellular space leads to a new ion gradient from the intravascular space across the intact BBB. This gradient leads to a fluid accumulation in the extracellular space, known as ionic edema, which is responsible for increased brain volume and intracranial pressure (Michinaga and Koyama 2015). Ionic edema appears immediately after cytotoxic edema when the BBB remains still intact. Excitotoxicity and oxidative stress elicit mitochondrial dysfunction and degradation of tight junctions in ECs, allowing the extravasation of proteins from the intravascular compartment to the extracellular space. This type of edema, called vasogenic edema, appears hours after the insult (Simard et al. 2007). The breakdown in the integrity of the BBB (see The Blood Barriers in the Central Nervous System section) allows the extravasation of all blood constituents, a process known as hemorrhagic transformation or hemorrhagic conversion, which appears in up to 30%–40% of ischemic strokes, increasing mortality (Stokum et al. 2016).

Signaling Molecules in Ischemia

DAMPs

DAMPs are released from dying cells in the core of the lesion and can stimulate the immune response in a nonspecific way (adjuvanticity). DAMPs have been divided into pathogen-associated molecular patterns (PAMPs) and alarmins, a term proposed to include endogenous molecules that signal tissue and cell damage (Bianchi 2007). Alarmins include both proteins—such as high-mobility group box 1 protein (HMGB1) and heat shock proteins—and non-protein molecules (i.e., ATP) (Bianchi 2007; Gülke et al. 2018). DAMPs activate local immune cells such as microglia and ECs through PRRs, which mainly belong to the toll-like receptor (TLR) family (Drieu et al. 2018; Gülke et al. 2018). Microglia (See Microglia Section) are rapidly activated by DAMPs and adopt a pro-inflammatory phenotype that releases pro-inflammatory cytokines into blood circulation, exacerbating the leukocyte transmigration across the CNS capillary vessels (Perego et al. 2011; Drieu et al. 2018).

ROS and RNS

Normal metabolic activities produce free radicals—mainly ROS and reactive nitrogen species (RNS)—that, under physiological conditions, are neutralized by endogenous antioxidants to maintain the redox balance. ROS include a wide range of signaling molecules such as superoxide ($O_2^{\bullet-}$), hydrogen peroxide (H_2O_2), and the hydroxyl radical ($OH^{\bullet}$). RNS include molecules such as peroxynitrite ($ONOO^-$), a potent oxidizing agent. Peroxynitrite results from the combination of nitric oxide (NO, produced by nitric oxide synthases [NOS]) with superoxide anions. ROS and RNS play physiological roles at low/moderate concentrations. Thus, the phagocytic isoform of nicotinamide adenine dinucleotide phosphate (NADPH) oxidase in activated macrophages and neutrophils can produce large amounts of superoxide, whose derivatives have antimicrobial and tumoricidal functions in an inflammatory environment. In this regard, eliciting an "oxidative burst" forms part of the first line of defense against environmental pathogens. In addition, the combined action of NADPH oxidase and myeloperoxidase (MPO) produces hypochlorous acid (hClO), one of the strongest physiological oxidants and a powerful antimicrobial agent (Dröge 2002; Jelinek et al. 2021; Ashok et al. 2022). Most cell types generate low ROS concentrations when stimulated by cytokines, growth factors, and hormones (Thannickal and Fanburg 2000). ROS generated by the action of these ligands can behave as true second messengers, mediating functions such as proliferation and programmed cell death (Valko et al. 2007; Zhang et al. 2016). However, the overproduction of reactive species leads to oxidative or nitrosative stress, which damages DNA and oxidizes lipids and proteins, impairing homeostasis and playing crucial roles in the inflammatory response (Stadtman 2004; Valko et al. 2007). In addition, dysfunctional mitochondria under oxidative stress could be involved in progressive neurodegeneration (Ashok et al. 2022).

Cytokines

Cytokines are small proteins acting as chemical messengers that play a major role in cell activation, proliferation, and differentiation. They include lymphokines, made by lymphocytes that attract immune cells such as macrophages; monokines, produced by monocytes that attract neutrophils; chemokines associated with chemotactic actions; and interleukins (ILs), made by leukocytes to communicate with other leukocytes. Growth factors, interferons (IFNs), and tumor necrosis factors (TNFs) are sometimes included as cytokines and made by more than one cell type. In contrast to hormones secreted by specialized cells and released into the bloodstream to act on distant cells, cytokines usually act locally in an autocrine or paracrine manner. However, they sometimes enter the bloodstream and act as hormones. Cytokines present pleiotropic effects because they act on different cell types. The same cytokine can regulate different functions, different cytokines can perform the same function (redundancy), and they are multifunctional (Viviani et al. 2004; Huang et al. 2006; Adibhatla et al. 2008; Jayarag et al. 2019).

Inflammation depends on the balance between pro-inflammatory cytokines, such as TNF-α, IL-1, IFN-γ, IL-12, and IL-18, and anti-inflammatory cytokines, such as IL-4, IL-10, IL-13, IFN-α, and transforming growth factor-ß (TGF-ß) (Stoll 2002). However, the classification of pro- and anti-inflammatory cytokines is considered too simplistic and does not mirror the complexity of the cytokine effects. Thus, some cytokines such as IL-6 can present pro- and anti-inflammatory properties. Other cytokines present pro- or anti-inflammatory effects depending on the activating signal, the amount of cytokine, the timing of the action, the experimental model, and other factors (Cavaillon 2001).

The expression of different cytokines is closely related. For example, TNF-α induces the expression of IL-1 and IL-6, and IL-1 can induce both TNF-α and IL-6 (Andre et al. 2005). After the CNS insult, the initial upregulation of cytokines results in secondary cytokine signaling (Lucas et al. 2006) and synergistic cooperation in different signaling pathways. For example, TNF-α, IL-1α, and IFN-γ cooperatively induce cell death in mouse primary cortical neuron/glia co-cultures (Jeohn et al. 1998).

The pro-inflammatory cytokines TNF-α and IL-1 play a crucial role in the ischemic pathway (Clausen et al. 2020). TNF-α is rapidly upregulated in the ischemic brain, reaches a peak 6–12 hours after the ischemic onset, and maintains its expression up to 24–78 hours. Interestingly, TNF-α levels in cerebrospinal fluid (CSF) and serum correlate with brain infarct volume (Feuerstein et al. 1994; Lovering and Zhang 2005). Among the TNF-α effects in stroke are the activation of endothelial and leukocyte molecules that promote leukocyte infiltration across the BBB (Feuerstein et al. 1994), upregulation of matrix metalloproteinases (MMPs) such as MMP-2 and MMP-9 (Horstmann et al. 2003), increased BBB permeability (Dickstein et al. 2000), and exacerbation of neurological damage (Barone et al. 1997). Two receptors for TNF-α (p55 and p75) appear upregulated after ischemia. p55 contains the death domain and is overexpressed in the first hours following ischemia, while p75 increases after 24 hours or later (Botchkina et al. 1997; Lambertsen et al. 2007). IL-1 is made of two agonist ligands, IL-1α and IL-1β, that bind to IL-1 type I receptor and trigger similar but not completely overlapping functions (Andre et al. 2005). IL-1β is rapidly upregulated after ischemia and is considered the main form of IL-1 contributing to ischemic injury. IL-1 receptor antagonist (IL-1ra) is a third member of the IL-1 family that blocks the effects of IL-1α and IL-1β. IL-1ra administration drastically reduces the infarct volume in the middle cerebral artery occlusion (MCAO) model (Boutin et al. 2001). Microglia release the IL-1ra and are responsible for the neuroprotective effects of this IL-1 antagonist (Pinteaux et al. 2006). Cell membrane lipids are also strongly affected by cytokines. Upregulation of both TNF-α and IL-1β after stroke alters phospholipid metabolism, stimulating hydrolysis, inhibiting the synthesis of phosphatidylcholine and sphingomyelin, and disrupting membrane integrity. These cytokines also initiate the arachidonic acid cascade after stroke, activating the cytosolic phospholipase A2 (cPLA2) and cyclooxygenase 2 (COX-2) in astrocytes (Adibhatla et al. 2008).

IL-6 is also upregulated following cerebral ischemia. Its role as pro- or anti-inflammatory molecule in ischemia is controversial. It has been proposed that IL-6 acts as an inflammatory mediator during the acute phase of inflammation and as a neurotrophic factor in subacute and later phases (Suzuki et al. 2009). Elevated levels of IL-6 in serum and CSF have also been correlated with increased infarct volume and worse outcomes (Smith et al. 2004). A role for this cytokine in regulating the body temperature has also been suggested since cerebral ischemia increases the expression of IL-6 in mice (Herrman et al. 2003).

Reperfusion and Excitotoxicity

The restoration of blood flow (reperfusion) is required for the survival of the neurons; however, reperfusion elicits new mechanisms of damage such as excitotoxicity and inflammation. Thus, blood flow reperfusion stimulates the release of the neurotransmitter glutamate by the dying cells, resulting in the prolonged stimulation of α-amino-3-hydroxy-5-methyl-4-isoxazolepropionic acid (AMPA) and N-methyl-D-aspartate (NMDA) glutamatergic receptors in the neurons, promoting a massive influx of Ca^{2+}, Na^{+}, and water into neurons (cytotoxic edema) as mentioned above. Ca^{2+} overload in the cells activates catabolic processes mediated by proteases, lipases, and nucleases (Ankarcrona et al. 1995). Activating Ca^{2+}-dependent enzymes such as neuronal nitric oxide synthase (nNOS) or phospholipase A2 (PLA2) leads to the production of arachidonic acid metabolites, ROS, and RNS. Furthermore, this excitotoxic response results in mitochondrial damage and elicits different types of programmed cell death such as apoptosis, necroptosis, or ferroptosis at different times and in distinct areas of the brain (Mehta et al. 2007; Sandoval and Witt 2008; Moskowitz et al. 2010; Khatri et al. 2012; Vieira et al. 2014; Font-Belmonte et al. 2019). For a detailed review of excitotoxicity, see Kirdajova et al. (2020).

Adhesion Molecules and Leukocyte Infiltration

The inflammatory response that follows stroke, and other types of CNS insults, includes the infiltration of different leukocytes, such as neutrophils and monocytes/macrophages, which produce ROS, proteases, and pro-inflammatory mediators that contribute to BBB damage, edema, microvessel obstruction, cellular necrosis, and tissue infarction (Abbot 2000; Huang et al. 2006; Kang et al. 2020). Leukocyte infiltration starts with the activation of ECs and platelets, which store P-selectin and von Willebrand factor (vWF) in the EC Weibel–Palade bodies and in platelet α-granules. Ischemia-dependent activation leads to the translocation of P-selectin to the surface membrane and the release of vWF, which promotes the rolling of leukocytes and platelets on ECs (Cambien and Wagner 2004; Dole et al. 2005; Borregaard 2010; De Meyer et al. 2016). Stimulation by hypoxia, cytokines, and other mediators induces the transcriptional expression of cell adhesion molecules (CAMs) such as E-selectin and intercellular cell adhesion molecule-1 (ICAM-1) that bind to the leukocyte integrin CD11b/CD18, allowing the firm adherence of leukocytes to the vascular endothelium (Huang et al. 2006). In addition, oxidative stress reduces the bioavailability of NO in ECs. Thus, the beneficial effects of NO, such as vasodilation and inhibition of platelet aggregation and leukocyte adhesion, decrease, aggravating the ischemic insult (Yilmaz and Granger 2010; Iadecola and Anrather 2011).

The accumulation of adherent leukocytes in cerebral venules begins a few minutes after reperfusion and increases progressively up to 48 hours after reperfusion. Four hours after reperfusion, most adherent leukocytes are neutrophils (~85%). After 24 hours, the number of adherent leukocytes is roughly double that observed at 4 hours; however, the number of neutrophils only accounts for 20% of adherent leukocytes. The remaining fraction of adherent leukocytes consists of monocytes and T lymphocytes (Yilmaz and Granger 2010). Neutrophils remain in the brain for days, but their presence seems to be masked by the accumulation of microglia/macrophages in the inflammatory region (Weston et al. 2007). The presence of neutrophils in the ischemic cortex of mice has been described at least 14 days after stroke, with a peak three days after the insult (Kang et al. 2020). Leukocytes may remain close to the capillaries, which impairs CBF, or may reach the brain parenchyma, where they release pro-inflammatory cytokines, chemokines, ROS, and NOS (Danton and Dietrich 2003; Amantea et al. 2008; Kang et al. 2020).

Cellular and molecular magnetic resonance image (MRI) allows exploring the spatiotemporal profile of neuroinflammation (see Stroke Imaging section). The best strategy for detecting circulating monocytes is the administration of iron oxide nanoparticles that can be detected on T2-weighted images (Shichinohe et al. 2012).

Upon infiltration, neutrophils produce inducible nitric oxide synthase (iNOS), generating toxic NO concentrations and releasing MMPs such as

MMP-9 and MPO responsible for the first disruption of the BBB (Justicia et al. 2003). Loss of ATP and oxygen leads to the activation of the transcription factor hypoxia-inducible factor-1α (HIF-1α), which results in MMP2 activation, while cytokines such as TNF-α and IL-1β activate MMP-3 and MMP-9. MMP-2 (gelatinase A) causes transient and reversible degradation of tight junction proteins several hours after reperfusion onset and, later, the release of MMP-3 and MMP-9 (gelatinase B), which degrade the basal lamina and tight junctions of ECs, leading to intense and irreversible damage (Yang and Rosenberg 2011). Degradation of tight junction proteins is a hallmark of BBB disruption in ischemic stroke (Abdullahi et al. 2018), which results in vasogenic edema (Yang and Rosenberg 2011). Resident macrophages and CNS-resident mast cells (MCs) are also activated. MCs secrete MMP-2, MMP-9, tryptases, and chymases, enhancing the degradation of the extracellular matrix (ECM) (Peruzzotti-Jametti et al. 2014). Infiltrated eosinophils secrete MMPs and elastases that contribute to the BBB disruption and ECM degradation (Jacobsen et al. 2007). Growth factors such as vascular endothelial growth factor (VEGF) and TGF-β are usually bound to the ECM as zymogens and activated as a consequence of ECM degradation (Zlokovic 2006). Growth factors, infiltrating immune cells, and mediators accumulated in the perivascular space stimulate astrocytes at the lesion border, and this early glial activation is crucial in the outcome after stroke (Peruzzotti-Jametti 2014).

Infiltrating T lymphocytes are considered detrimental and present cytotoxic activity unrelated to adaptive immunity or thrombus formation (Kleinschnitz et al. 2010). Natural killer (NK) cells and γδ T lymphocytes also contribute to ischemic injury, and cytolytic activity of NK cells on ischemic neurons has also been suggested (Gelderblom et al. 2012; Gan et al. 2014). Enhanced migration of regulatory T cells (Tregs) across the BBB could be protective, since these cells may inactivate MMP-9 limiting BBB breakdown (Li et al. 2013). However, the role of Tregs on BBB integrity is still uncertain (Liesz and Kleinschnitz 2016).

The Subacute Phase of Inflammation in Stroke

The subacute phase involves the resolution of inflammation (Drieu et al. 2018), a mechanism mediated by several overlapping processes with a complex regulation that drives tissue healing (Serhan et al. 2008). These processes include reduction or cessation of extravasation across the BBB, blocking the effect of pro-inflammatory mediators, replacing pro-survival signaling by RCD signaling in neutrophils to be phagocytosed by macrophages (efferocytosis), modification of the macrophage phenotype (from pro- to anti-inflammatory), and the return to the blood or lymph of cells not committed to RCD (Sugimoto et al. 2016). The resolution of inflammation also involves changes in signaling that include the release of anti-inflammatory and pro-resolving mediators. While anti-inflammatory mediators inhibit inflammation (for example, blocking cell infiltration), pro-resolving mediators stimulate processes addressed to the resolution of inflammation (for example, promoting RCD or efferocytosis) (Sugimoto et al. 2016). Pro-resolving mediators include a variety of molecules such as lipids (lipoxins, resolvins, protectins, or marexins), proteins, gases, and small molecules (Headland and Norling 2015).

Neutrophil Depletion

The depletion of neutrophils, a process in which macrophages play a crucial role, is the key to the resolution of inflammation and contrasts with the presence of extravascular accumulation of neutrophils, considered the hallmark of acute inflammation (Ortega-Gómez et al. 2013; Sugimoto et al. 2016). The resolution of inflammation requires stopping the recruitment of new neutrophils to the inflamed area, followed by RCD of extravascular neutrophils. Most of the literature indicates apoptosis as the RCD of neutrophils (Fox et al. 2010; Ortega-Gómez et al. 2013; Sugimoto et al. 2016); however, other RCD subroutines for neutrophils have been reported, including NETosis, necroptosis, or pyroptosis (Pérez-Figueroa et al. 2021).

Chemokines play crucial roles in neutrophil recruitment; thus, chemokine cleavage or chemokine sequestration is essential to block neutrophil tissue infiltration. In this regard, cleavage of the glutamic acid–leucine–arginine (ELR) motif of CXC chemokines (chemokines with two N-terminal cysteines separated by an amino acid) by MMP-12, for example, blocks their binding to their neutrophil receptors and prevents neutrophil recruitment (Dean et al. 2008). In addition, sequestering CC chemokines (chemokines with two N-terminal adjacent cysteines) and CCX pro-inflammatory chemokines—for example, by decoy receptors expressed in ECs—decreases the neutrophil recruitment (Gardner et al. 2004; Mantovani et al. 2006).

Neutrophils contribute to the resolution of inflammation and tissue repair by promoting their removal and releasing anti-inflammatory and pro-resolving mediators such as annexin or lipoxin A4 (Kolaczkowska and Kubes 2013). Thus, the role of neutrophils in ischemic stroke has two sides: the harmful effects promoted by pro-inflammatory neutrophils and the reparative effects on post-stroke inflammation (Chen et al. 2021). Neutrophil apoptosis is activated by different stimuli such as Fas-ligand and TNF-α released by activated macrophages (van den Berg et al. 2001), and dying neutrophils release various mediators that contribute to the resolution of inflammation (Ortega-Gomez et al. 2013; Sugimoto et al. 2016; Chen et al. 2021). For example, resting neutrophils present annexin A1 in the cytosol that, after activation, is translocated to the membrane, contributing to moderate leukocyte adhesion and migration and promoting neutrophil apoptosis and clearance of neutrophils by macrophages (Scannell et al. 2007). Similarly, pro-resolving mediator lipoxin A4 inhibits neutrophil transmigration (Maddox et al. 1997) and promotes chemotaxis in monocytes and macrophages (Maddox et al. 1997; József et al. 2002). Dying neutrophils present *find me* and *eat me* signals that attract microglia and macrophages to the injury site (Davalos et al. 2005). Major *find me* signals include lysophosphatidylcholine, sphingosine 1-phosphate, the chemokine fractalkine CX3XL1, and nucleotides such as ATP and uridine triphosphate (UTP), whose gradients attract phagocytic cells to the dead cell. *Eat me* signals such as phosphatidylserine identify a dying cell for efferocytosis (Ortega-Gomez et al. 2013).

Despite the detrimental effects of neutrophils in the ischemic area, these cells also promote reparative functions. Thus, neutrophil gelatinase-associated lipocalin polarizes macrophages toward a reparative phenotype (Carbone et al. 2020). In this regard, neutrophil accumulation in the brain above a certain level has been suggested to change from a pro-inflammatory phenotype (N1) to an anti-inflammatory phenotype (N2) (Easton 2013), which is related to the alleviation of cerebral infarction and could present protective effects in stroke (Cuartero et al. 2013; Chen et al. 2021). However, whether the different roles of neutrophils result from different neutrophil subsets requires further confirmation (Chen et al. 2021).

Resolution-Phase Macrophages

Macrophages integrate signals from multiple sources such as phagocytosed cells, microvesicles, and molecules in the ECM via endocrine and paracrine signaling. Furthermore, macrophages interact with tissue-resident cell populations, immune cells recruited during injury, and extracellular proteins. Therefore, macrophages play diverse roles in tissue injury and the repair response (Watanabe et al. 2019). After efferocytosis, macrophages switch from the release of pro-inflammatory mediators to anti-inflammatory mediators such as IL-10 and TGF-β (Fadok et al. 1998) involved in the clearance of inflammatory cells and return to homeostasis. These resolution-phase macrophages also activate pro-resolving mechanisms, such as stimulating phagocytic activities not accompanied by the release of pro-inflammatory mediators (Sugimoto et al. 2016). The recovery of spinal cord injury after injection of "alternatively activated" blood macrophages (Rapalino et al. 1998) showed the potential beneficial effect of these cells in CNS repair, and subsequent studies have allowed distinguishing different functional responses between resident-activated microglia and infiltrating monocyte-derived macrophages (Schwartz et al. 2013). Blood-derived macrophages recruited to the injured site after the insult become monocyte-derived macrophages, which present a beneficial effect, mediated by IL-10, on the spinal cord (Shechter et al. 2009), regulating microglia and contributing to the resolution of the inflammation and scar formation (Shechter et al. 2009; Schwartz et al. 2013). In physiological conditions, tissue-resident macrophages eliminate dead cells, toxins, particulates, or pathogens from the local microenvironment and produce many mediators that interact with fibroblasts and immune, epithelial, endothelial, and stem cells, contributing to homeostasis. Monocyte-derived macrophages present a strong inflammatory response during injury and can undergo apoptosis or survive by self-renewal. Tissue-resident macrophages show a weak inflammatory response during injury and can die or repopulate the niche by self-renewal. Finally, phenotypes of tissue-resident and monocyte-derived macrophage populations become similar (Watanabe et al. 2019).

Adaptive Immune Response

The damage elicited by stroke generates novel brain antigens that stimulate B and T lymphocytes. Resolution-phase macrophages secrete T and B cell chemoattractants that promote the repopulation of resolving inflammation sites with NK cells and lymphocytes such as B1, $\gamma\delta$T, $CD4^{+}CD25^{+}$, and B2 cells, which, although dispensable for resolution, have been suggested to be involved in a protective role in the resolution phase. Several days after stroke, T lymphocytes migrate to the ischemic region in a way not dependent on antigens. Tregs reduce astrogliosis, eliminate the astroglial neurotoxic phenotype, and promote functional recovery, but the infarct volume is unaffected. Regulatory B lymphocytes also present a protective role and enhance the beneficial effects of Tregs (Rajakariar et al. 2008; Ren et al. 2011; Bodhankar et al. 2013; Iadecola et al. 2020).

The Late Phase of Inflammation in Stroke

Tissue repair and reestablishment of functionality are complex processes that occur in the late phase of inflammation, where macrophages, stem cells, and stromal cells cooperate to prevent, as much as possible, the ineffective or inappropriate tissue function resulting from fibrosis or the glial scar. In particular, anti-inflammatory activated macrophages play a crucial role in the reparative process, releasing mediators such as IL-1ra, IL-10, TGF-β, and VEGF (Ortega-Gómez et al. 2013).

In the CNS, the late phase of inflammation includes different processes such as matrix remodeling, neurogenesis, axon sprouting, dendritogenesis, and oligodendrogenesis addressed to restore tissue integrity and initiate an extensive glial response called reactive gliosis (Peruzzotti-Jametti et al. 2014; Drieu et al. 2018). Activated astrocytes will form the glial scar by secreting chondroitin sulfate proteoglycans such as neurocan, phosphacan, or versican into the ECM, enhancing the expression of vimentin and glial fibrillary acidic protein (GFAP). The glial scar limits extravasated leukocytes in perivascular clusters and prevents the infiltration of immune cells into the CNS parenchyma. The glial scar in the spinal cord has been widely studied, characterizing different roles for its components. In this regard, resident astrocytes and ependymal neural stem cell (NSC)-derived astrocytes participate in glial scar formation and play different functions (Peruzzotti-Jametti et al. 2014). Ependymal NSC-derived astrocytes comprise the core of the scar, surrounded by resident astrocytes (Barnabé-Heider et al. 2010) that seem to be involved in restricting the infiltration of inflammatory cells (Okada et al. 2006; Herrmann et al. 2008) and the inhibition of neutrophil degranulation (Xie et al. 2010). In contrast, ependymal NSC-derived astrocytes reinforce the injured spinal cord (Sabelström et al. 2013).

The glial scar impedes axonal regrowth and other regenerative mechanisms (Silver and Miller 2004); therefore, recovery of the damaged CNS requires some degree of ECM remodeling and astroglial modulation (Zuo et al. 1998). Different cells seem to contribute to sorting out the glial scar limitations. Thus, MCs secrete a protease able to degrade cytokines associated with inflammation and reduce astrogliosis (Nelissen et al. 2014); complement-dependent cell-mediated cytotoxicity of astrocytes might be amplified by eosinophils (Zhang and Verkman 2013); and M2 macrophages could also remodel the glial scar to make it more permissive for axonal regrowth (Shechter et al. 2009).

Atherosclerosis and Stroke

Inflammation, Atherosclerosis, and Large Artery Stroke

Atherosclerosis is a progressive disease where the accumulation of lipids and fibrous elements in the wall of large arteries gives rise to atheromatous plaques (Lusis 2000). Anatomopathological, laboratory, epidemiological, genetic, and imaging studies have demonstrated that large vessel atherosclerosis presents an inflammatory response that chronically affects the arterial wall (Muir et al. 2007). Destabilization of an atherosclerotic plaque may elicit severe clinical effects such as ischemic episodes in the heart and the brain. Because inflammation plays a crucial role in the onset and evolution of atherosclerotic plaque, many inflammatory proteins have been analyzed as possible markers of cardiovascular diseases in clinical and public health practice (Pearson et al. 2003). Different inflammation-associated proteins appear to be involved in destabilizing atheromatous plaque. For example, myeloid-related protein (Mrp)-8 and Mrp-14, expressed in inflammatory cells such as neutrophils, monocytes, and macrophages, form Mrp-8/Mrp-14 complexes after cell activation related to an increased risk of cardiovascular events (Ionita et al. 2010). Other markers, such as MMP-1, MMP-7, tissue inhibitor of metalloproteinase (TIMP)-1, TNF-α, and IL-8, increase in patients with unstable plaques (Pelisek et al. 2009).

The onset of arteriosclerosis is caused by damage in the endothelium due to aggressive stimuli such as elevated low-density lipoprotein (LDL) cholesterol concentrations, free radicals (caused by smoking and diabetes), elevated blood pressure levels, infections by microorganisms such as herpes virus or *Chlamydia*, and hemodynamic alterations in certain anatomical segments (Ross 1999; Fan and Watanabe 2003; Blanco et al. 2006; Di Napoli and Papa 2006; Fisher et al. 2012). In normal conditions, circulating blood cells do firmly adhere to ECs. However, noxious stimuli promote the expression of CAMs, such as vascular cell adhesion protein 1 (VCAM-1), E-selectin, and P-selectin, allowing the adhesion of neutrophils, monocytes, and T lymphocytes to the endothelium, followed by their migration through the endothelial wall. Monocytes in the arterial intima acquire the morphological characteristics of macrophages and express receptors for LDL, absorbing them to form foam cells that contribute to establishing the necrotic nucleus of the atherosclerotic lesion. Simultaneously, macrophages, as a result of the action of monocyte chemotactic protein 1 (MCP-1), differentiate into the pro-inflammatory M1 phenotype and express pro-inflammatory cytokines, such as IL-1β and TNF-α, amplifying the local inflammatory response. Other cytokines (platelet-derived growth factors) stimulate the migration of smooth muscle cells of the vascular wall from the adventitia and media to the intima, where they form the layers of atheromatous plaques. These fibrous layers suffer erosion and rupture due to cytokines and MMPs released by macrophages, leading to the plaque rupture. Macrophages also produce tissue factor, which reaches the blood after plaque rupture and induces the coagulation cascade, leading to thrombus formation. Thrombus embolization can cause an ischemic cerebrovascular event (Libby 2002, Libby et al. 2019).

Several epidemiological studies support the relationship between inflammation and the risk of cerebrovascular disease, with a correlation between common inflammatory markers (cytokines, TNF-α, and C-reactive protein [CRP]) and the development of vascular disease. A comprehensive study with more than 1.1 million people and approximately 70,000 recorded cardiovascular events concluded that CRP concentrations are associated with the risk of coronary heart disease, ischemic stroke, and other pathologies (ERFC 2010). Similarly, in the Framingham study, during 12–14 years of follow-up, men and women with CRP in the highest quartile had more than a 2-fold increased risk of ischemic stroke than those with CRP in the lowest quartile (Rost et al. 2001). Other proatherogenic cytokines, such as IL-6 and TNF-α, have also been associated with an increased risk of stroke in both epidemiological (Cesari et al. 2003) and genetic studies (Georgakis et al. 2020; Yuan et al. 2020).

Imaging techniques (see Imagen Stroke section) are also used to evaluate atherosclerotic plaque vulnerability related to inflammatory activity. For example, positron emission tomography (PET) using tracers such as ^{18}F-fluorodeoxyglucose (FDG) and ^{18}F-sodium fluoride (NaF) allow visualizing carotid wall inflammation and microcalcification, respectively. FDG-PET studies provide information about the inflammatory part of carotid atherosclerosis, while NaF-PET seems to predict long-term consequences of ongoing inflammation suggesting clinically significant carotid atherosclerosis (Piri et al. 2020). Moreover, FDG uptake in atherosclerotic plaques from patients with symptomatic carotid stenosis improves the prediction of recurrent stroke risk compared with risk stratification using only the degree of stenosis (Kelly et al. 2020).

Inflammation in Small Vessel Disease

Small vessel disease (SVD) has been related to alterations in the permeability of the BBB, giving rise to enlarged Virchow–Robin perivascular spaces, subcortical white matter lesions, lacunar infarcts, and brain microbleeds, and can activate ECs and the monocyte-macrophage system. Patients with a high degree of SVD present high levels of CRP, neopterin, and CAMs such as E- and P-selectins (Rouhl et al. 2012). Inflammation is a risk factor in SVD, although the underlying mechanisms and causal pathways remain unclear. A recent systematic review has evidenced the association between inflammatory markers and radiological findings related to SVD. The authors classified inflammatory markers as systemic inflammation (CRP, IL-6, and fibrinogen) or vascular inflammation/endothelial dysfunction (homocysteine and vWF) and seem to be differentially related to two different forms of SVD. Thus, markers of systemic inflammation seem to be associated with cerebral amyloid angiopathy-related vascular damage, such as the centrum semiovale, while vascular inflammatory markers appear in SVD in areas characteristic of hypertensive arteriopathy, such as the basal ganglia (Low et al. 2019).

Anti-Inflammatory Therapies in the Prevention of Stroke

Some of the main drugs used to prevent ischemic cerebrovascular disease have anti-inflammatory properties. Aspirin (an antithrombotic agent), angiotensin II inhibitors (a hypotensive agent), statins (lipid-lowering agents), and other anti-inflammatory agents act at different levels and are used in various diseases. Corticosteroids, COX inhibitors, colchicine, methotrexate, and anti-TNF agents are included in this pharmacological category, and their preventive capacity has been reviewed recently.

For example, high doses of aspirin inhibit inducible COX-2, resulting in decreased prostaglandin synthesis in response to inflammatory cytokines. However, the main therapeutic effect of low doses of aspirin commonly used for stroke prevention is probably mediated by a reduction in platelet lifespan, due to the inhibition of COX-1 and thromboxane A2 (Awtry and Loscalzo 2000). Aspirin is effective in the secondary prevention of stroke; however, its benefits in the primary prevention of stroke are controversial (Lei et al. 2016).

Angiotensin II promotes atherogenic inflammation by upregulating endothelial adhesion molecules (E-selectin and VCAM-1), MCP-1, and IL-6, increasing the adhesion and recruitment of monocytes. In spontaneously hypertensive rats, blocking the angiotensin II AT1 receptor reduces the infiltration of microvascular macrophages and IL-1β. Conversely, stimulating the angiotensin II AT1 receptor enhances TNF-α and intracellular adhesion molecule expression (Ando et al. 2004).

The JUPITER trial in more than 17,000 healthy men and women with LDL cholesterol < 130 mg/dL and high-sensitivity CRP > 2.0 mg/L showed that treatment with rosuvastatin (20 mg daily) resulted in a 48% relative risk reduction for the first stroke, a 50% reduction in LDL cholesterol levels, and a 37% reduction in high-sensitivity CRP. However, the JUPITER study could not determine whether these effects are specifically attributable to anti-inflammatory effects (Ridker et al. 2008).

Several recombinant engineered antibodies that interact with the immune system have been developed, some of them targeted toward cytokines involved in the inflammatory pathway. The main targets are TNF-α (infliximab and adalimumab), IL-1 (canakinumab and anakinra), and IL-2 (daclizumab). Canakinumab is an anti-human IL-1 monoclonal antibody. The CANTOS clinical trial evaluated the clinical effect of canakinumab on the incidence of cardiovascular events in patients with previous myocardial infarction and elevated ultrasensitive CRP (≥ 2 mg/L), demonstrating that the reduction in inflammation targeting IL-1β is associated with a reduction in cardiovascular events. This study also showed that a 150 mg dose of canakinumab reduced the incidence of cardiovascular events to a similar magnitude in diabetics, pre-diabetics, and non-diabetics. However, the high cost of canakinumab and its most unfavorable risk (fatal sepsis) has led to its use not being recommended in clinical practice (Ridker et al. 2017).

Colchicine, a potent inhibitor of cell cytoskeletal microtubule polymerization, mitosis, and inflammatory cell motility, has emerged as a potential drug for arthritis and inflammatory conditions because it inhibits inflammasome assembly and IL-1β activation (Leung et al. 2015; Angelidis et al. 2018). In a model of atherosclerotic plaque in rabbit aorta, colchicine treatment seems to stabilize atherosclerotic plaque by reducing its inflammatory component without reducing its size or lipid content (Cecconi et al. 2021). Several trials using low-dose colchicine have shown its usefulness in preventing cardiovascular events (Nidorf et al. 2013), reducing the risk for total myocardial infarction (Hemkens et al. 2016; Tardif et al. 2019; Nidorf et al. 2020). A phase 3 trial to study the possible effects of using colchicine to prevent vascular inflammation in non-cardioembolic stroke is currently under way (Kelly et al. 2021).

Stroke Imaging

Several non-invasive techniques have increased the tools to detect stroke-derived brain damage. For example, computed tomography (CT, also known as CT scan) combines X-rays and computer software to generate images of the inside of the body, allowing clinicians to observe bones, muscle, fat, and blood vessels and differentiate brain parenchyma. Computed tomography angiography (CTA) highlights blood vessels by intravenous injection of a contrast agent dye, usually iodine-based contrast. The wide availability, execution speed, and proven efficacy in detecting ischemia of CT and CTA are essential in the initial study of patients with suspected stroke (Figure 1). In addition, other techniques such as computed tomography perfusion (CTP) (Figure 1), which uses an intravascular tracer that can be followed in CT serial images, magnetic resonance imaging (MRI), and PET can demonstrate salvageable tissue (penumbra) and allow extending the therapeutic window after stroke (Hetts and Khangura 2019; Kawahara and Nagata 2021; Dong et al. 2022).

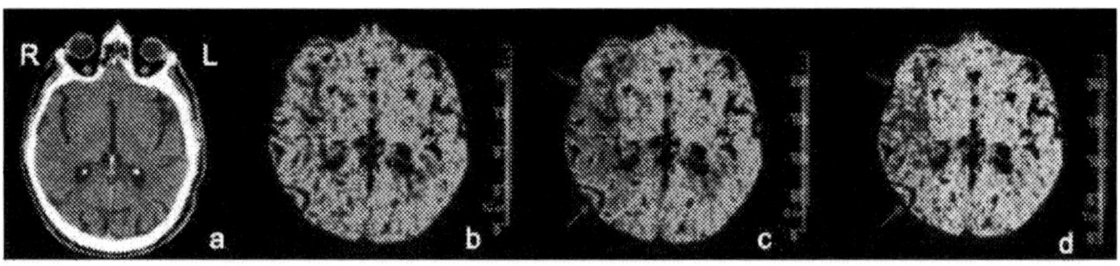

Figure 1. Computed tomography (CT) and computed tomography perfusion (CTP) of a patient with acute ischemic stroke in right hemisphere 2 hours after its onset. Non-contrast CT scan (a); CTP with no significant abnormal areas in cerebral blood volume (CBV) (b), diminished cerebral blood flow (CBF, arrows) (c), and delayed time to peak (TTP, arrows) (d), indicating the penumbra and potentially recoverable tissue.

CTP allows measuring the blood flow through the neural parenchyma (Figure 2). The CTP raw data are displayed in parameter maps, including CBF (the volume of blood flow per minute per 100 mL of tissue), cerebral blood volume (CBV, the volume of blood in a given amount of brain tissue, usually milliliters of blood per 100 g of brain tissue), the mean transit time (MTT, the average transit time for a tracer particle to traverse the capillary bed), and time to peak (TTP, the time at which the maximal contrast concentration can be observed). Core infarctions present reduced CBF and CBV, while the penumbra has prolonged MTT or TTP and normal CBV Worldwide, CTP is the most used technique to determine the penumbra. Nevertheless, CTP usually relies on predefined software characteristics that may not take into account patient peculiarities (Heiss et al. 2000; Wintermark et al. 2008; Demeestere et al. 2020).

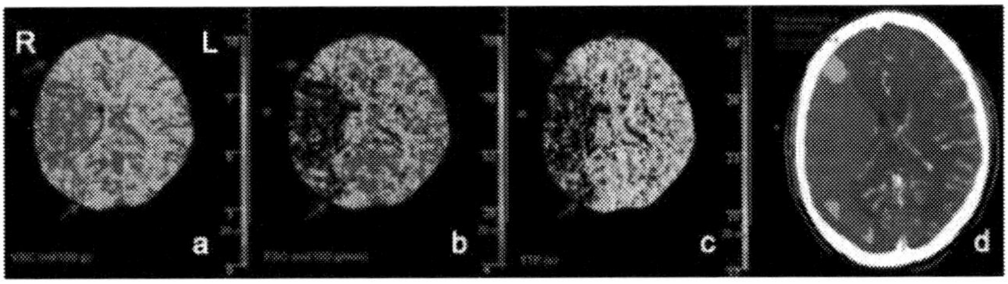

Figure 2. Computed tomography perfusion (CTP) of a stroke patient.
The images are from a 54-year-old woman who awoke with right hemispheric symptoms. The right frontoparietal region shows cerebral blood volume (CBV) (a) and cerebral blood flow (CBF) reduction (b), and delayed time to peak (TTP) (c). Summary image (d) shows a large area of tissue necrosis (red) and a small penumbra (green), unfavorable for endovascular thrombectomy.

Although MRI scanning takes a long time, it provides useful functional information from different contrast images (Figure 3). T1-weighted[1] images enhance the fat tissue and suppress the water signal, while T2-weighted images enhance the water signal (Kawahara and Nagata 2021). MRI can also be used to characterize the core and penumbra. Thus, the lowest diffusion-weighted imaging (DWI)[2] coefficients allow delimiting the central tissue of the infarct that is irreversibly damaged, while perfusion-weighted imaging (PWI)[3] provides information about the infarct core and the surrounding hypoperfused tissue. A PWI/DWI mismatch (PDM) ratio can be obtained by

[1] T1-weighted images are produced using a short time to echo (TE, the time between the delivery of the external radio frequency pulse, and the receipt of the signal) and a short repetition time (TR, the amount of time between successive pulse sequences applied to the same slide). In contrast, T2-weighted images are obtained by using long TE and TR times. CSF appears dark in T1-weighted images and bright in T2-weighted images, allowing clinicians to distinguish easily between T1- and T2-weighted images. Using very long TE and TR times, the sequence called fluid attenuated inversion recovery (FLAIR) provides T2-weighted images where normal CSF appears dark and abnormalities appear bright. FLAIR makes it easier to differentiate between CSF and abnormalities.

[2] DWI is a method based on the differences in Brownian motion. It is designed to detect the random movements of water protons and to generate signal contrast, allowing the evaluation of molecular functions and microarchitecture of the tissues (Baliyan et al. 2016).

[3] PWI includes hemodynamic measurements such as CBV, CBF, and MTT.

combining both sequences, where the penumbra is represented by a PDM ratio ≥ 1.2. PDM is an extraordinarily quantitative method to assess the penumbra, although not widely available (Singer et al. 2004; Ford et al. 2014).

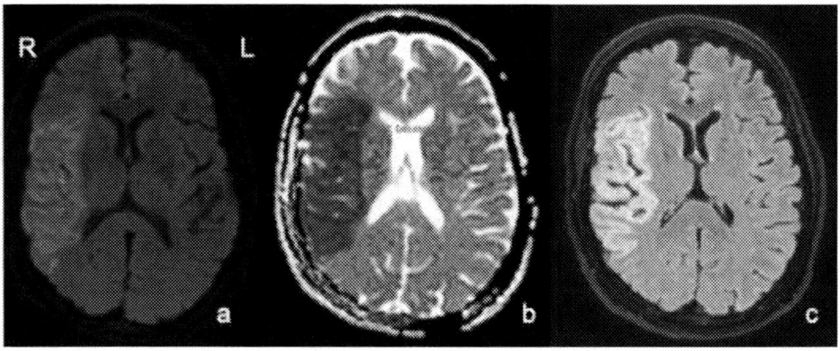

Figure 3. Magnetic resonance imaging (MRI) in a patient with right hemispheric infarction. Right hemispheric hypersignal in diffusion-weighted image (DWI) (a), hyposignal in attenuation diffusion coefficient (ADC) image (b), and hypersignal in fluid-attenuated inversion recovery (FLAIR) sequence (c) with similar extension indicating subacute evolution and tissue necrosis.

Some MRI-based imaging modalities allow defining different metabolic regions. Magnetic resonance spectroscopy (MRS) can detect differences in the main brain metabolites with potential value for clinical stroke assessment, such as lactate and *N*-acetyl aspartate (tNAA). The tNAA concentration in the core and penumbra may decrease below the detection limit from 6 hours after ischemic stroke, which is related to a serious clinical syndrome. On the other hand, lactate increases immediately after the ischemic event, associated with the final core size. Although these techniques are promising, they are not suitable for clinical use because of the long period of sequence acquisition (Lu et al. 2021).

Oxygen challenge imaging is an MRI-based technique based on blood oxygen levels. It reflects changes in blood oxygen saturation from the core to the penumbra over time due to the paramagnetic effect of O_2. Using 100% normobaric hyperoxia, T2* sequences show high signal intensity in the penumbra and low or absent signal intensity in the infarct core. Although not clinically proven yet, this method is considered one of the most promising metabolic techniques (Muehllehner and Karp 2006; Shen et al. 2016; Deuchar et al. 2019).

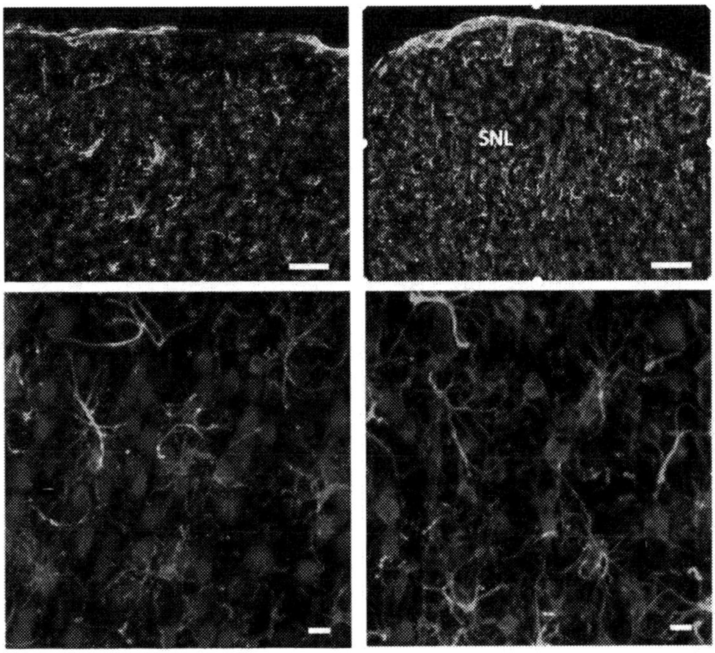

Figure 4. Cellular changes after ischemia/reperfusion in confocal microscopy. Triple labeling for glial fibrillary acid protein (GFAP) in astroglia (green), NeuN in neurons (blue), and ionized calcium-binding adapter molecule 1 (Iba-1) in microglia (red) in contralateral (a, c) and ipsilateral (b, d) rat brain 48 hours after medial cerebral artery occlusion (MCAO). Notice in (b) the area with selective neuronal loss (SNL) with increased expression of microglia and surrounded by astroglia enriched in GFAP, in contrast to the distribution of astroglia in the contralateral hemisphere (a). In (d), details of the neuronal loss, increased expression of microglia, as well as increased in the size and deramification of microglia can be observed compared with the contralateral hemisphere (c). Scale bar is 100 μm in (a) and (b) and 10 μm in (c) and (d). Images kindly provided by Santos-Galdiano, University of León, Spain.

PET uses a radioactive substance (tracer) as a maker whose ionizing radiation is detected in a scintillator, which converts a fraction of this energy into visible or ultraviolet photons. This light pulse is detected by a photodetector, which converts it into an electrical signal (Melcher 2000). Different tracers can be used, but the ^{15}O radiotracer allows PET to assess CBF, the oxygen extraction fraction (OEF), and the cerebral metabolic rate of oxygen, among other parameters. Basically, the penumbra is defined by decreased CNS blood flow and increased OEF. The mismatch between CBF and oxygen metabolism is considered a penumbra hallmark, making PET the gold standard technique for determining the penumbra. However, it has several limitations, such as technical difficulty, exposure to radioactivity, and high cost, all of which prevent it from being clinically acceptable. Newly developed PET ligands have been explored to delineate disease in preclinical and clinical research to make the use of PET in clinics more suitable. For example, areas with reduced perfusion, but still alive, can bind ^{11}C-flumazenil (FMZ), indicating the possible benefits of reperfusion therapy, whereas areas without FMZ binding indicate permanent lesions. Radiolabeled fluoromisonidazole and copper-based radiopharmaceuticals have also been explored preclinically (Lee et al. 2015; Rojas et al. 2011).

The use of histological techniques is very common to assess brain damage in animal models of stroke. In the MCAO model, the delayed progression of the ischemic damage can be easily studied in the cerebral cortex (Carmichael 2005), and areas of selective neuronal loss (SNL) (Figure 4) that progress from partial infarction to pan-necrosis can be observed (Santos Galdiano et al. 2018).

The Blood Barriers in the Central Nervous System

Three main sites of interface barriers can be distinguished in the CNS: the BBB located in the brain microvessels, the epithelium of the choroid plexus, and the epithelium of the arachnoid mater, which covers the outer brain surface above the layer of subarachnoid CSF. The choroid plexus and arachnoid form the blood–cerebrospinal fluid barrier (BCSFB) (Abbot et al. 2010). The tight junctions between adjacent cells in these sites restrict the diffusion of polar solutes between the CNS parenchyma and blood cells through the gaps between the barrier cells (paracellular pathway). Thus, the trafficking of small solutes across these barriers is controlled by solute carriers located in both apical and basal lamina of barrier cells, together with endoenzymes and exoenzymes, while the trafficking of larger molecules (peptides, proteins) is regulated by adsorptive and receptor-mediated transcytosis. These barriers are also involved in the recruitment and transmigration of leukocytes and therefore take part in regulating the innate immune response. Thus, the CNS presents physical, transport, enzymatic (metabolic), and immunological barriers regulated by many signals from both blood and the CNS. These barriers are very susceptible to pathological modification (Abbot and Friedman 2012).

Essentially, the BBB includes ECs, the glycocalyx surrounding the vessel lumen, the basal lamina containing pericytes, and the astrocytic end-feet

(Figure 5). In the current view, the CNS endothelium forms part of a cellular complex, called the neurovascular unit (NVU) composed of a capillary segment including its associated pericytes, the corresponding basal laminas, perivascular astrocytes, and microglia supporting a small number (typically < 8) of neurons within that particular NVU module (Iadecola and Nedergaard 2007; Abbott et al. 2010; Mäe et al. 2011; Abbot and Friedman 2012).

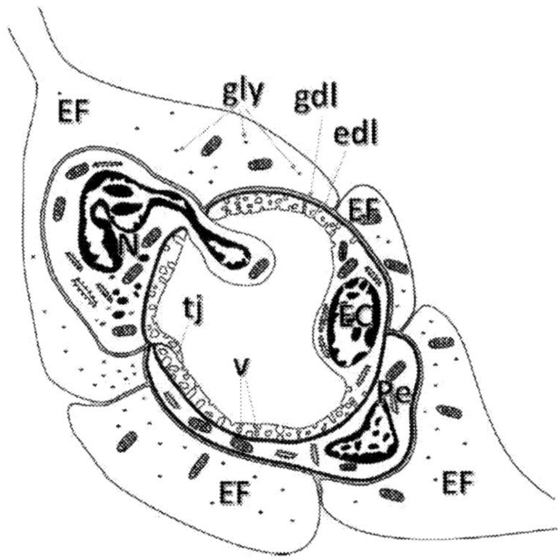

Figure 5. The blood-brain barrier. The light of the vessel is edged by endothelial cells (EC) whose tight junctions (tj) limit the diffusion of the blood components between the cells (paracellular pathway). Thus, the traffic between the blood and the nervous parenchyma is controlled by the ECs and mainly carried out through vesicles (v) of macropinocytosis and transcytosis. The abluminal surface of ECs is recovered by the endothelial-derived layer (edl, dark gray). This layer also recovers the pericytes (Pe) that wrap most of the vessel. The basal lamina presents an additional glial-derived layer (gdl, light gray) formed by the end-feet (EF) of the astrocytes that wrap the vessel contributing to the barrier. EF contain glycogen granules (gly). Neutrophils (N) and other leukocytes migrate through the vessel between the egl and edl of the basal lamina (see details in the text).

The glycocalyx is secreted by ECs and acts as a molecular sieve, limiting the diffusion of molecules ≥ 40 kDa (Kutuzov et al. 2018). The CNS glycocalyx is thicker and less permeable than the glycocalyx in other body organs. Furthermore, it presents a negative charge that blocks negatively charged plasma proteins (Yuan et al. 2010). Pro-inflammatory molecules can reduce the thickness of the glycocalyx (Fitzgerald et al. 2000), and MMPs secreted by rolling leukocytes or ECs degrade some of the glycocalyx components (Taraboletti et al. 2002), facilitating leukocyte interactions with ECs and the subsequent transmigration across the endothelium (Galea 2021).

ECs in the BBB present some differences compared with other body ECs, such as tight junctions, more mitochondria, less macropinocytosis and caveolar transcytosis, the absence of fenestrae (Banks et al. 2021), as well as many different transporters to control trafficking between the intravascular compartment and the CNS parenchyma (Morris et al. 2017). The continuous band around the capillaries formed by tight junctions acts as a barrier impeding small molecules from diffusing down concentration gradients between the ECs (paracellular pathway). Occludins, claudins, and junctional adhesion molecules assemble in complexes to form tight junctions and attach to the endothelial cytoskeleton by zonula occludens proteins (Galea 2021). BBB ECs also present receptors for pro-inflammatory mediators such as PRRs that bind to DAMPs (Wilhelm et al. 2017).

The basal lamina is 30–40 nm thick and wraps around the endothelium, anchoring the cellular components of the BBB, mediating their crosstalk, and providing microvascular stability (Pandit et al. 2019). The basal lamina is formed from two juxtaposed layers derived from ECs and astroglia. The endothelial-derived layer contains laminin-411 and laminin-511, while the glial-derived layer contains laminin-111 and laminin-112 (Sixt et al. 2001). A potential perivascular space exists between these layers where CD-163-positive macrophages reside and scavenge the BBB (Mato et al. 1996). These macrophages play an important role as antigen-presenting cells to lymphocytes (Hickey and Kimura 1988). Leukocytes can also be observed in this space under inflammatory conditions (Mato et al. 1996). The endothelial layer presents areas with low laminin-511 expression described as exit points for T cell extravasation in postcapillary venules in the lymph nodes. Leukocytes tend to be held up in the perivascular space (Zhang et al. 2020). The selective cleavage of dystroglycan, the transmembrane receptor that binds astrocyte end-feet with the glial basement lamina, by MMP-2 and MMP9, is required for leukocytes to cross the glial layer (Agrawal et al. 2006). Thus, the glial-derived layer of the basal lamina prevents leukocyte infiltration more strictly than its endothelial counterpart (Galea 2021).

Pericytes derived from neural crests cover about 40% of ECs, representing the higher pericyte-to-EC ratio of the body. They are wrapped by the endothelial basal lamina and present thousands of cytoplasmic extensions into EC invaginations, whose function is unknown (Galea 2021). The main role of pericytes is to maintain BBB integrity by inhibiting transcytosis and by inducing the expression of tight junction proteins (Armulik et al. 2010). In addition, pericytes regulate blood flow by controlling the diameter of capillaries (Peppiatt 2006). Thus, pericytes regulate the BBB surface area and blood flow to control the barrier in a region-specific manner (Galea 2021).

Astrocytic end-feet interdigitate and overlap, covering the CNS capillaries and forming the innermost layer of the BBB (Mathiisen et al. 2010). Astrocytic end-feet do not present tight junctions, but in some areas, they appear as a barrier that limits the diffusion of molecules > 500 Da (Nuriya et al. 2013). Astrocytic end-feet release molecules such as angiopoietin-1 that takes part in the control of occludin recruitment at tight junctions and its stabilization, contributing to the maintenance of the BBB (Siddiqui et al. 2015). Astrocytic end-feet also express AQP-4, which plays a crucial role in the water flux across the BBB and edema formation (Song et al. 2016).

Stroke induces BBB permeability in a biphasic open-close-open process, but recent reports propose that biphasic peaks do not present BBB closure between openings (Liu P et al. 2018). The first opening occurs in the acute phase of stroke—within 6 hours after stroke onset in both animals (Lin et al. 2008) and humans (Merali et al. 2017)—due to hypoxia and early BBB disruption (Abdullahi et al. 2018). A second permeability peak occurs in the subacute phase of stroke (Lin et al. 2008; Durukan et al. 2009). Furthermore, high BBB permeability after 1 week has been reported (Merali et al. 2017). Thus, the BBB has been suggested to stay open during subacute and late phases of stroke, and the late opening would be correlated with the regenerative processes leading to tissue repair (Bernardo-Castro 2020).

Microglia

Microglia are the resident immune cells of the CNS and, in contrast to other populations of the mononuclear phagocyte system, come from embryonic yolk sac precursors. The microglial population is maintained by self-renewal and self-differentiation (Ginhoux et al. 2010; Ginhoux and Guilliams 2016; Li and Barres 2017; Askew et al. 2017). The characteristics of resting microglial cells include a small cell soma and wide branches projecting out, and they present low expression of cluster of differentiation (CD)45, CD80, CD86, CD11c, and major histocompatibility complex II (MHCII) (Ma et al. 2017).

In the past, researchers had associated microglial functions with their rapid responses to injury and disease, particularly in controlling the inflammatory response in brain diseases. However, the current view is that microglia perform normal homeostatic functions throughout life (Schafer and

Stevens 2015). Thus, microglia play different roles throughout development, including the regulation of the number of neural precursor cells (Cunningham et al. 2013), wiring modulation (Squarzoni et al. 2014), and synaptic pruning (Paolicelli et al. 2011). In addition, microglia regulate adult neurogenesis (Sierra et al. 2013) and monitor the functional state of synapses (Wake et al. 2009). Overall, microglial processes constantly monitor CNS activity in their environment, in both the developing and adult CNS (Schafer and Stevens 2015; Frost and Schafer 2016; Li and Barres 2017), which represents a survey of the microenvironment scanning in the entire brain parenchyma every few hours (Nimmerjahn et al. 2005). More recently, a new role for microglia in regulating neurovascular structure and function has been included in the multiple functions of this cell population (Bisht et al. 2021; Kisler et al. 2021).

Microglia, the main effectors of the innate immune response to stroke, are activated in minutes after cerebral ischemia and can remain activated for weeks (Lalancette-Héber 2007). Microglial activation is characterized by morphological changes such as decreases in the length and number of microglial branches (Santos-Galdiano et al. 2018), increases in the size of the soma, and upregulation of surface markers such as CD45, CD68, and MHCII (Ransohoff and Perry 2009). Microglia and recruited macrophages activated by stroke can polarize into pro-inflammatory (M1) and anti-inflammatory (M2) phenotypes, which are involved in tissue damage and repair, respectively (Gordon 2003; Perry et al. 2010; Tang and Le 2016; Jiang et al. 2020). M1 microglia release IL-6, IL-1β, NO, and TNF-α, all of which exacerbate brain damage, while M2 microglia secrete IL-4, IL-10, and TGF-β, which promote brain repair (Ma et al. 2017; Zhang et al. 2018). However, the classification into two phenotypes of activated microglia represents an oversimplification, and a range of different "activated" states can be recognized (see below). In fact, the terms resting and activated microglia are too simplistic because in the healthy CNS, microglia enter into activated states (Cherry et al. 2014; Ma et al. 2017).

Ischemia/hypoxia activates transcription factors, such as members of the signal transducers and activators of transcription (STAT) family and the nuclear factor kappa light chain enhancer of activated B cells (NF-κB) pathway, in microglia leading to the pro-inflammatory M1 phenotype. This microglial subtype expresses iNOS, which can produce ROS and RNS; proteases such as MMP-9 and MMP-3; and pro-inflammatory mediators such as IL-1β, IL-6, IFN-γ, TNF-α, CCL2, and CXCL10 (Ma et al. 2017; Jiang et al. 2020; Xin et al. 2021). The M1 phenotype is geared toward presenting antigens and killing intracellular pathogens, denoted by upregulation of the membrane proteins MHCII and CD86, which are involved in crosstalk with other immune cells (Taylor et al. 2005; Yenari et al. 2010; Cherry et al. 2014; Ma et al. 2017). Surface markers for M1 microglia (and also for macrophages) include integrin alpha-M (CD11b), CD16, CD32, and CD86 (Jiang et al. 2020). Ionized calcium-binding adapter molecule 1 (Iba1) is also expressed by M1 microglia and macrophages (Imai et al. 1996), and it is still a challenge to distinguish between resident microglia and blood-derived macrophages (Jiang et al. 2020).

In contrast, anti-inflammatory activated macrophages (the M2 phenotype) express receptors and release pro-angiogenic and anti-inflammatory mediators such as IL-10, IL-4, IL-13, TGF-β, insulin-like growth factor, and VEGF, which inhibit inflammation and promote tissue repair (Jiang et al. 2020). M2 microglia can be activated by nuclear factor erythroid 2-related factor 2 (Nrf2) and peroxisome proliferator-activated receptor γ (PPARγ), a transcription factor with anti-inflammatory properties (Liu R et al. 2018; Jiang et al. 2020). One of the hallmarks of the M2 phenotype is arginase 1 (Arg1), which converts arginine to ornithine and then to polyamines (putrescine, spermidine, and spermine), and proline that contributes to tissue regeneration, cell proliferation, matrix deposition, and reduced inflammation (Munder et al. 2009). Other markers for the M2 phenotype include the heparin-binding lectin Ym1, a cysteine-rich secreted protein called FIZZ1 (found in the inflammatory zone), which promotes deposition of ECM, and CD206, a mannose receptor (Cherry et al. 2014).

The M2 phenotype has been subdivided into three sub-classes—M2a, M2b and M2c—based on the cytokines that induce them (Cherry et al. 2014). M2a microglia, characterized by the expression of Arg1, Ym1, IGF-1, CD206, chitinase 3-like proteins, and FIZZ1 (Latta et al. 2015), suppress inflammation and are induced by IL-4 or IL-13 (Cherry et al. 2014; Ma et al. 2017).

The M2b phenotype presents an increased expression of IL1-ra, CD86, and SOCS3, but it does not express Arg1, Ym1, and Fizz1 (Mantovani et al. 2004; Cherry et al. 2014). M2b microglia present high levels of MHCII and CD86, which support their ability to stimulate T cells. They are considered regulatory macrophages with immune-suppressive functions and are generated in response to immune complexes and TLR stimulation (Cherry et al. 2014; Headland and Norling 2015).

The M2c phenotype is known as "deactivated microglia" and can be induced by TGF-β, IL-10, and glucocorticoids (Chhor et al. 2013; Mecha et al. 2015). This phenotype seems to be involved in tissue regeneration when the inflammatory response decreases and is induced by IL-10, glucocorticoids, and TGF-β (Mantovani et al. 2004; Cherry et al. 2014).

Ischemia and subsequent reperfusion are major factors in damaged tissue favoring M1 phenotype activity (Hu et al. 2012). The M1 phenotype, neutrophils, and macrophages contribute to the inflammatory cascade and expand cell death beyond the initial ischemic region (Cherry et al. 2014). Despite the dominant pro-inflammatory state, certain anti-inflammatory activity exists in an attempt to control inflammation (Hu et al. 2012). In fact, the lack of ability to promote M2 microglial induction in mice worsens the outcome after cerebral ischemia (Xiong et al. 2011), highlighting the importance of the M2 response to counteract inflammation and to repair tissue damage. In this regard, the lack of an appropriate M2 response might be an important mechanism underlying neurodegeneration, and there is a growing recognition of the importance of M1/M2 dynamics in diseases that involve chronic neuroinflammation (Cherry et al. 2014).

PET imaging can detect microglial activation by using ^{11}C-vinpocetine as a radiotracer of the 18 kDa translocator protein, which increases after ischemic stroke. Nevertheless, the interpretation of these techniques is still challenging and presents additional concerns, such as the toxicity of MRI contrast agents (Gulyás et al. 2012).

Several microRNAs (miRNAs) have been reported to be involved in the activation and polarization of microglia in CNS pathologies, including stroke, which modulates microglial polarization and its role in brain injury and tissue repair (Ma et al. 2017). In physiological conditions, non-activated microglia express high levels of miR-124, while in pathological conditions, M1 microglia present low miR-124 levels. In experimental autoimmune encephalomyelitis, transfection with miR-124 reduces microglial activation and leukocyte infiltration and alleviates clinical symptoms, while repression of miR-124 leads to microglial activation. Thus, miR-124 seems to maintain the quiescent phenotype of microglia (Ponomarev et al. 2011, 2013) and seems to be a putative target for treating inflammation or microglial activation–associated diseases, including ischemic stroke (Ma et al. 2017). In contrast, miR-155 is accepted as a pro-inflammatory miRNA and seems to be crucial for M1 polarization (Guedes et al. 2013). miR-155 inhibition also appears as a tool for treating neurological diseases such as ischemic stroke (Ma et al. 2017). Other miRNAs, such as miR-Let7a, modulate microglial polarization toward the M2 phenotype and promote microglial autophagy (Louafi et al. 2010; Cho et al. 2015). Ischemia and inflammation upregulate miR-Let7c-5p in microglia, while miR-Let7c-5p overexpression inhibits microglial activation, suppressing the caspase-3 pathway. These findings support miR-Let7c-5p as a putative target to inhibit microglia following cerebral ischemia (Ni et al. 2015). Another potential inhibitor of microglia activation is miR-181c, which reduces the production of TNF-α by microglia and apoptosis after hypoxia-ischemia (Zhang et al. 2012).

Astroglia

Astrocytes, the most abundant glial cell type, play a crucial role in controlling CNS homeostasis at different organizational levels in developmental and adult neurogenesis. Astrocytic control at a molecular level includes the supply of energy substrates and neurotransmitter precursors to neurons, ion transport, and clearance of released neurotransmitters and ROS. Furthermore, astrocytic processes enwrap synaptic terminals, regulating the formation, maturation, function, and elimination of synapses, thus modulating neuronal activity. Vascular astrocytic end-feet constitute another type of astrocytic process; they cover blood vessels and actively control trafficking between blood and the CNS parenchyma. Finally, astrocytes are also involved in the defensive system of the CNS. Several excellent reviews on astroglia provide details on astrocyte properties (Sofroniew and Vinters 2010; Clarke and Barres 2013; Khakh and Sofroniew 2015; Allen and Eroglu 2017; Verkhratsky and Nedergaard 2018; Sofroniew 2020; Patabendige et al. 2021).

Pathological situations induce changes in the morphology and functions of astrocytes, a process known as reactive astrogliosis; the main characteristics include cellular hypertrophy, proliferation, and strong GFAP expression (Patabendige et al. 2021). The increase in GFAP-positive cells derives from GFAP synthesis and condensation of glial filaments rather than from the generation of new astrocytes (Sofroniew and Vinters 2010). Although calcium-binding protein B (S100B) is not specific for astrocytes, the release of this protein is considered a marker of astrocytic activation (Gonçalves et al. 2008), as well as the increased expression of aldehyde dehydrogenase 1 family member L1 (ALDH1A1) (Matias et al. 2019).

Two subtypes of reactive astrocytes, A1 and A2, have been described (Liddelow et al. 2017). IL-1α, TNFα, and complement component 1q (C1q), released by activated microglia, induce the A1 subtype, which contributes to the death of neurons and oligodendrocytes. In contrast, A2 reactive astrocytes release neurotrophic factors and promote tissue repair and neuronal survival. Complement component C3 is upregulated in A1 but not A2 astrocytes and can be used as a marker to differentiate both subtypes (Liddelow and Barres 2017). During ischemia, astroglia present morphological changes modulated by direct cell-cell interactions through Notch signaling (Acaz-Fonseca et al. 2019).

After ischemic stroke, astrocytes play different roles (Patabendige et al. 2021). One of the earliest responses to cerebral ischemia is astrocytic swelling (cytotoxic edema) due to the expression of AQP-4 on the cell surface and increased uptake of glutamate and glucose. Astrocytes swell in ischemic stroke while the BBB is still intact, preventing brain tissue from swelling (Steiner et al. 2012), compressing cerebral vessels, and reducing the blood flow (Syková 2001). Activated astrocytes present upregulated MMP-9 expression (Qiu et al. 2010) and release IL-1β, IL-6, IL-10, IFN-γ, and TGF-β, which can play neurodegenerative or neuroprotective roles (Buffo et al. 2010). Astrocytes also modulate the immune response by blocking monocyte activation and inhibiting T cells (Priego and Valiente 2019). They can also become non-professional phagocytes, contributing to eliminating debris in the infarct area (Morizawa et al. 2017). Astrocytes are also involved in glial scar formation, whose controversial role in tissue repair has been mentioned above. The high secretory activity of astrocytes (Verkhratsky et al. 2016) is involved in many physiological and pathological functions. Thus, astrocytes release signaling molecules and many neurotrophic factors with neurorestorative effects after stroke (Buffo et al. 2010), as well as axon guidance molecules such as netrins, ephrins, and semaphorins (Poskanzer and Molofsky 2018). Other molecules secreted by astrocytes, such as proteoglycans and tenascins, contribute to ECM formation (Wiese et al. 2012) or their degradation by metalloproteases (Qiu et al. 2010). Finally, extracellular vesicles released by astrocytes have been reported to suppress autophagy and to reduce neuronal damage in ischemic stroke (Pei et al. 2019).

References

Abbott NJ. 2000. Inflammatory mediators and modulation of blood-brain barrier permeability. *Cell Mol. Neurobiol* 20(2):131–147.

Abbott NJ, Friedman A. 2012. Overview and introduction: the blood-brain barrier in health and disease. *Epilepsia* 53 Suppl 6(0 6):1-6.

Abbott NJ, Patabendige AA, Dolman DE, Yusof SR, Begley DJ. 2010. Structure and function of the blood-brain barrier. *Neurobiol Dis* 37(1):13-25.

Abdullahi W, Tripathi D, Ronaldson PT. 2018. Blood-brain barrier dysfunction in ischemic stroke: targeting tight junctions and transporters for vascular protection. *Am J Physiol Cell Physiol* 315:C343-56.

Acaz-Fonseca E, Ortiz-Rodriguez A, Azcoitia I, Garcia-Segura LM, Arevalo MA. 2019. Notch signaling in astrocytes mediates their morphological response to an inflammatory challenge. *Cell Death Discov* 5:85.

Adibhatla RM, Dempsy R, Hatcher JF. 2008. Integration of cytokine biology and lipid metabolism in stroke. *Front Biosci* 13:1250-70.

Agrawal S, Anderson P, Durbeej M, van Rooijen N, Ivars F, Opdenakker G, Sorokin LM. 2006. Dystroglycan is selectively cleaved at the parenchymal basement membrane at sites of leukocyte extravasation in experimental autoimmune encephalomyelitis. *J Exp Med* 203(4):1007-19.

Allen NJ, Eroglu C. 2017. Cell biology of astrocyte-synapse interactions. *Neuron* 96(3):697-708.

Amantea D, Nappi G, Bernardi G, Bagetta G, Corasaniti MT. 2008. Post-ischemic brain damage: pathophysiology and role of inflammatory mediators. *FEBS J* 276(1):13–26.

Ando H, Zhou J, Macova M, Imboden H, Saavedra JM. 2004. Angiotensin II AT1 receptor blockade reverses pathological hypertrophy and inflammation in brain microvessels of spontaneously hypertensive rats. *Stroke* 35(7):1726-31.

Andre R, Pinteaux E, Kimber I, Rothwell NJ. 2005. Differential actions of IL-1 alpha and IL-1 beta in glial cells share common IL-1 signalling pathways. *Neuroreport* 16(2):153-7.

Angelidis C, Kotsialou Z, Kossyvakis C, Vrettou AR, Zacharoulis A, Kolokathis F, Kekeris V, Giannopoulos G. 2018. Colchicine pharmacokinetics and mechanism of action. *Curr Pharm Des* 24(6):659-63.

Ankarcrona M, Dypbukt JM, Bonfoco E, Zhivotovsky B, Orrenius S, Lipton SA, Nicotera P. 1995. Glutamate-induced neuronal death: a succession of necrosis or apoptosis depending on mitochondrial function. *Neuron* 15:961-73.

Anrather J, Iadecola C. 2016. Inflammation and stroke: An overview. *Neurotherapeutics* 13(4):661-70.

Armulik A, Genové G, Mäe M, Nisancioglu MH, Wallgard E, Niaudet C, He L, Norlin J, Lindblom P, Strittmatter K, Johansson BR, Betsholtz C. 2010. Pericytes regulate the blood-brain barrier. *Nature* 468(7323):557-61.

Ashok A, Andrabi SS, Mansoor S, Kuang Y, Kwon BK, Labhasetwar V. 2022. Antioxidant therapy in oxidative stress-induced neurodegenerative diseases: Role of nanoparticle-based drug delivery systems in clinical translation. *Antioxidants* (Basel) 11(2):408.

Askew K, Li K, Olmos-Alonso A, Garcia-Moreno F, Liang Y, Richardson P, Tipton T, Chapman MA, Riecken K, Beccari S, Sierra A, Molnár Z, Cragg MS, Garaschuk O, Perry VH, Gomez-Nicola D. 2017. Coupled proliferation and apoptosis maintain the rapid turnover of microglia in the adult brain. *Cell Rep* 18(2):391-405.

Astrup J, Siesjo BK, Symon L. 1981. Thresholds in cerebral ischemia—The ischemic penumbra. *Stroke* 12, 723-25.

Awtry EH, Loscalzo J. 2000. Aspirin. *Circulation* 101(10):1206-18.

Baliyan V, Das CJ, Sharma R, Gupta AK. 2016. Diffusion weighted imaging: Technique and applications. *World J Radiol* 8(9):785-98.

Banks WA, Reed MJ, Logsdon AF, Rhea EM, Erickson MA. 2021. Healthy aging and the blood-brain barrier. *Nat Aging* 1(3):243-54.
Barnabé-Heider F, Göritz C, Sabelström H, Takebayashi H, Pfrieger FW, Meletis K, Frisén J. 2010. Origin of new glial cells in intact and injured adult spinal cord. *Cell Stem Cell* 7(4):470-82.
Baron JC. 1999. Mapping the ischaemic penumbra with PET: implications for acute stroke treatment. *Cerebrovasc Dis* 9:193–201.
Baron JC. 2018. Protecting the ischaemic penumbra as an adjunct to thrombectomy for acute stroke. *Nature Rev Neurol* 14:325-37.
Barone FC, Arvin B, White RF, Miller A, Webb CL, Willette RN, Lysko PG, Feuerstein GZ. 1997. Tumor necrosis factor-alpha. A mediator of focal ischemic brain injury. *Stroke* 28(6):1233-44.
Bernardo-Castro S, Sousa JA, Brás A, Cecília C, Rodrigues B, Almendra L, Machado C, Santo G, Silva F, Ferreira L, Santana I, Sargento-Freitas J. 2020. Pathophysiology of blood-brain barrier permeability throughout the different stages of ischemic stroke and its implication on hemorrhagic transformation and recovery. *Front Neurol* 11:594672.
Bianchi ME. 2007 DAMPs, PAMPs and alarmins: all we need to know about danger. *J Leukoc Biol* 81(1):1-5.
Bisht K, Okojie KA, Sharma K, Lentferink DH, Sun Y-Y, Chen H-R, Uweru JO, Amancherla S, Calcuttawala Z, Campos-Salazar AB, Corliss B, Jabbour L, Benderoth J, Friestad B, Mills III WA, Isakson BE, Tremblay M-E, Kuan C-Y, Eyo UB. 2021. Capillary-associated microglia regulate vascular structure and function through PANX1-P2RY12 coupling in mice. *Nat Commun* 12:5289.
Blanco M, Castellanos M, Rodríguez-Yáñez M., Sobrino T, Leira R, Vivancos J, Lizasoain I, Serena J, Dávalos A, Castillo J. 2006. High blood pressure and inflammation are associated with poor prognosis in lacunar infarctions. *Cerebrovasc Dis* 22:123-29.
Bodhankar S, Chen Y, Vandenbark AA, Murphy SJ, Offner H. 2013. IL-10-producing B-cells limit CNS inflammation and infarct volume in experimental stroke. *Metab Brain Dis* 28(3):375-86.
Borregaard N. 2010. Neutrophils, from marrow to microbes. *Immunity* 33 (5):657-70.
Botchkina GI, Meistrell ME, Botchkina IL, Tracey KJ. 1997. Expression of TNF and TNF receptors (p55 and p75) in the rat brain after focal cerebral ischemia. *Mol Med* 3:765-81.
Boutin H, LeFeuvre RA, Horai R, Asano M, Iwakura Y, Rothwell NJ. 2001. Role of IL-1alpha and IL-1beta in ischemic brain damage. *J Neurosci* 21(15):5528-34.
Buffo A, Rolando C, Ceruti S. 2010. Astrocytes in the damaged brain: molecular and cellular insights into their reactive response and healing potential. *Biochem Pharmacol* 79(2):77-89.
Cambien B, Wagner DD. 2004. A new role in hemostasis for the adhesion receptor P-selectin. *Trends Mol Med* 10(4):179-86.
Carbone F, Bonaventura A, Montecucco F. 2020. Neutrophil-related oxidants drive heart and brain remodeling after ischemia/reperfusion injury. *Front Physiol* 10:1587.
Carmichael ST. 2005. Rodent models of focal stroke: size, mechanism, and purpose. *NeuroRx* 2(3):396-409.

Carmichael ST. 2016 The 3 Rs of stroke biology: radial, relayed, and regenerative. *Neurotherapeutics* 13:348–59.

Cavaillon JM. 2001. Pro-versus anti-inflammatory cytokines: myth or reality. *Cell Mol Biol* (Noisy-le-grand) 47(4):695-702.

Cecconi A, Vilchez-Tschischke JP, Mateo J, Sanchez-Gonzalez J, España S, Fernandez-Jimenez R, Lopez-Melgar B, Fernández Friera L, López-Martín GJ, Fuster V, Ruiz-Cabello J, Ibañez B. 2021. Effects of colchicine on atherosclerotic plaque stabilization: a multimodality imaging study in an animal model. *J Cardiovasc Transl Res* 14(1):150-60.

Cesari M, Penninx BW, Newman AB, Kritchevsky SB, Nicklas BJ, Sutton-Tyrrel K, Rubin SM, Ding J, Simonsick EM, Harris TB, Pahor M. 2003. Inflammatory markers and onset of cardiovascular events: results from the Health ABC study. *Circulation* 108 (19):2317-22.

Chen R, Zhang X, Gu L, Zhu H, Zhong Y, Ye Y, Xiong X, Jian Z. 2021. New insight into neutrophils: a potential therapeutic target for cerebral ischemia. *Front Immunol* 12:692061.

Cherry JD, Olschowka JA, O'Banion MK. 2014. Neuroinflammation and M2 microglia: the good, the bad, and the inflamed. *J Neuroinflammation* 11:98.

Chhor V, Le Charpentier T, Lebon S, Oré MV, Celador IL, Josserand J, Degos V, Jacotot E, Hagberg H, Sävman K, Mallard C, Gressens P, Fleiss B. 2013. Characterization of phenotype markers and neuronotoxic potential of polarised primary microglia in vitro. *Brain Behav Immun* 32:70-85.

Cho KJ, Song J, Oh Y, Lee JE. 2015. MicroRNA-Let-7a regulates the function of microglia in inflammation. *Mol Cell Neurosci* 68:167-76.

Clarke LE, Barres BA. 2013. Emerging roles of astrocytes in neural circuit development. *Nat Rev Neurosci* 14(5):311-21.

Clausen BH, Wirenfeldt M, Høgedal SS, Frich LH, Nielsen HH, Schrøder HD, Østergaard K, Finsen B, Kristensen BW, Lambertsen KL. 2020. Characterization of the TNF and IL-1 systems in human brain and blood after ischemic stroke. *Acta Neuropathol Commun* 8(1):81.

Cuartero MI, Ballesteros I, Moraga A, Nombela F, Vivancos J, Hamilton JA, Corbí ÁL, Lizasoain I, Moro MA. 2013. N2 neutrophils, novel players in brain inflammation after stroke: modulation by the PPARγ agonist rosiglitazone. *Stroke* 44(12):3498-508.

Cunningham C. 2013. Microglia and neurodegeneration: the role of systemic inflammation. *Glia* 61(1):71-90.

Dalby T, Wohl E, Dinsmore M, Unger Z, Chowdhury T, Venkatraghavan L. 2020. Pathophysiology of cerebral edema-a comprehensive review. *J Neuroanaesth Crit Care* 32(3):256-62.

Danton GH, Dietrich WD. 2003. Inflammatory mechanisms after ischemia and stroke. *J Neuropathol Exp Neurol* 62:127-36.

Davalos D, Grutzendler J, Yang G, Kim JV, Zuo Y, Jung S, Littman DR, Dustin ML, Gan WB. 2005. ATP mediates rapid microglial response to local brain injury in vivo. *Nat Neurosci* 8(6):752-8.

Davis SM, Donnan GA. 2021. Ischemic penumbra: A personal view. *Cerebrovasc Dis* 50:656-65.

De Meyer SF, Denorme F, Langhauser F, Geuss E, Fluri F, Kleinschnitz, C. 2016. Thromboinflammation in stroke brain damage. *Stroke* 47(4):1165-72.

Dean RA, Cox JH, Bellac CL, Doucet A, Starr AE, Overall CM. 2008. Macrophage-specific metalloelastase (MMP-12) truncates and inactivates ELR+ CXC chemokines and generates CCL2, -7, -8, and -13 antagonists: potential role of the macrophage in terminating polymorphonuclear leukocyte influx. *Blood* 112(8):3455-64.

Demeestere J, Wouters A, Christensen S, Lemmens R, Lansberg MG. 2020. Review of perfusion imaging in acute ischemic stroke: from time to tissue. *Stroke* 51(3):1017-24.

Deuchar GA, van Kralingen JC, Work LM, Santosh C, Muir KW, McCabe C, Macrae IM. 2019. Preclinical validation of the therapeutic potential of glasgow oxygen level dependent (GOLD) technology: a theranostic for acute stroke. *Transl Stroke Res* 10(5):583-95.

Di Napoli M, Papa F. 2006. Systemic inflammation, blood pressure, and stroke outcome. *J Clin Hypertens* 8(3):187-94.

Dickstein JB, Moldofsky H, Hay JB. 2000. Brain-blood permeability: TNF-alpha promotes escape of protein tracer from CSF to blood. *Am J Physiol Regul Integr Comp Physiol* 279(1):R148-51.

Dole VS, Bergmeier W, Mitchell HA, Eichenberger SC, Wagner DD. 2005. Activated platelets induce Weibel-Palade-body secretion and leukocyte rolling in vivo: role of P-selectin. *Blood* 106(7):2334-39.

Dong T, Li M, Gao F, Wei P, Wang J. 2022. Construction and imaging of a neurovascular unit model. *Neural Regen Res* 17(8):1685-94.

Doyle KP, Simon RP, Stenzel-Poore MP. 2008. Mechanisms of ischemic brain damage. *Neuropharmacology* 55(3):310-8.

Drieu A, Levard D, Vivien D, Rubio M. 2018. Anti-inflammatory treatments for stroke: from bench to bedside. *Ther Adv Neurol Disord* 11:1756286418789854.

Dröge, W. 2002. Free radicals in the physiological control of cell function. *Physiol Rev* 82:47–95.

Durukan A, Marinkovic I, Strbian D, Pitkonen M, Pedrono E, Soinne L, Abo-Ramadan U, Tatlisumak T. 2009. Post-ischemic blood-brain barrier leakage in rats: one-week follow-up by MRI. *Brain Res* 1280:158–65.

Easton AS. 2013. Neutrophils and stroke - can neutrophils mitigate disease in the central nervous system? *Int Immunopharmacol* 17(4):1218-25.

ERFC. Emerging Risk Factors Collaboration, Kaptoge S, Di Angelantonio E, Lowe G, Pepys MB, Thompson SG, Collins R, Danesh J. 2010. C-reactive protein concentration and risk of coronary heart disease, stroke, and mortality: an individual participant meta-analysis. *Lancet* 375(9709):132-40.

Fadok VA, Bratton DL, Konowal A, Freed PW, Westcott JY, Henson PM. 1998. Macrophages that have ingested apoptotic cells in vitro inhibit proinflammatory cytokine production through autocrine/paracrine mechanisms involving TGF-beta, PGE2, and PAF. *J Clin Invest* 101:890-98.

Fan J, Watanabe T. 2003. Inflammatory reactions in the pathogenesis of atherosclerosis. *J Atheroscler Thromb* 10(2):63-71.

Feuerstein GZ, Liu T, Barone FC. 1994. Cytokines, inflammation, and brain injury: role of tumor necrosis factor-alpha. *Cerebrovasc Brain Metab Rev* 6(4):341-60.

Fisher M, Vasilevko V, Cribbs DH. 2012. Mixed cerebrovascular disease and the future of stroke prevention. *Transl Stroke Res* 3(Suppl 1):39-51.

Fitzgerald ML, Wang Z, Park PW, Murphy G, Bernfield M. 2000. Shedding of syndecan-1 and -4 ectodomains is regulated by multiple signaling pathways and mediated by a Timp-3–sensitive metalloproteinase. *J Cell Biol* 148:811–24.

Font-Belmonte E, Ugidos IF, Santos-Galdiano M, González-Rodríguez P, Anuncibay-Soto B, Pérez-Rodríguez D, Gonzalo-Orden JM, Fernández-López A. 2019. Post-ischemic salubrinal administration reduces necroptosis in a rat model of global cerebral ischemia. *J Neurochem* 151(6): 777-94.

Ford AL, An H, Kong L, Zhu H, Vo KD, Powers WJ, Lin W, Lee JM. 2014. Clinically relevant reperfusion in acute ischemic stroke: MTT performs better than Tmax and TTP. *Transl Stroke Res* 5(3):415-21.

Fox S, Leitch AE, Duffin R, Haslett C, Rossi AG. 2010. Neutrophil apoptosis: relevance to the innate immune response and inflammatory disease. *J Innate Immun* 2(3):216-27.

Frost JL, Schafer DP. 2016. Microglia: Architects of the developing nervous system. *Trends Cell Biol* 26(8):587-97.

Galea I. 2021. The blood-brain barrier in systemic infection and inflammation. *Cell Mol Immunol* 18(11):2489-501.

Gan Y, Liu Q, Wu W, Yin J-X, Bai X-F, Shen R, Wang Y, Chen J, La Cava A, Poursine-Laurent J, Yokoyama W, Shi F-D. 2014. Ischemic neurons recruit natural killer cells that accelerate brain infarction. *Proc Natl Acad Sci USA* 111:2704-09.

Gardner L, Patterson AM, Ashton BA, Stone MA, Middleton J. 2004. The human Duffy antigen binds selected inflammatory but not homeostatic chemokines. *Biochem Biophys Res Commun* 321(2):306-12.

GBD 2016 Lifetime Risk of Stroke Collaborators, Feigin VL, Nguyen G, Cercy K, Johnson CO, Alam T, Parmar PG, Abajobir AA, Abate KH, Abd-Allah F, Abejie AN, Abyu GY, Ademi Z, Agarwal G, Ahmed MB, Akinyemi RO, Al-Raddadi R, Aminde LN, Amlie-Lefond C, Ansari H, Asayesh H, Asgedom SW, Atey TM, Ayele HT, Banach M, Banerjee A, Barac A, Barker-Collo SL, Bärnighausen T, Barregard L, Basu S, Bedi N, Behzadifar M, Béjot Y, Bennett DA, Bensenor IM, Berhe DF, Boneya DJ, Brainin M, Campos-Nonato IR, Caso V, Castañeda-Orjuela CA, Rivas JC, Catalá-López F, Christensen H, Criqui MH, Damasceno A, Dandona L, Dandona R, Davletov K, de Courten B, deVeber G, Dokova K, Edessa D, Endres M, Faraon EJA, Farvid MS, Fischer F, Foreman K, Forouzanfar MH, Gall SL, Gebrehiwot TT, Geleijnse JM, Gillum RF, Giroud M, Goulart AC, Gupta R, Gupta R, Hachinski V, Hamadeh RR, Hankey GJ, Hareri HA, Havmoeller R, Hay SI, Hegazy MI, Hibstu DT, James SL, Jeemon P, John D, Jonas JB, Jóźwiak J, Kalani R, Kandel A, Kasaeian A, Kengne AP, Khader YS, Khan AR, Khang YH, Khubchandani J, Kim D, Kim YJ, Kivimaki M, Kokubo Y, Kolte D, Kopec JA, Kosen S, Kravchenko M, Krishnamurthi R, Kumar GA, Lafranconi A, Lavados PM, Legesse Y, Li Y, Liang X, Lo WD, Lorkowski S, Lotufo PA, Loy CT, Mackay MT, Abd El Razek HM, Mahdavi M, Majeed A, Malekzadeh R, Malta DC, Mamun AA, Mantovani LG, Martins SCO, Mate KK, Mazidi M, Mehata S, Meier T, Melaku YA, Mendoza W, Mensah GA, Meretoja A,

Mezgebe HB, Miazgowski T, Miller TR, Ibrahim NM, Mohammed S, Mokdad AH, Moosazadeh M, Moran AE, Musa KI, Negoi RI, Nguyen M, Nguyen QL, Nguyen TH, Tran TT, Nguyen TT, Anggraini Ningrum DN, Norrving B, Noubiap JJ, O'Donnell MJ, Olagunju AT, Onuma OK, Owolabi MO, Parsaeian M, Patton GC, Piradov M, Pletcher MA, Pourmalek F, Prakash V, Qorbani M, Rahman M, Rahman MA, Rai RK, Ranta A, Rawaf D, Rawaf S, Renzaho AM, Robinson SR, Sahathevan R, Sahebkar A, Salomon JA, Santalucia P, Santos IS, Sartorius B, Schutte AE, Sepanlou SG, Shafieesabet A, Shaikh MA, Shamsizadeh M, Sheth KN, Sisay M, Shin MJ, Shiue I, Silva DAS, Sobngwi E, Soljak M, Sorensen RJD, Sposato LA, Stranges S, Suliankatchi RA, Tabarés-Seisdedos R, Tanne D, Nguyen CT, Thakur JS, Thrift AG, Tirschwell DL, Topor-Madry R, Tran BX, Nguyen LT, Truelsen T, Tsilimparis N, Tyrovolas S, Ukwaja KN, Uthman OA, Varakin Y, Vasankari T, Venketasubramanian N, Vlassov VV, Wang W, Werdecker A, Wolfe CDA, Xu G, Yano Y, Yonemoto N, Yu C, Zaidi Z, El Sayed Zaki M, Zhou M, Ziaeian B, Zipkin B, Vos T, Naghavi M, Murray CJL, Roth GA. 2018. Global, regional, and country-specific lifetime risks of stroke, 1990 and 2016. *N Engl J Med.* 379(25):2429-37.

Gelderblom M, Weymar A, Bernreuther C, Velden J, Arunachalam P, Steinbach K, Orthey E, Arumugam TV, Leypoldt F, Simova O, Thom V, Friese MA, Prinz I, Hölscher C, Glatzel M, Korn T, Gerloff C, Tolosa E, Magnus T. 2012. Neutralization of the IL-17 axis diminishes neutrophil invasion and protects from ischemic stroke. *Blood* 120(18):3793-802.

Georgakis MK, Malik R, Gill D, Franceschini N, Sudlow CLM, Dichgans M; INVENT Consortium, CHARGE Inflammation Working Group. 2020. Interleukin-6 signaling effects on ischemic stroke and other cardiovascular outcomes: a mendelian randomization study. *Circ Genom Precis Med* 13(3):e002872.

Ginhoux F, Greter M, Leboeuf M, Nandi S, See P, Gokhan S, Mehler MF, Conway SJ, Ng LG, Stanley ER, Samokhvalov IM, Merad M. 2010. Fate mapping analysis reveals that adult microglia derive from primitive macrophages. *Science* 330(6005):841-5.

Ginhoux F, Guilliams M. 2016. Tissue-resident macrophage ontogeny and homeostasis. *Immunity* 44(3):439-49.

Gonçalves CA, Leite MC, Nardin P. 2008. Biological and methodological features of the measurement of S100B, a putative marker of brain injury. *Clin Biochem* 41(10-11):755-63.

Gordon S. 2003. Alternative activation of macrophages. *Nat Rev Immunol* 3: 23-35.

Gorelick PB. 2019. The global burden of stroke: persistent and disabling. *Lancet Neurol* 18(5):417-18.

Guedes J, Cardoso AL, Pedroso de Lima MC. 2013. Involvement of microRNA in microglia-mediated immune response. *Clin Dev Immunol* 2013:186872.

Gülke E, Gelderblom M, Magnus T. 2018. Danger signals in stroke and their role on microglia activation after ischemia. *Ther Adv Neurol Disord* 11: 175628641877425.

Gulyás B, Tóth M, Schain M, Airaksinen A, Vas A, Kostulas K, Lindström P, Hillert J, Halldin C. 2012. Evolution of microglial activation in ischaemic core and peri-infarct regions after stroke: a PET study with the TSPO molecular imaging biomarker [((11))C]vinpocetine. *J Neurol Sci* 320(1-2):110-7.

Headland SE, Norling LV. 2015. The resolution of inflammation: Principles and challenges. *Semin Immunol* 27(3):149-60.

Heiss WD. 2000. Ischemic penumbra: evidence from functional imaging in man. *J Cereb Blood Flow Metab* 20(9):1276-93.

Hemkens LG, Ewald H, Gloy VL, Arpagaus A, Olu KK, Nidorf M, Glinz D, Nordmann AJ, Briel M. 2016. Colchicine for prevention of cardiovascular events. *Cochrane Database Syst Rev* 2016(1):CD011047.

Herrmann JE, Imura T, Song B, Qi J, Ao Y, Nguyen TK, Korsak RA, Takeda K, Akira S, Sofroniew MV. 2008. STAT3 is a critical regulator of astrogliosis and scar formation after spinal cord injury. *J Neurosci* 28(28):7231-43.

Herrmann O, Tarabin V, Suzuki S, Attigah N, Coserea I, Schneider A, Vogel J, Prinz S, Schwab S, Monyer H, Brombacher F, Schwaninger M. 2003. Regulation of body temperature and neuroprotection by endogenous interleukin-6 in cerebral ischemia. *J Cereb Blood Flow Metab* 23(4):406-15.

Hetts S, Khangura R. 2019. Imaging of acute stroke: current state. *Radiol Clin North Am* 57(6):1083-91.

Hickey WF, Kimura H. 1988. Perivascular microglial cells of the CNS are bone marrow-derived and present antigen in vivo. *Science* 239(4837):290-2.

Horstmann S, Kalb P, Koziol J, Gardner H, Wagner S. 2003. Profiles of matrix metalloproteinases, their inhibitors, and laminin in stroke patients: influence of different therapies. *Stroke* 34(9):2165-70.

Hu X, Li P, Guo Y, Wang H, Leak RK, Chen S, Gao Y, Chen J. 2012. Microglia/ macrophage polarization dynamics reveal novel mechanism of injury expansion after focal cerebral ischemia. *Stroke* 43: 3063-70.

Huang J, Upadhyay UM, Tamargo RJ. 2006. Inflammation in stroke and focal cerebral ischemia. *Surg Neurol* 66(3):232-45.

Iadecola C, Anrather J. 2011. The immunology of stroke: from mechanisms to translation. *Nat Med* 17(7):796-808.

Iadecola C, Buckwalter MS, Anrather J. 2020. Immune responses to stroke: mechanisms, modulation, and therapeutic potential. *J Clin Invest* 130(6):2777-88.

Iadecola C, Nedergaard M. 2007. Glial regulation of the cerebral microvasculature. *Nat Neurosci* 10:1369-76.

Imai Y, Ibata I, Ito D, Ohsawa K, Kohsaka S. 1996. A novel gene iba1 in the major histocompatibility complex class III region encoding an EF hand protein expressed in a monocytic lineage. *Biochem Biophys Res Commun* 224(3):855-62.

Ionita MG, Catanzariti LM, Bots ML, de Vries JP, Moll FL, Kwan Sze S, Sze Kwan S, Pasterkamp G, de Kleijn DP. 2010. High myeloid-related protein: 8/14 levels are related to an increased risk of cardiovascular events after carotid endarterectomy. *Stroke* 41: 2010-15.

Jacobsen EA, Taranova AG, Lee NA, Lee JJ. 2007. Eosinophils: singularly destructive effector cells or purveyors of immunoregulation? *J Allergy Clin Immunol* 119(6): 1313-20.

Jayaraj RL, Azimullah S, Beiram R, Jalal FY, Rosenberg GA. 2019. Neuroinflammation: friend and foe for ischemic stroke. *J Neuroinflammation* 16:142.

Jelinek M, Jurajda M, Duris K. 2021. Oxidative stress in the brain: basic concepts and treatment strategies in stroke. *Antioxidants* (Basel) 10(12):1886.

Jeohn GH, Kong LY, Wilson B, Hudson P, Hong JS. 1998. Synergistic neurotoxic effects of combined treatments with cytokines in murine primary mixed neuron/glia cultures. *J Neuroimmunol* 85(1):1-10.

Jiang CT, Wu WF, Deng YH, Ge JW. 2020. Modulators of microglia activation and polarization in ischemic stroke. *Mol Med Rep* 21:2006-18.

József L, Zouki C, Petasis NA, Serhan CN, Filep JG. 2002. Lipoxin A4 and aspirin-triggered 15-epi-lipoxin A4 inhibit peroxynitrite formation, NF-kappa B and AP-1 activation, and IL-8 gene expression in human leukocytes. *Proc Natl Acad Sci USA* 99(20):13266-71.

Justicia C, Panés J, Solé S, Cervera A, Deulofeu R, Chamorro A, Planas AM. 2003. Neutrophil infiltration increases matrix metalloproteinase-9 in the ischemic brain after occlusion/reperfusion of the middle cerebral artery in rats. *J Cereb Blood Flow Metab* 23(12):1430-40.

Kang L, Yu H, Yang X, Zhu Y, Bai X, Wang R, Cao Y, Xu H, Luo H, Lu L, Shi MJ, Tian Y, Fan W, Zhao BQ. 2020. Neutrophil extracellular traps released by neutrophils impair revascularization and vascular remodeling after stroke. *Nat Commun* 11(1):2488.

Kawahara D, Nagata Y. 2021. T1-weighted and T2-weighted MRI image synthesis with convolutional generative adversarial networks. *Rep Pract Oncol Radiother* 26(1):35-42.

Kelly P, Weimar C, Lemmens R, Murphy S, Purroy F, Arsovska A, Bornstein NM, Czlonkowska A, Fischer U, Fonseca AC, Forbes J, Hill MD, Jatuzis D, Kõrv J, Kruuse C, Mikulik R, J Nederkoorn P, O'Donnell M, Sandercock P, Tanne D, Tsivgoulis G, Walsh C, Williams D, Zedde M, Price CI. 2021. Colchicine for prevention of vascular inflammation in Non-CardioEmbolic stroke (CONVINCE) - study protocol for a randomised controlled trial. *Eur Stroke* J 6(2):222-28.

Kelly PJ, Camps-Renom P, Giannotti N, Martí-Fàbregas J, McNulty JP, Baron JC, Barry M, Coutts SB, Cronin S, Delgado-Mederos R, Dolan E, Fernández-León A, Foley S, Harbison J, Horgan G, Kavanagh E, Marnane M, McCabe J, McDonnell C, Sharma VK, Williams DJ, O'Connell M, Murphy S. 2020. A risk score including carotid plaque inflammation and stenosis severity improves identification of recurrent stroke. *Stroke* 51(3):838-45.

Khakh BS, Sofroniew MV. 2015. Diversity of astrocyte functions and phenotypes in neural circuits. *Nat Neurosci* 18(7):942-52.

Khatri R, McKinney AM, Swenson B, Janardhan V. 2012. Blood-brain barrier, reperfusion injury, and hemorrhagic transformation in acute ischemic stroke. *Neurology* 79 (Suppl. 13):S52–7.

Kirdajova DB, Kriska J, Tureckova J, Anderova M. 2020. Ischemia-triggered glutamate excitotoxicity from the perspective of glial cells. *Front Cell Neurosci* 14:51.

Kisler K, Nikolakopoulou AM, Zlokovic BV. 2021. Microglia have a grip on brain microvasculature. *Nat Commun* 12(1):5290.

Kleinschnitz C, Schwab N, Kraft P, Hagedorn I, Dreykluft A, Schwarz T, Austinat M, Nieswandt B, Wiendl H, Stoll G. 2010. Early detrimental T-cell effects in experimental cerebral ischemia are neither related to adaptive immunity nor thrombus formation. *Blood* 115(18):3835-42.

Kolaczkowska E, Kubes P. 2013. Neutrophil recruitment and function in health and inflammation. *Nat Rev Immunol* 13(3):159-75.

Kutuzov N, Flyvbjerg H, Lauritzen M 2018. Contributions of the glycocalyx, endothelium, and extravascular compartment to the blood-brain barrier. *Proc Natl Acad Sci USA* 115(40):E9429-38.

Lalancette-Hébert M, Gowing G, Simard A, Weng YC, Kriz J. 2007. Selective ablation of proliferating microglial cells exacerbates ischemic injury in the brain. *J Neurosci* 27(10):2596-605.

Lambertsen KL, Clausen BH, Fenger C, Wulf H, Owens T, Dagnaes-Hansen F. 2007. Microglia and macrophages express tumor necrosis factor receptor p75 following middle cerebral artery occlusion in mice. *Neuroscience* 144:934-49.

Latta CH, Sudduth TL, Weekman EM, Brothers HM, Abner EL, Popa GJ, Mendenhall MD, Gonzalez-Oregon F, Braun K, Wilcock DM. 2015. Determining the role of IL-4 induced neuroinflammation in microglial activity and amyloid-β using BV2 microglial cells and APP/PS1 transgenic mice. *J Neuroinflammation* 12:41.

Lee GH, Kim JS, Oh SJ, Kang DW, Kim JS, Kwon SU. 2015. (18)F-fluoromisonidazole (FMISO) positron emission tomography (PET) predicts early infarct growth in patients with acute ischemic stroke. *J Neuroimaging* 25(4):652-5.

Lei H, Gao Q, Liu SR, Xu J. 2016. The benefit and safety of aspirin for primary prevention of ischemic stroke: a meta-analysis of randomized trials. *Front Pharmacol* 7:440.

Leung YY, Yao Hui LL, Kraus VB. 2015. Colchicine–Update on mechanisms of action and therapeutic uses. *Semin Arthritis Rheum* 45(3):341-50.

Li P, Gan Y, Sun BL, Zhang F, Lu B, Gao Y, Liang W, Thomson AW, Chen J, Hu X. 2013. Adoptive regulatory T-cell therapy protects against cerebral ischemia. *Ann Neurol* 74(3):458-71.

Li Q, Barres B. 2017. Microglia and macrophages in brain homeostasis and disease. *Nat Rev Immunol* 18, 225-42.

Liang D, Bhatta S, Gerzanich V, Simard JM. 2007. Cytotoxic edema: mechanisms of pathological cell swelling. *Neurosurg Focus* 22(5):E2.

Libby P. 2002. Inflammation in atherosclerosis. *Nature* 420(6917):868-74.

Libby P, Buring JE, Badimon L, Hansson GK, Deanfield J, Bittencourt MS, Tokgözoğlu L, Lewis EF. 2019. Atherosclerosis. *Nat Rev Dis Primers* 5(1):56.

Liddelow S.A., Barres B.A. 2017. Reactive astrocytes: production, function, and therapeutic potential. *Immunity* 46:957-67.

Liddelow SA, Guttenplan KA, Clarke LE, Bennett FC, Bohlen CJ, Schirmer L, Bennett ML, Münch AE, Chung WS, Peterson TC, Wilton DK, Frouin A, Napier BA, Panicker N, Kumar M, Buckwalter MS, Rowitch DH, Dawson VL, Dawson TM, Stevens B, Barres BA. 2017. Neurotoxic reactive astrocytes are induced by activated microglia. *Nature* 541(7638):481-87.

Liesz A, Kleinschnitz C. 2016. Regulatory T cells in post-stroke immune homeostasis. *Transl Stroke Res* 7(4):313-21.

Lin CY, Chang C, Cheung WM, Lin MH, Chen JJ, Hsu CY, Chen JH, Lin TN. 2008. Dynamic changes in vascular permeability, cerebral blood volume, vascular density, and size after transient focal cerebral ischemia in rats: evaluation with contrast-enhanced magnetic resonance imaging. *J Cereb Blood Flow Metab* 28:1491–501.

Liu P, Zhang R, Liu D, Wang J, Yuan C, Zhao X, Li Y, Ji X, Chi T, Zou L. 2018. Time-course investigation of blood–brain barrier permeability and tight junction protein changes in a rat model of permanent focal ischemia. *J Physiol Sci* 68:121–7.

Liu R, Diao J, He S, Li B, Fei Y, Li Y, Fang W. 2018. XQ-1H protects against ischemic stroke by regulating microglia polarization through PPARγ pathway in mice. *Int Immunopharmacol* 57:72-81.

Louafi F, Martinez-Nunez RT, Sanchez-Elsner T. 2010. MicroRNA-155 targets SMAD2 and modulates the response of macrophages to transforming growth factor-(beta). *J Biol Chem* 285(53):41328-36.

Lovering F, Zhang Y. 2005. Therapeutic potential of TACE inhibitors in stroke. *Curr Drug Targets CNS Neurol Disord* 4:161-68.

Low A, Mak E, Rowe JB, Markus HS, O'Brien JT. 2019. Inflammation and cerebral small vessel disease: A systematic review. *Ageing Res Rev* 53:100916.

Lu J, Mei Q, Hou X, Manaenko A, Zhou L, Liebeskind DS, Zhang JH, Li Y, Hu Q. 2021. Imaging acute stroke: From one-size-fit-all to biomarkers. *Front Neurol* 12:697779.

Lucas SM, Rothwell NJ, Gibson RM. 2006. The role of inflammation in CNS injury and disease. *Br J Pharmacol* 147 Suppl 1():S232-40.

Lusis, AJ. 2000. Atherosclerosis. *Nature.* 407 (6801): 233-41.

Ma Y, Wang J, Wang Y, Yang G-Y. 2017. The biphasic function of microglia in ischemic stroke. *Prog Neurobiol* 157:247-72.

Maddox JF, Hachicha M, Takano T, Petasis NA, Fokin VV, Serhan CN. 1997. Lipoxin A4 stable analogs are potent mimetics that stimulate human monocytes and THP-1 cells via a G-protein-linked lipoxin A4 receptor. *J Biol Chem* 272(11):6972-8.

Mäe M, Armulik A, Betsholtz C. 2011. Getting to know the cast –cellular interactions and signaling at the neurovascular unit. *Curr Pharm Des* 17:2750-54.

Mantovani A, Sica A, Sozzani S, Allavena P, Vecchi A, Locati M. 2004. The chemokine system in diverse forms of macrophage activation and polarization. *Trends Immunol* 25: 677-86.

Mathiisen TM, Lehre KP, Danbolt NC, Ottersen OP. 2010. The perivascular astroglial sheath provides a complete covering of the brain microvessels: an electron microscopic 3D reconstruction. *Glia* 58(9):1094-103.

Matias I, Morgado J, Gomes FCA. 2019. Astrocyte heterogeneity: impact to brain aging and disease. *Front Aging Neurosci* 11:59.

Mato M, Ookawara S, Sakamoto A, Aikawa E, Ogawa T, Mitsuhashi U, Masuzawa T, Suzuki H, Honda M, Yazaki Y, Watanabe E, Luoma J, Yla-Herttuala S, Fraser I, Gordon S, Kodama T. 1996. Involvement of specific macrophage-lineage cells surrounding arterioles in barrier and scavenger function in brain cortex. *Proc Natl Acad Sci USA* 93(8):3269-74.

Mecha M, Feliú A, Carrillo-Salinas FJ, Rueda-Zubiaurre A, Ortega-Gutiérrez S, de Sola RG, Guaza C. 2015. Endocannabinoids drive the acquisition of an alternative phenotype in microglia. *Brain Behav Immun* 49:233-45.

Mehta SL, Manhas N, Raghubir R. 2007. Molecular targets in cerebral ischemia for developing novel therapeutics. *Brain Res Rev* 54(1):34-66.

Melcher CL. 2000. Scintillation crystals for PET. *J Nucl Med* 41(6):1051-5.

Merali Z, Huang K, Mikulis D, Silver F, Kassner A. 2017. Evolution of blood-brain-barrier permeability after acute ischemic stroke. *PLoS ONE* 12:e0171558.

Michinaga S, Koyama Y. 2015. Pathogenesis of brain edema and investigation into anti-edema drugs. *Int J Mol Sci.* 2015;16(5):9949-75.

Montaño A, Hanley DF, Hemphill JC 3rd. 2021. Hemorrhagic stroke. *Handb Clin Neurol* 176:229-48.

Morizawa YM, Hirayama Y, Ohno N, Shibata S, Shigetomi E, Sui Y, Nabekura J, Sato K, Okajima F, Takebayashi H, Okano H, Koizumi S. 2017. Reactive astrocytes function as phagocytes after brain ischemia via ABCA1-mediated pathway. *Nat Commun* 8:28.

Morris ME, Rodriguez-Cruz V, Felmlee MA. 2017. SLC and ABC transporters: expression, localization, and species differences at the blood-brain and the blood-cerebrospinal fluid barriers. *AAPS J* 19(5):1317-31.

Moskowitz MA, Lo EH, Iadecola C. 2010. The science of stroke: mechanisms in search of treatments. *Neuron* 67(2):181-98.

Muehllehner G, Karp JS. 2006. Positron emission tomography. *Phys Med Biol* 51(13):R117-37.

Muhammad S, Chaudhry SR, Kahlert UD, Niemelä M, Hänggi D. 2021. Brain immune interactions-novel emerging options to treat acute ischemic brain injury. *Cells* 10(9):2429.

Muir KW, Tyrrell P, Sattar N, Warburton E. 2007. Inflammation and ischaemic stroke. *Curr Opin Neurol* 20(3):334-42.

Munder M. 2009. Arginase: an emerging key player in the mammalian immune system. *Br J Pharmacol* 158: 638-51.

Nelissen S, Vangansewinkel T, Geurts N, Geboes L, Lemmens E, Vidal PM, Lemmens S, Willems L, Boato F, Dooley D, Pehl D, Pejler G, Maurer M, Metz M, Hendrix S. 2014. Mast cells protect from post-traumatic spinal cord damage in mice by degrading inflammation-associated cytokines via mouse mast cell protease 4. *Neurobiol Dis* 62:260-72.

Netea MG, Balkwill F, Chonchol M, Cominelli F, Donath MY, Giamarellos-Bourboulis EJ, Golenbock D, Gresnigt MS, Heneka MT, Hoffman HM, Hotchkiss R, Joosten LAB, Kastner DL, Korte M, Latz E, Libby P, Mandrup-Poulsen T, Mantovani A, Mills KHG, Nowak KL, O'Neill LA, Pickkers P, van der Poll T, Ridker PM, Schalkwijk J, Schwartz DA, Siegmund B, Steer CJ, Tilg H, van der Meer JWM, van de Veerdonk FL, Dinarello CA. 2017. A guiding map for inflammation. *Nat Immunol* 18(8):826-31.

Ni J, Wang X, Chen S, Liu H, Wang Y, Xu X, Cheng J, Jia J, Zhen X. 2015. MicroRNA let-7c-5p protects against cerebral ischemia injury via mechanisms involving the inhibition of microglia activation. *Brain Behav Immun* 49:75–85.

Nidorf SM, Eikelboom JW, Budgeon CA, Thompson PL. 2013. Low-dose colchicine for secondary prevention of cardiovascular disease. *J Am Coll Cardiol* 61(4):404-10.

Nidorf SM, Fiolet ATL, Mosterd A, Eikelboom JW, Schut A, Opstal TSJ, The SHK, Xu XF, Ireland MA, Lenderink T, Latchem D, Hoogslag P, Jerzewski A, Nierop P, Whelan A, Hendriks R, Swart H, Schaap J, Kuijper AFM, van Hessen MWJ, Saklani P, Tan I, Thompson AG, Morton A, Judkins C, Bax WA, Dirksen M, Alings M,

Hankey GJ, Budgeon CA, Tijssen JGP, Cornel JH, Thompson PL; LoDoCo2 Trial Investigators. 2020. Colchicine in patients with chronic coronary disease. *N Engl J Med* 383(19):1838-47.

Nimmerjahn A., Kirchhoff F, Helmchen F. 2005. Resting microglial cells are highly dynamic surveillants of brain parenchyma in vivo. *Science* 308:1314-18.

Nuriya M, Shinotsuka T, Yasui M. 2013. Diffusion properties of molecules at the blood-brain interface: potential contributions of astrocyte endfeet to diffusion barrier functions. *Cereb Cortex* 23(9):2118-26.

Okada S, Nakamura M, Katoh H, Miyao T, Shimazaki T, Ishii K, Yamane J, Yoshimura A, Iwamoto Y, Toyama Y, Okano H. 2006. Conditional ablation of Stat3 or Socs3 discloses a dual role for reactive astrocytes after spinal cord injury. *Nat Med* 12(7): 829-34.

Ortega-Gomez A, Perretti M, Soehnlein O. 2013. Resolution of inflammation: an integrated view. *EMBO Mol Med* 5(5):661–74.

Pandit R, Chen L, Götz J. 2019. The blood-brain barrier: physiology and strategies for drug delivery. *Adv Drug Deliv Rev* 165-166:1-14.

Paolicelli RC, Bolasco G, Pagani F, Maggi L, Scianni M, Panzanelli P, Giustetto M, Ferreira TA, Guiducci E, Dumas L, Ragozzino D, Gross CT. 2011. Synaptic pruning by microglia is necessary for normal brain development. *Science* 333: 1456-58.

Papadopoulos MC, Verkman AS. 2013. Aquaporin water channels in the nervous system. *Nat. Rev. Neurosci* 14:265-77.

Parmet S, Glass TJ, Glass RM. 2004. Hemorrhagic stroke. *JAMA* 292(15):1916.

Patabendige A, Singh A, Jenkins S, Sen J, Chen R. 2021. Astrocyte activation in neurovascular damage and repair following ischaemic stroke. *Int J Mol Sci* 22(8):4280.

Pearson TA, Mensah GA, Alexander RW, Anderson JL, Cannon RO 3rd, Criqui M, Fadl YY, Fortmann SP, Hong Y, Myers GL, Rifai N, Smith SC Jr, Taubert K, Tracy RP, Vinicor F; Centers for Disease Control and Prevention; American Heart Association. 2003. Markers of inflammation and cardiovascular disease: application to clinical and public health practice: A statement for healthcare professionals from the Centers for Disease Control and Prevention and the American Heart Association. *Circulation* 107(3):499-511.

Pei X, Li Y, Zhu L, Zhou Z. 2019. Astrocyte-derived exosomes suppress autophagy and ameliorate neuronal damage in experimental ischemic stroke. *Exp Cell Res* 382(2):111474.

Pelisek J, Rudelius M, Zepper P, Poppert H, Reeps C, Schuster T, Eckstein HH. 2009. Multiple biological predictors for vulnerable carotid lesions. *Cerebrovasc Dis* 28(6):601-10.

Peppiatt CM, Howarth C, Mobbs P, Attwell D. 2006. Bidirectional control of CNS capillary diameter by pericytes. *Nature* 443(7112):700-4.

Perego C, Fumagalli S, De Simoni MG. 2011. Temporal pattern of expression and colocalization of microglia/macrophage phenotype markers following brain ischemic injury in mice. *J Neuroinflammation* 8:174.

Pérez-Figueroa E, Álvarez-Carrasco P, Ortega E, Maldonado-Bernal C. 2021. Neutrophils: many ways to die. *Front Immunol* 12:631821.

Perretti, M. 1997. Endogenous mediators that inhibit the leukocyte-endothelium interaction. *Trends in Pharmacol Sci* 18(4):418-25.

Perry VH, Nicoll JA, Holmes C. 2010. Microglia in neurodegenerative disease. *Nat Rev Neurol* 6(4):193-201.

Peruzzotti-Jametti L, Donegá M, Giusto E, Mallucci G, Marchetti B, Pluchino S. 2014. The role of the immune system in central nervous system plasticity after acute injury. *Neuroscience* 283:210-21.

Pinteaux E, Rothwell NJ, Boutin H. 2006. Neuroprotective actions of endogenous interleukin-1 receptor antagonist (IL-1ra) are mediated by glia. *Glia* 53(5):551-6.

Piri R, Gerke O, Høilund-Carlsen PF. 2020. Molecular imaging of carotid artery atherosclerosis with PET: a systematic review. *Eur J Nucl Med Mol Imaging* 47(8): 2016-25.

Ponomarev ED, Veremeyko T, Barteneva N, Krichevsky AM, Weiner HL. 2011. MicroRNA-124 promotes microglia quiescence and suppresses EAE by deactivating macrophages via the C/EBP-alpha-PU.1 pathway. *Nat Med* 17:64–70.

Ponomarev ED, Veremeyko T, Weiner HL. 2013. MicroRNAs are universal regulators of differentiation, activation, and polarization of microglia and macrophages in normal and diseased CNS. *Glia* 61:91–103.

Poskanzer KE, Molofsky AV. 2018. Dynamism of an astrocyte in vivo: perspectives on identity and function. *Annu Rev Physiol* 80:143-57.

Priego N, Valiente M. 2019. The potential of astrocytes as immune modulators in brain tumors. *Front Immunol* 10:1314.

Qiu J, Xu J, Zheng Y, Wei Y, Zhu X, Lo EH, Moskowitz MA, Sims JR. 2010. High-mobility group box 1 promotes metalloproteinase-9 upregulation through Toll-like receptor 4 after cerebral ischemia. *Stroke* 41(9):2077-82.

Rajakariar R, Lawrence T, Bystrom J, Hilliard M, Colville-Nash P, Bellingan G, Fitzgerald D, Yaqoob MM, Gilroy DW 2008. Novel biphasic role for lymphocytes revealed during resolving inflammation. *Blood* 111(8):4184-92.

Ransohoff RM, Perry VH. 2009. Microglial physiology: unique stimuli, specialized responses. *Annu Rev Immuno* 27:119-45.

Rapalino O, Lazarov-Spiegler O, Agranov E, Velan GJ, Yoles E, Fraidakis M, Solomon A, Gepstein R, Katz A, Belkin M, Hadani M, Schwartz M. 1998. Implantation of stimulated homologous macrophages results in partial recovery of paraplegic rats. *Nat Med* 4:814-21.

Ren X, Akiyoshi K, Dziennis S, Vandenbark AA, Herson PS, Hurn PD, Offner H. 2011. Regulatory B cells limit CNS inflammation and neurologic deficits in murine experimental stroke. *J Neurosci* 31(23):8556-63.

Ridker PM, Danielson E, Fonseca FA, Genest J, Gotto AM Jr, Kastelein JJ, Koenig W, Libby P, Lorenzatti AJ, MacFadyen JG, Nordestgaard BG, Shepherd J, Willerson JT, Glynn RJ; JUPITER Study Group. 2008. Rosuvastatin to prevent vascular events in men and women with elevated C-reactive protein. *N Engl J Med* 359(21):2195-207.

Ridker PM, Everett BM, Thuren T, MacFadyen JG, Chang WH, Ballantyne C, Fonseca F, Nicolau J, Koenig W, Anker SD, Kastelein JJP, Cornel JH, Pais P, Pella D, Genest J, Cifkova R, Lorenzatti A, Forster T, Kobalava Z, Vida-Simiti L, Flather M, Shimokawa H, Ogawa H, Dellborg M, Rossi PRF, Troquay RPT, Libby P, Glynn RJ; CANTOS

Trial Group. 2017. Antiinflammatory therapy with canakinumab for atherosclerotic disease. *N Engl J Med* 377(12):1119-31.

Rock KL, Latz E, Ontiveros F, Kono H. 2010. The sterile inflammatory response. *Annu Rev Immunol* 28:321-42.

Roh JS, Sohn DH. 2018. Damage-associated molecular patterns in inflammatory diseases. *Immune Netw* 18(4):e27.

Rojas S, Martín A, Pareto D, Herance JR, Abad S, Ruíz A, Flotats N, Gispert JD, Llop J, Gómez-Vallejo V, Planas AM. 2011. Positron emission tomography with 11C-flumazenil in the rat shows preservation of binding sites during the acute phase after 2 h-transient focal ischemia. *Neuroscience* 182:208-16.

Rosamond W, Flegal K, Friday G, Furie K, Go A, Greenlund K, Haase N, Ho M, Howard V, Kissela B, Kittner S, Lloyd-Jones D, McDermott M, Meigs J, Moy C, Nichol G, O'Donnell CJ, Roger V, Rumsfeld J, Sorlie P, Steinberger J, Thom T, Wasserthiel-Smoller S, Hong Y, American Heart Association Statistics Committee and Stroke Statistics Subcommittee. 2007. Heart disease and stroke statistics-2007 update: a report from the American Heart Association Statistics Committee and Stroke Statistics Subcommittee. *Circulation* 115(5):e69-171.

Ross R. 1999. Atherosclerosis is an inflammatory disease. *Am Heart J* 138(5 Pt 2):S419-20.

Rost NS, Wolf PA, Kase CS, Kelly-Hayes M, Silbershatz H, Massaro JM, D'Agostino RB, Franzblau C, Wilson PW. 2001. Plasma concentration of C-reactive protein and risk of ischemic stroke and transient ischemic attack: the Framingham study. *Stroke* 32(11):2575-9.

Rouhl RP, Damoiseaux JG, Lodder J, Theunissen RO, Knottnerus IL, Staals J, Henskens LH, Kroon AA, de Leeuw PW, Tervaert JW, van Oostenbrugge RJ. 2012. Vascular inflammation in cerebral small vessel disease. *Neurobiol Aging* 33(8):1800-6.

Sabelström H, Stenudd M, Réu P, Dias DO, Elfineh M, Zdunek S, Damberg P, Göritz C, Frisén J. 2013. Resident neural stem cells restrict tissue damage and neuronal loss after spinal cord injury in mice. *Science* 342(6158):637-40.

Sandoval KE, Witt KA. 2008. Blood-brain barrier tight junction permeability and ischemic stroke. *Neurobiol Dis* 32:200-19.

Santos-Galdiano M, Pérez-Rodríguez D, Anuncibay-Soto B, Font-Belmonte E, Ugidos IF, Pérez-García CC, Fernández-López A. 2018. Celecoxib treatment improves neurological deficit and reduces selective neuronal loss and glial response in rats following transient middle cerebral artery occlusion. *J Pharmacol Exp Ther* 367(3): 528-42.

Scannell M, Flanagan MB, deStefani A, Wynne KJ, Cagney G, Godson C, Maderna P. 2007. Annexin-1 and peptide derivatives are released by apoptotic cells and stimulate phagocytosis of apoptotic neutrophils by macrophages. *J Immunol* 178(7):4595-605.

Schafer DP, Stevens B. 2015. Microglia function in central nervous system development and plasticity. *Cold Spring Harb Perspect Biol* 7(10):a020545.

Schwartz M, Kipnis J, Rivest S, Prat A. 2013. How do immune cells support and shape the brain in health, disease, and aging? *J Neurosci* 33(45):17587-96.

Serhan C, Savill, J. 2006. Resolution of inflammation: the beginning programs the end. *Nat Immunol* 6:1191-97.

Serhan CN, Chiang N, Van Dyke TE. 2008. Resolving inflammation: dual anti-inflammatory and pro-resolution lipid mediators. *Nat Rev Immunol* 8(5):349-61

Shechter R, London A, Varol C, Raposo C, Cusimano M, Yovel G, Rolls A, Mack M, Pluchino S, Martino G, Jung S, Schwartz M. 2009. Infiltrating blood-derived macrophages are vital cells playing an anti-inflammatory role in recovery from spinal cord injury in mice. *PLoS Med* 6(7):e1000113.

Shen Q, Huang S, Duong TQ. 2016. T2*-weighted fMRI time-to-peak of oxygen challenge in ischemic stroke. *J Cereb Blood Flow Metab* 36(2):283-91.

Shi K, Tian DC, Li ZG, Ducruet AF, Lawton MT, Shi FD. 2019. Global brain inflammation in stroke. *Stoll Lancet Neurol* 18(11):1058-66.

Shichinohe H, Kuroda S, Kudo K, Ito M, Kawabori M, Miyamoto M, Nakanishi M, Terae S, Houkin K. 2012. Visualization of the superparamagnetic iron oxide (SPIO)-labeled bone marrow stromal cells using a 3.0-T MRI-a pilot study for clinical testing of neurotransplantation. *Transl Stroke Res* 3(1):99-106.

Siddiqui MR, Mayanil CS, Kim KS, Tomita T. 2015. Angiopoietin-1 regulates brain endothelial permeability through PTPN-2 mediated tyrosine dephosphorylation of occludin. *PLoS One* 10(6):e0130857.

Sierra A, Encinas JM, Deudero JJ, Chancey JH, Enikolopov G, Overstreet-Wadiche LS, Tsirka SE, Maletic-Savatic M. 2010. Microglia shape adult hippocampal neurogenesis through apoptosis-coupled phagocytosis. *Cell Stem Cell* 7:483-95.

Silver J, Miller JH. 2004. Regeneration beyond the glial scar. *Nat Rev Neurosci* 5(2):146-56.

Simard JM, Kent TA, Chen M, Tarasov KV, Gerzanich V. 2007. Brain oedema in focal ischaemia: molecular pathophysiology and theoretical implications. *Lancet Neurol* 6(3):258-68.

Singer OC, Du Mesnil De Rochemont R, Foerch C, Stengel A, Sitzer M, Lanfermann H, Neumann-Haefelin T. 2004. Early functional recovery and the fate of the diffusion/perfusion mismatch in patients with proximal middle cerebral artery occlusion. *Cerebrovasc Dis* 17(1):13-20.

Sixt M, Engelhardt B, Pausch F, Hallmann R, Wendler O, Sorokin LM. 2001. Endothelial cell laminin isoforms, laminins 8 and 10, play decisive roles in T cell recruitment across the blood-brain barrier in experimental autoimmune encephalomyelitis. *J Cell Biol* 153(5):933-46.

Smith CJ, Emsley HC, Gavin CM, Georgiou RF, Vail A, Barberan EM, del Zoppo GJ, Hallenbeck JM, Rothwell NJ, Hopkins SJ, Tyrrell PJ. 2004. Peak plasma interleukin-6 and other peripheral markers of inflammation in the first week of ischaemic stroke correlate with brain infarct volume, stroke severity and long-term outcome. *BMC Neurol* 4:2.

Sofroniew MV, Vinters HV. 2010. Astrocytes: biology and pathology. *Acta Neuropathol* 119:7-35.

Sofroniew MV. 2020. Astrocyte reactivity: subtypes, states, and functions in CNS innate immunity. *Trends Immunol* 41(9):758-70.

Song TT, Bi YH, Gao YQ, Huang R, Hao K, Xu G, Tang JW, Ma ZQ, Kong FP, Coote JH, Chen XQ, Du JZ. 2016. Systemic pro-inflammatory response facilitates the development of cerebral edema during short hypoxia. *J Neuroinflammation* 13(1):63.

Spite M, Serhan CN. 2010. Novel lipid mediators promote resolution of acute inflammation: impact of aspirin and statins. *Circulation Res* 107(10):1170-84.

Squarzoni P, Oller G, Hoeffel G, Pont-Lezica L, Rostaing P, Low D, Bessis A, Ginhoux F, Garel S. 2014. Microglia modulate wiring of the embryonic forebrain. *Cell Rep* 8(5):1271-9.

Stadtman ER. 2004. Role of oxidant species in aging. *Curr Med Chem* 11:1105-12.

Steiner E, Enzmann GU, Lin S, Ghavampour S, Hannocks MJ, Zuber B, Rüegg MA, Sorokin L, Engelhardt B. 2012. Loss of astrocyte polarization upon transient focal brain ischemia as a possible mechanism to counteract early edema formation. *Glia* 60(11):1646-59.

Stokum JA, Gerzanich V, Simard JM. 2016. Molecular pathophysiology of cerebral edema. *J Cereb Blood Flow Metab* 36(3):513-38.

Stoll G, Jander S, Schroeter M. 2002. Detrimental and beneficial effects of injury-induced inflammation and cytokine expression in the nervous system. *Adv Exp Med Biol* 513:87-113.

Sugimoto MA, Sousa LP, Pinho V, Perretti M, Teixeira MM. 2016. Resolution of inflammation: what controls its onset? *Front Immunol* 7:160.

Suzuki S, Tanaka K, Suzuki N. 2009. Ambivalent aspects of interleukin-6 in cerebral ischemia: inflammatory versus neurotrophic aspects. *J Cereb Blood Flow Metab* 29(3):464-79.

Syková E. 2001. Glial diffusion barriers during aging and pathological states. *Prog Brain Res* 132:339-63.

Tang Y, Le W. 2016. Differential roles of M1 and M2 microglia in neurodegenerative diseases. *Mol Neurobiol* 53:1181-94.

Taraboletti G, D'Ascenzo S, Borsotti P, Giavazzi R, Pavan A, Dolo V. 2002. Shedding of the matrix metalloproteinases MMP-2, MMP-9, and MT1-MMP as membrane vesicle-associated components by endothelial cells. *Am J Pathol* 160:673–80.

Tardif JC, Kouz S, Waters DD, Bertrand OF, Diaz R, Maggioni AP, Pinto FJ, Ibrahim R, Gamra H, Kiwan GS, Berry C, López-Sendón J, Ostadal P, Koenig W, Angoulvant D, Grégoire JC, Lavoie MA, Dubé MP, Rhainds D, Provencher M, Blondeau L, Orfanos A, L'Allier PL, Guertin MC, Roubille F. 2019. Efficacy and safety of low-dose colchicine after myocardial infarction. *N Engl J Med* 381(26):2497-505.

Taylor PR, Martinez-Pomares L, Stacey M, Lin HH, Brown GD, Gordon S. 2005. Macrophage receptors and immune recognition. *Annu Rev Immunol* 23: 901-44.

Thannickal VJ, Fanburg BL. 2000. Reactive oxygen species in cell signaling. *Am J Physiol Lung Cell Mol Physiol* 279:L1005-28.

Valko M, Leibfritz D, Moncol J, Cronin MT, Mazur M, Telser J. 2007. Free radicals and antioxidants in normal physiological functions and human disease. *Int J Biochem Cell Biol* 39(1):44-84.

van den Berg JM, Weyer S, Weening JJ, Roos D, Kuijpers TW. 2001. Divergent effects of tumor necrosis factor alpha on apoptosis of human neutrophils. *J Leukoc Biol* 69:467-73.

Verkhratsky A, Matteoli M, Parpura V, Mothet JP, Zorec R. 2016. Astrocytes as secretory cells of the central nervous system: idiosyncrasies of vesicular secretion. *EMBO J* 35(3):23.

Verkhratsky A, Nedergaard M. 2018. Physiology of astroglia. *Physiol Rev* 98(1):239-389.

Vieira M, Fernandes J, Carreto L, Anuncibay-Soto B, Santos M, Han J, Fernández-López A, Duarte CB, Carvalho AL, Santos AE. 2014. Ischemic insults induce necroptotic cell death in hippocampal neurons through the up-regulation of endogenous RIP3. *Neurobiol Dis* 68:26-36.

Viviani B, Bartesaghi S, Corsini E, Galli CL, Marinovich M. 2004. Cytokines role in neurodegenerative events. *Toxicol Lett* 149(1-3):85-9.

Wake H, Moorhouse AJ, Jinno S, Kohsaka S, Nabekura J. 2009. Resting microglia directly monitor the functional state of synapses in vivo and determine the fate of ischemic terminals. *J Neurosci* 29(13):3974-80.

Watanabe S, Alexander M, Misharin AV, Budinger GRS. 2019. The role of macrophages in the resolution of inflammation. *J Clin Invest* 129(7):2619-28.

Weston RM, Jones NM, Jarrott B, Callaway JK. 2007. Inflammatory cell infiltration after endothelin-1-induced cerebral ischemia: Histochemical and myeloperoxidase correlation with temporal changes in brain injury. *J. Cereb. Blood Flow. Metab* 27: 100-14.

Wiese S, Karus M, Faissner A. 2012. Astrocytes as a source for extracellular matrix molecules and cytokines. *Front Pharmacol* 3:120.

Wilhelm I, Nyúl-Tóth Á, Kozma M, Farkas AE, Krizbai IA. 2017. Role of pattern recognition receptors of the neurovascular unit in inflamm-aging. *Am J Physiol Heart Circ Physiol* 313(5):H1000-12.

Wintermark M, Albers GW, Alexandrov AV, Alger JR, Bammer R, Baron JC, Davis S, Demaerschalk BM, Derdeyn CP, Donnan GA, Eastwood JD, Fiebach JB, Fisher M, Furie KL, Goldmakher GV, Hacke W, Kidwell CS, Kloska SP, Köhrmann M, Koroshetz W, Lee TY, Lees KR, Lev MH, Liebeskind DS, Ostergaard L, Powers WJ, Provenzale J, Schellinger P, Silbergleit R, Sorensen AG, Wardlaw J, Wu O, Warach S. 2008. Acute stroke imaging research roadmap. *Stroke* 39(5):1621-28.

Xie L, Poteet EC, Li W, Scott AE, Liu R, Wen Y, Ghorpade A, Simpkins JW, Yang SH. 2010. Modulation of polymorphonuclear neutrophil functions by astrocytes. *J Neuroinflammation* 7:53.

Xin WQ, Wei W, Pan YL, Cui BL, Yang XY, Bähr M, Doeppner TR. 2021. Modulating poststroke inflammatory mechanisms: Novel aspects of mesenchymal stem cells, extracellular vesicles and microglia. *World J Stem Cells* 13(8):1030-48.

Xiong X, Barreto GE, Xu L, Ouyang YB, Xie X, Giffard RG. 2011. Increased brain injury and worsened neurological outcome in interleukin-4 knockout mice after transient focal cerebral ischemia. *Stroke* 42:2026-32.

Yang Y, Rosenberg GA. 2011. Blood-brain barrier breakdown in acute and chronic cerebrovascular disease. *Stroke* 42(11):3323-8.

Yenari MA, Kauppinen TM, Swanson RA. 2010. Microglial activation in stroke: therapeutic targets. *Neurotherapeutics* 7(4):378-91.

Yilmaz G, Granger DN. 2010. Leukocyte recruitment and ischemic brain injury. *Neuromolecular Med* 12:193-204.

Yuan S, Carter P, Bruzelius M, Vithayathil M, Kar S, Mason AM, Lin A, Burgess S, Larsson SC. 2020. Effects of tumour necrosis factor on cardiovascular disease and cancer: A two-sample Mendelian randomization study. *EBioMedicine* 59:102956.

Yuan W, Li G, Zeng M, Fu BM. 2010. Modulation of the blood–brain barrier permeability by plasma glycoprotein orosomucoid. *Microvascular Res* 80:148-57.

Zhang H, Verkman AS. 2013. Eosinophil pathogenicity mechanisms and therapeutics in neuromyelitis optica. *J Clin Invest* 123(5):2306-16.

Zhang J, Wang X, Vikash V, Ye Q, Wu D, Liu Y, Dong W. 2016. ROS and ROS-mediated cellular signaling. *Oxid Med Cell Longev* 2016:4350965.

Zhang L, Dong LY, Li YJ, Hong Z, Wei WS. 2012. The microRNA miR-181c controls microglia-mediated neuronal apoptosis by suppressing tumor necrosis factor. *J Neuroinflammation* 9: 211.

Zhang L, Zhang J, You Z. 2018. Switching of the microglial activation phenotype is a possible treatment for depression disorder. *Front Cell Neurosci* 12:306.

Zhang X, Wang Y, Song J, Gerwien H, Chuquisana O, Chashchina A, Denz C, Sorokin L. 2020. The endothelial basement membrane acts as a checkpoint for entry of pathogenic T cells into the brain. *J Exp Med* 217(7):e20191339.

Zlokovic BV. 2006. Remodeling after stroke. *Nat Med* 12(4):390-1.

Zuo J, Neubauer D, Dyess K, Ferguson TA, Muir D. 1998. Degradation of chondroitin sulfate proteoglycan enhances the neurite-promoting potential of spinal cord tissue. *Exp Neurol* 154 (2):654-62.

Contents of Earlier Volumes

Horizons in Neuroscience Research. Volume 47

Horizons in Neuroscience Research. Volume 46

Horizons in Neuroscience Research. Volume 45

Horizons in Neuroscience Research. Volume 43

Index